Cases on Medical Nutrition Therapy for Gastrointestinal Disorders

Elham Abbas Aljaaly
King Abdulaziz University, Saudi Arabia

Nahlaa Abdelwahab Khalifa
King Abdulaziz University, Saudi Arabia

Rouba Khalil Naaman
King Abdulaziz University, Saudi Arabia

Manar Abduljalil Bakhsh
King Abdulaziz University, Saudi Arabia

A volume in the Advances in
Medical Diagnosis, Treatment, and
Care (AMDTC) Book Series

IGI Global
PUBLISHER of TIMELY KNOWLEDGE

Published in the United States of America by
IGI Global
Medical Information Science Reference (an imprint of IGI Global)
701 E. Chocolate Avenue
Hershey PA, USA 17033
Tel: 717-533-8845
Fax: 717-533-8661
E-mail: cust@igi-global.com
Web site: http://www.igi-global.com

Library of Congress Cataloging-in-Publication Data

Names: Aljaaly, Elham Abbas, 1962- editor. | Khalifa, Nahlaa Abdelwahab, 1964- editor. | Naaman, Rouba Khalil, 1986- editor. | Bakhsh, Manar Abduljalil, 1987- editor.
Title: Cases on medical nutrition therapy for gastrointestinal disorders / Elham Abbas Aljaaly, Nahlaa Abdelwahab Khalifa, Rouba Khalil Naaman and Manar Abduljalil Bakhsh, editors.
Description: Hershey, PA : Medical Information Science Reference, [2021] | Includes bibliographical references and index. | Summary: "This nutrition-related clinical education book reports real case studies conducted by research professionals sharing their expertise in the field of nutrition and dietetics. Through nutrition assessment and reassessment it provides a systematic approach for obtaining and analyzing information to identify nutrition-related problems and their causes"-- Provided by publisher.
Identifiers: LCCN 2020017061 | ISBN 9781799838029 (hardcover) | ISBN 9781799838036 (ebook)
Subjects: MESH: Gastrointestinal Diseases--diet therapy | Nutrition Therapy--methods | Case Reports
Classification: LCC RC806 | NLM WI 195 | DDC 616.3/30654--dc23
LC record available at https://lccn.loc.gov/2020017061

This book is published in the IGI Global book series Advances in Medical Diagnosis, Treatment, and Care (AMDTC) (ISSN: 2475-6628; eISSN: 2475-6636)

British Cataloguing in Publication Data
A Cataloguing in Publication record for this book is available from the British Library.

Advances in Medical Diagnosis, Treatment, and Care (AMDTC) Book Series

ISSN:2475-6628
EISSN:2475-6636

MISSION

Advancements in medicine have prolonged the life expectancy of individuals all over the world. Once life-threatening conditions have become significantly easier to treat and even cure in many cases. Continued research in the medical field will further improve the quality of life, longevity, and wellbeing of individuals.

The **Advances in Medical Diagnosis, Treatment, and Care (AMDTC)** book series seeks to highlight publications on innovative treatment methodologies, diagnosis tools and techniques, and best practices for patient care. Comprised of comprehensive resources aimed to assist professionals in the medical field apply the latest innovations in the identification and management of medical conditions as well as patient care and interaction, the books within the AMDTC series are relevant to the research and practical needs of medical practitioners, researchers, students, and hospital administrators.

COVERAGE

- Cancer Treatment
- Patient-Centered Care
- Alternative Medicine
- Medical Testing
- Medical Procedures
- Experimental Medicine
- Disease Management
- Internal Medicine
- Critical Care
- Emergency Medicine

IGI Global is currently accepting manuscripts for publication within this series. To submit a proposal for a volume in this series, please contact our Acquisition Editors at Acquisitions@igi-global.com or visit: http://www.igi-global.com/publish/.

The Advances in Medical Diagnosis, Treatment, and Care (AMDTC) Book Series (ISSN 2475-6628) is published by IGI Global, 701 E. Chocolate Avenue, Hershey, PA 17033-1240, USA, www.igi-global.com. This series is composed of titles available for purchase individually; each title is edited to be contextually exclusive from any other title within the series. For pricing and ordering information please visit http://www.igi-global.com/book-series/advances-medical-diagnosis-treatment-care/129618. Postmaster: Send all address changes to above address.

Titles in this Series

For a list of additional titles in this series, please visit:
https://www.igi-global.com/book-series/advances-medical-diagnosis-treatment-care/129618

Handbook of Research on Disease Prediction Through Data Analytics and Machine Learning
Geeta Rani (Manipal University Jaipur, India) and Pradeep Kumar Tiwari (Manipal University Jaipur, India)
Medical Information Science Reference • © 2021 • 586pp • H/C (ISBN: 9781799827429) • US $395.00

Handbook of Research on Evidence-Based Perspectives on the Psychophysiology of Yoga and Its Applications
Shirley Telles (Patanjali Research Foundation, India) and Ram Kumar Gupta (Patanjali Research Foundation, India)
Medical Information Science Reference • © 2021 • 577pp • H/C (ISBN: 9781799832546) • US $345.00

New Developments in Diagnosing, Assessing, and Treating ADHD
Rejani Thudalikunnil Gopalan (Mahatma Gandhi Medical College and Hospital, India)
Medical Information Science Reference • © 2021 • 419pp • H/C (ISBN: 9781799854951) • US $265.00

Handbook of Research on Oncological and Endoscopical Dilemmas in Modern Gynecological Clinical Practice
Konstantinos Dinas (2nd Department of Obstetrics and Gynaecology, Aristotle University of Thessaloniki, Greece) Stamatios Petousis (2nd Department of Obstetrics and Gynaecology, Aristotle University of Thessaloniki, Greece) Matthias Kalder (Department of Obstetrics and Gynaecology, Philipps-University of Marburg, Germany) and George Mavromatidis (2nd Department of Obstetrics and Gynaecology, Aristotle University of Thessaloniki, Greece)
Medical Information Science Reference • © 2021 • 460pp • H/C (ISBN: 9781799842132) • US $385.00

IGI Global
PUBLISHER of TIMELY KNOWLEDGE

701 East Chocolate Avenue, Hershey, PA 17033, USA
Tel: 717-533-8845 x100 • Fax: 717-533-8661
E-Mail: cust@igi-global.com • www.igi-global.com

Table of Contents

Detailed Table of Contents

This chapter discusses a gastroesophageal reflux disease (GERD) case. GERD is a common disorder affecting the gastrointestinal tract. It results from the relaxation of the lower esophageal sphincter, which leads to stomach acid reflux, which in turn causes heartburn and discomfort. Certain lifestyle factors and dietary choices aggravate this condition, leading to serious tissue damage. Management of GERD usually requires medications and lifestyle and dietary modifications. This case involves the symptoms and aggravating factors of GERD. It also shows the role of medical nutrition therapy in managing GERD symptoms. Moreover, it will allow dietetic professionals to assess GERD symptoms to plan for nutrition interventions and educate patients about the dietary manipulation required to reduce gastric acid secretions and relieve pain.

This chapter will discuss a peptic ulcer disease (PUD) case. PUD is a common gastrointestinal tract disease (GIT) that affects the stomach and duodenum. It is characterized by deep lesions into the mucosal thickness. Various dietary and behavioral choices could aggravate the epigastric pain associated with PUD and interfere with the healing process leading to complications. Management of PUD includes medical treatment with medications along with behavioral and nutritional changes. This case presents a complication of PUD, and choices exacerbating the condition. It will also discuss the role of medical nutrition therapy in minimizing the symptoms and promoting ulcer healing. Additionally, it will allow the dietetic professional to methodically assess the elements in the case that are relevant for planning the nutrition intervention; in addition to, educating the patient about dietary modifications to improve the patient's quality of life.

This chapter will discuss a case of diarrhea/constipation. Diarrhea and constipation are functional bowel disorders (FBDs) of the mid or lower gastrointestinal (GI) tract. These FBDs result from intestinal motility dysfunction and/or changes in intestinal fluid absorption, which in turn leads to bloating, discomfort, and occasionally, abdominal pain. Certain dietary choices aggravate these conditions, leading to serious complications. Management of diarrhea/constipation usually requires the use of medications and/or lifestyle modifications. The presently discussed case involved factors that exacerbated the conditions of diarrhea/constipation. This case serves as an example of the role of medical nutrition therapy in managing FBDs (particularly diarrhea and constipation). Moreover, this case will allow the dietetic professional to assess the causes of diarrhea/constipation in order to plan for the nutrition intervention and educate the patient about the dietary manipulations required to reduce their symptoms.

This chapter reveals and discusses a case involving celiac disease (CD). CD is a common, lifelong, genetically-based autoimmune disorder that causes inflammation of the proximal small intestine. This disease is triggered by eating foods containing gluten, which causes intestinal discomfort. Gluten is a protein that is found naturally in wheat, barley, and rye and is common in foods such as bread, pasta, cookies, and cakes. Many pre-packaged foods, lip balms and lipsticks, hair and skin products, toothpaste and vitamin and nutrient supplements contain gluten, although it is rarely found in medicine. The key to living with CD is to follow a gluten-free diet. This case shows the role of medical nutrition therapy in managing and preventing the undesirable symptoms of CD. Moreover, it allows dietetic professionals to assess celiac patients' conditions and provide them with relief from undesirable symptoms, while also establishing an effective follow-up plan with each patient.

This chapter presents a case scenario of lactose intolerance. Lactose intolerance is the inability to digest and absorb lactose, which is the sugar in milk, due to deficiency of the enzyme lactase. This condition commonly occurs after weaning, and it results in various gastrointestinal symptoms such as diarrhea. In addition, it may result in nutritional deficiencies. Management of lactose intolerance requires diet manipulations. This case study provides the needed information to implement the appropriate intervention such as patient's details and case history. Moreover, the case analysis section discusses in detail the disease pathophysiology and the medical nutrition therapy goals. This comprehensive analysis will allow the dietetic professional to follow the nutrition care process (NCP) framework (assessment, diagnosis, intervention, and monitoring and evaluation) to properly intervene and deal with the case. This case study will show the importance of the medical nutrition therapy for the management of lactose intolerance.

The proposed case will discuss irritable bowel syndrome. Individualized medical nutrition therapy is critical in the disease management. In this case, the learner will be provided with details to conceptualize the case and will be able to conduct a comprehensive nutrition assessment to evaluate the nutritional status. After identifying and prioritizing nutrition problems, the learner will determine the nutrition diagnoses and write proper statements. Based on the collected data, the learner will develop a nutrition care plan with appropriate goals, interventions, and strategies for monitoring and evaluation. Unspecified-IBS encounter challenges with food as it triggers the symptoms. Thus, the learner will evaluate the nutrient composition of dietary history and provide a substitute considering individual tolerance and severity of the symptoms. In addition, FODMAP will be applied. It also teaches patients what foods or eating patterns would be best (or best to avoid) for their day-to-day activities through self-awareness of symptoms and dietary food log.

Weight management offers patients with liver cirrhosis significant health benefits. This case study describes the treatment of liver cirrhosis through dietary interventions. A 48-year-old male presented at Doctor Soliman Fakeeh Hospital in Saudi Arabia, Jeddah. The patient was suffering from morbid obesity (BMI= 43.76 kg/m2), non-alcoholic steatohepatitis, and chronic hepatitis B viral infection. Sleeve gastrectomy surgery was not possible due to the patient having liver fibrosis (stage 4). Alternatively, he was offered a healthy lifestyle intervention involving advisement regarding dietary habits and the initiation of a regular exercise routine. FibroScan was repeated seven months after the dietary intervention, where it was observed that the liver fibrosis improved from stage 4 to stage 3 post-treatment. Additionally, the patient lost almost 29% of his original body weight. In this case, weight management through following a healthy, balanced diet and increasing physical activity for one year produced remarkable improvement in the patient's liver cirrhosis related to non-alcoholic steatohepatitis.

Preface

Over the last few years there have been numerous positive developments in clinical education in the field of nutrition and dietetics, including the use of a problem-based approaches that draw on real and simulated data to facilitate more effective learning.

Amongst the many works that have contributed to the development of clinical education in dietetics is the handbook *Cases on Medical Nutrition Therapy for GI Disorders*. Edited by Elham A. Aljaaly, Ph.D., Nahlaa A. Khalifa, Ph.D., Rouba K. Naaman, Ph.D., and Manar A. Bakhsh, MSc, the handbook provides readers with a number of case studies that can in turn guide health providers' approaches to managing gastrointestinal (GI) disorders. This nutrition-related clinical education handbook reports real case studies conducted by the editors as well other experts in the field of nutrition and dietetics.

The editors of this book are all academic staff in the field of nutrition and dietetics with many years of experience in both research and practice. The editors are mostly clinicians who are involved in clinical education and training. Dr. Khalifa is the founder of the second clinical nutrition program at King Abdulaziz University in Saudi Arabia. She is also a *ThinkBuzan Licensed Instructor* (TLI) in Mind Mapping and thus utilizes mind mapping as an effective multisensory method in medical education. Dr. Aljaaly is an associate professor and consultant in clinical nutrition (CLN) and has previously headed the CLN program at King Abdul Aziz University. She is the first Saudi registered clinical dietitian. She also coordinates and delivers courses in clinical education. Dr. Naaman and Mrs. Bakhsh are graduates of the first cohort of the same program. Both are academic staff and registered dietitians who deliver theoretical and training courses on 'medical nutrition therapy', or MNT.

The term 'medical nutrition therapy', was first used by the American Dietetic Association in 1994 to better state the nutrition therapy process. It is defined as the use of specific nutrition services to treat an illness, condition, or injury. It includes two phases: 1) the assessment of the nutritional status and 2) treatment which includes nutrition therapy, counselling, and the use of specialized nutritional supplements. Many textbooks and case-based approach books are based on MNT to manage and report nutrition therapy for diseases.

Each editor therefore has a wealth of expertise and is therefore well-equipped to write comprehensively about their chosen topics in this book. The interpretations communicated in this book are explanations by the authors of each chapter or the reports of each case in their areas of specialty and practice. Some users of the book might have views that differ from those presented here, however differences of opinion are commonplace and it is important that health workers for nutrition-related disorders have the right to draw on up-to-date MNT resources such as this handbook in their trainings.

MNT is a specific application of the Nutrition Care Process (NCP) in clinical settings that focuses on the management of diseases through individualized nutritional assessment. NCP is a standardized problem-solving method used by nutrition and dietetics professionals to improve the nutritional care provided. The use of NCP has been associated with several benefits in clinical settings as well as in research. This includes the standardization of the process used to provide the nutritional care, improve dietitians' critical thinking when making decisions, and the incorporation of evidence-based practice. NCP consists of four steps applied by dietitians, namely: nutrition-related assessment, diagnosis, intervention and monitoring and evaluation.

Generally, the specific scope of medical practice identification including GI problems, has some limitations for medical practitioners. Previous reports showed a dearth of available data specific to gastroenterology. In response to the previous calls, the editors of this book introduce cases to inspire practitioners to action in writing their experience by collecting and sharing data of case studies and its management based on their practice in the scope of gastroenterology.

The chapters of this handbook are organized into two sections. The first section serves as an introduction chapter while the second section covers eleven case studies. These case studies look at the most recent research and evidenced-based literature, with each case study telling one part of the overall story.

The book called for international contributors in the dietetics practice and academics from various educational institutions. Medical practitioners in the scope of GI disorders were also invited to participate in writing case studies that involved the use of MNT. Contributors who reported their conducted case studies include academic staff who are clinically based; clinicians involved with the training process in universities, including those providing clinical nutrition-related programs. Clinicians such as adult and pediatric gastroenterologists, as well as gastroenterology surgeons also participated in providing and reporting case studies. Other contributors included registered dietitians and academic staff who are clinicians as well.

Readers of this book can therefore use it to perform developed levels of practice. Case reports include upper and lower GI tract disorders as: dysphagia, gastroesophageal reflux disease GERD), peptic ulcer disease, diarrhea/constipation, celiac disease, lactose intolerance, inflammatory bowel diseases (Crohn's disease

& ulcerative colitis), Irritable bowel syndrome (IBS), and small bowel obstruction. In addition, a liver-related disorder includes a case study of liver cirrhosis.

The Introduction presents an overview about the book and all used approaches to guide conduct and reports of case scenarios related to GI disorders. This include MNT, NCP and mind mapping (MM) to illustrate the MNT and NCP of each case study starting from the pathophysiology and how a disease starts and works and end with the management of the presented case. All mind maps were done by the editor Nahlaa Khalifa, which is specialist in this approach and all authors were given the chance to have their chapters after concluded to be illustrated by MM. Most case reports, especially those written by or involve registered dietitians (RD) or registered dietitian nutritionist (RDN) are reported using ADIME, which include Assessment, Diagnosis, Intervention, and Monitoring/Evaluation. The ADIME approach is used by nutrition experts for the secure of high-quality nutrition care to patients and clients. The chapter was written by all the editors of the book.

Chapter 1 presents a case scenario dysphagia and its considered nutritional intervention. Dysphagia is a complex disorder which requires an interdisciplinary collaborative approach to achieve optimal health outcomes. This chapter describes dysphagia from the perspective of the speech-language pathologist. It attempts to facilitate an understanding of how the mechanical aspects of normal and disordered swallowing factor into considerations for appropriate nutritional recommendations. Through a better understanding of normal and disordered swallowing function, dietetics professionals have more information on which to base clinical decisions for people in all stages of illness and recovery.

Chapter 2 presents a case scenario that provides an extensive overview about the gastroesophageal reflux disease (GERD) including the disease epidemiology, pathophysiology, risk factors, signs, symptoms and diagnosis. The chapter then discusses approaches of GERD management including medical and surgical interventions, in addition to lifestyle and dietary modifications. The chapter applies the information presented in a case study which highlights the role of nutrition in the management of GERD.

Chapter 3 provides a detailed background about the peptic ulcer disease (PUD), which is a common disease that many registered dietitians may come across. Also, the chapter is discussing a real-life case study bases on scientific evidence through a case scenario followed by a detailed, standardized case analysis using the NCP procedure and reported using ADIME. Thus, allows the reader to utilize the needed information to provide a practical and evidenced-based MNT for PUD including: case summary, patient's health/medical history, demographic, medical diagnosis, anthropometric assessment, biochemical data, nutrition-focused physical examination, food and nutrition history including a 24-hour recall, and medications.

Chapter 4 is about diarrhea and constipation. Constipation and diarrhea are considered symptomatic disorders rather than serious diseases. Nonetheless, they can interfere with everyday individuals' activities by reducing their quality of life through social effects and the necessity of medical treatments. A comprehensive evaluation is necessary to determine the underlying cause of either diarrhea and/or constipation. Since the medical nutrition therapy for either condition is unique for each individual, a dietitian should assess the causes of diarrhea/constipation carefully to identify the dietary and/or other factors that might be impacting these symptoms and furthermore providing the right nutritional intervention.

Chapter 5 reveals and discusses a case involving celiac disease (CD). This disease is triggered by eating foods containing gluten, which causes intestinal discomfort. The key to living with CD is to follow a gluten-free diet. This case shows the role of MNT in managing and preventing the undesirable symptoms of CD. Moreover, it allows dietetic professionals to assess celiac patients' conditions and provide them with relief from undesirable symptoms, while also establishing an effective follow-up plan with each patient.

Chapter 6 presents a case scenario about lactose intolerance, which is a common gastrointestinal problem; in some regions, lactose intolerance affects almost all individuals. It can be misdiagnosed and easily confused with other gastrointestinal diseases. This condition causes symptoms that can be stressful and might affect a person's quality of life. It can also result in other negative health consequences. Treatment mainly involves dietary changes that alleviate or eliminate symptoms. Therefore, it is crucial for health practitioners and specifically dietetic professionals to better understand and review updated evidence about this condition that might be bewildering.

Chapter 7 reflects on the practice of clinical dietitians who are dealing with patients diagnosed with inflammatory bowel diseases (IBD). It will allow the readers to assess the symptoms and associated nutritional complications and develop a nutrition support intervention plan. Moreover, readers would be able to critically evaluate and apply the most recent evidence and guidelines concerned with IBD nutritional therapy.

Chapter 8 presents a pediatric case study of ulcerative colitis (UC) with extra intestinal manifestations in different forms. Pediatric UC is broad and severe at the diagnosis, treatment and follow-up and has been inadequately reported. Additionally, there is a dearth of information on the extra-intestinal manifestations and their impact on the disease of UC. For better health and nutrition outcomes, the disease needs a comprehensive evidenced-based management by an integrated multidisciplinary. Therefore, the case was aiming for an interprofessional collaboration, which mainly include a RD and a radiologist who is a medical doctor and specialized in diagnosing and treating disease and injury. This facilitate the use of some medical imaging techniques. The case is significantly reflecting medical care with prescribed drugs, diagnostic procedures, and nutrition interventions. Incorporation of evidence-based guidelines was considered throughout the case management, to improves health and nutrition outcomes of the disease in children. Consequently, the case was not only managed to follow the nutrition care process but also evaluated the most current literature in managing the disease.

Chapter 9 presents a case study of irritable bowel syndrome (IBS), which is one of the common intestinal disorders. Its prevalence is increasing with unknown causes. Diet plays a very crucial role in the disease exacerbation as it acts as inducers of gastrointestinal symptoms. This chapter discusses the individualized MNT approach which is a critical component in the medical management of the disease.

Chapter 10 explains the authors' experience in medically and nutritionally handling a case of an overweight patient with liver cirrhosis and the success in changing the patient's lifestyle. It presents the used techniques in convincing the patient to manage his weight without using a surgical intervention and to manage patient's liver disease at the same time. Authors' key massage through this chapter is that providing patients with good support and excellent communication might help them control their lifestyle and extra weight with challenging issues accomplished of their goals.

Elham Abbas Aljaaly
King Abdulaziz University, Saudi Arabia

Acknowledgment

The editors of this book would like to thank all the authors who contributed in this book. A special thank for the reviewers for their thoughtful comments and valuable suggestions. The editors would also like to express their thankfulness to Siham El-Kafafi for her very dearly loved time and opinions about what could be done about a situation. We are also thankful to Eric Whalen for his consultation and following up in finalizing this book. Without all supports and despite difficult circumstances during COVID 19, this book would not have been possible.

Elham Abbas Aljaaly
King Abdulaziz University, Saudi Arabia

Nahlaa Abdelwahab Khalifa
King Abdulaziz University, Saudi Arabia

Rouba Khalil Naaman
King Abdulaziz University, Saudi Arabia

Manar Abduljalil Bakhsh
King Abdulaziz University, Saudi Arabia

Introduction

The key objective of *Cases on Medical Nutrition Therapy for GI Disorders* handbook is to provide both dietetics professionals and health professionals more generally with practical guidelines in nutritional management of several GI disorders.

The use of case studies in the process of learning has gained growing interest in both academia and clinical practice (Kris-Etherton et al., 2014; Shaterjalali et al., 2018) as it facilitates group learning and allows students to learn from one another by encouraging students to engage in discussions in order to solve nutrition-related problems. Moreover, the use of case studies is extensively essential to dietitians and nutritionists since this approach could help in improving students' nutritional knowledge through the application of MNT. It could also help them to be skilled in taking actions to prevent and control GI disorders in a unified manner.

In the context of clinical education for dietetics students, the problem-based approach to learning is the main method of teaching and training used at the King Abdulaziz University (Aljaaly, 2019). This approach enhances students' learning by facilitating the application of theories within real-life or simulation-based settings.

This book therefore can serve to guide students who are applying for a placement in hospitals who are providing MNT services. In addition, this book can help dietetics practitioners to nutritionally manage patients with GI disorders using MNT (Lacey & Pritchett, 2003). The MNT approach has a central role in the management of nutrition-related disorders (Swan et al., 2019). This includes reducing disease risk, slowing disease progression, monitoring of nutritional status, limiting the effects of reduced organs' function, and treating complications. Several dietary elements usually require consideration and may change over time. Nutritional approach for patients with nutrition-related diseases is highly important in maintaining adequate nutrition of those patients (Shao et al., 2017).

Some international associations for Dietetics such as the Academy of Nutrition and Dietetics have called on dieticians to use the NCP and to adapt its standardized language for nutrition diagnosis. This is because in many countries there are still no uniform nutrition and dietetic practices to manage different GI diseases and disorders, particularly in Arab countries. In many dietetics' educational programs in Arab countries, junior students learn the NCP and continue to learn about this process and its components throughout the dietetic program. However, when they come to practice and fieldwork, they continue to apply other traditional care models (Charney, 2010). This could be referred to the applied hospitals' policies where the students practice their profession. Students might also be lacking in confidence to implement the NCP and its components or use its standardized language such as Nutrition Diagnosis.

Therefore, it is essential for all dietetics students to be exposed to the NCP steps extensively. This is in order to facilitate their understanding and application of the NCP steps on real cases in the future.

In 2003, the Academy of Nutrition and Dietetics formerly known as the American Dietetic association has approved the use of the NCP locally and internationally. The NCP is defined as a systematic problem-solving process used by dietitians to improve the nutritional care provided (Lacey & Pritchett, 2003).

Using the NCP has been associated with several benefits in clinical settings as well as in research. This includes the standardization of the process used to provide nutritional care, improving dietitians' critical thinking when making decisions, and the incorporation of evidence-based practice (Swan et al., 2017). The NCP consists of four main steps that are carried out by dietetics professionals only including: Nutrition assessment and reassessment, nutrition diagnosis, nutrition intervention and nutrition monitoring and evaluation. A screening-referral system is a supporting step but not a core one as it may be applied by other health care professionals.

Nutrition assessment and reassessment is a methodical approach for acquiring and analyzing information to identify nutritional problems and their causes. This process is continuous as it involves initial data collection as well as following-up interactions to reassess the patient/client. Types of data collected during this step are classified into five groups: Food and nutrition-related history, anthropometric measurements, biochemical data, medical tests and procedures, nutrition-focused physical examination, and client history.

Food and nutrition related history depends on information about food intake, food administration, alternative/complementary medicine use, nutritional-related principles and views, food accessibility, nutrition quality of life, in addition to physical activity. Some of the most frequently used dietary assessment methods in this category are the 24-hour recall, food frequency questionnaire, weighed food record, and records using an electronic gadget like a mobile phone or camera (Fkub, 2013).

Anthropometric measurements comprise measuring the weight, height, body mass index (BMI), growth pattern, waist circumference, fat mass, fat-free mass, and the weight history. Examples of the tools used here are weighing scales, stadiometers, calipers, and bioelectrical impedance analysis devices. Dietitians should be trained in using these tools, and in choosing the suitable anthropometries for each patient/client depending on the health status and outcomes (Madden & Hoffman, 2019).

Biochemical data is basically laboratory data such as glucose, lipids, vitamins, and electrolytes. Such data sets are important in assessing the status of nutrients and in monitoring various clinical conditions like diabetes mellitus, cardiovascular diseases, and renal diseases. Examples of medical tests and procedures include X-rays, gastric emptying time, and resting metabolic rate (Madden & Hoffman, 2019).

The Nutrition-focused physical findings are used to evaluate physical changes of the patient/client from head-to-toe like fat loss, muscle wasting, edema, swallow function, skin integrity, and dentition. As this will help in the early detection of nutritional abnormalities like malnutrition, nutrient deficiencies, or nutrient toxicities (Litchford, 2015).

Client history relates to personal, medical/health, surgical, family, and social history as well the patient's history of using complementary or alternative medicines. This category is essential in determining the correct diagnosis and intervention (Fkub, 2013).

For the assessment/reassessment step, however, dietitians should employ strong critical thinking skills in order to collect, select, and interpret data related to the patient or client as this will lead to a successful nutritional assessment methodology. Related critical thinking skills might include determining proper data to collect, deciding the need for supplementary information, choosing suitable tools and procedures, applying assessment techniques correctly, and interpreting the data (Skipper, 2008).After the completion of this step and based on its findings, a nutrition-related problem may be identified, and this will help in making a nutrition diagnosis.

Nutrition Diagnosis is the second step in the NCP, where nutrition-related problems are identified and described. Unlike medical diagnosis, the issue here is expected to improve or be treated after nutritional intervention. Nutrition diagnosis is documented using a specific format: Problem, etiology, and signs/symptoms (PES). The problem (P) describes alterations in nutritional status. Standardized diagnostic terms are used to cover the following domains: intake, clinical, and behavioral/environmental problems. The etiology (E) is defined as the underlying cause of the nutritional problem. The term "related to" is used here to link (E) to (P). The signs/symptoms (S) are the proof that the nutrition problem exists. The term "as evidenced by" is used to link (S) to (E). The following sentence is an example of the PES statement format: High energy intake (P) related to frequent consumption of junk-food (E) as evidenced by 10 Kg weight gain during the past 12 months (S) (Mathieu et al., 2005).

Critical thinking skills are required by the dietitian in nutrition diagnosis in order to make sure that the PES statement clarifies the nutrition diagnosis and that the nutrition assessment data supports the nutrition problem, etiology, and signs and symptoms (Hakel-Smith et al., 2005). It is important to note that dietitians could find several nutrition diagnoses and write more than one PES statement. However, the focus should be on a single problem in each statement.

Nutrition Intervention is a designed action used to manage the causes of the nutrition-related problem. It involves two phases: planning phase, where intervention goals are identified and prioritized; and intervention phase whereby the appropriate intervention is implemented. The selected nutrition intervention intends primarily to resolve the nutrition diagnosis, particularly the etiology of the problem. Evidence-based nutrition guidelines or other evidence libraries are the ideal resources for the applied interventions. When planning the intervention, prioritizing and feasibility should be considered. After that, comes the implementation of the planned intervention, and it should be based on teamwork between the healthcare team and the patient/client. For the intervention goals, they should be set in consideration of time and frequency of follow-ups. Thereafter, according to the patient/client response, the intervention can be modified as needed (Mahan et al., 2012). The terminology used at this step is organized in the following five domains: 1) food and/or nutrient delivery, 2) nutrition education, 3) nutrition counseling, 4) coordination of nutrition care, and 5) population based nutrition action (Swan et al., 2019).

Monitoring and Evaluation is the last step in the NCP. This step is critical because it measures the progress towards solving the nutritional problem and determines if the patient/client is achieving the nutrition intervention goals. Monitoring is the re-examination of the patient/client's status by collecting new data. It includes two distinct steps involving progress monitoring by checking the compliance with the plan and outcomes/indicators measuring. Evaluation is the assessment of patient's current health status in comparison to previous findings or to reference standards. The terms used during this step are similar to those used during the assessment step as the two steps are closely related. They are organized in the following four domains: 1) food/nutrition-related history outcomes, 2) anthropometric measurement outcomes, 3) biochemical data, medical tests, and procedure outcomes, and 4) nutrition-focused physical findings outcomes (Swan et al., 2019).

The approaches used in the handbook *Cases on Medical Nutrition Therapy for GI Disorders* require case reporters for each case to review the pathophysiology of the disease, and the assessment of risk factors to help diagnose the underlying causes of the problem. Case reports also include nutritional assessment of the disease, medical nutritional therapy and complementary & alternative medicine (CAM) - if applicable - in the management of diseases.

The book uses up-to-date information and practices, shares ideas from experts in the field, and provides dietetic and other health practitioners in the clinical dietetic practice with guidelines in managing disease in the scope of GI disorders by using an relatively straight forward method known as 'mind mapping' (MM) to conclude the MNT for each case study with a greater level of interrelated information.

Mind Mapping (MM) is a nonlinear, multisensory learning and teaching method which has been increasingly used in higher education settings to improve students' analytical thinking and assist learners manage greater volumes of interconnected information (Pudelko et al., 2012). It is not uncommon for medical students to be challenged by information overload, with their learnings made all the more challenging by their limited time to study and recall all this information when needed, which in turn ultimately contributes to lower levels of success through the examination period (Yusoff et al., 2013). This problem isn't helped by the fact that most medical educators use traditional teaching and learning methods, such as PowerPoint slides. Text slides like these are purely linear representations that unfortunately fail to adequately reveal the rich inter-connectedness between the medical ideas and concepts. Because of the shortcomings of such traditional educational tools and techniques, many researchers have recognized the necessity for substituting learning and teaching techniques which will allow medical students to memorize large amounts of information, gain critical thinking competencies, and solve various clinical problems.

MM is one such tool that can be used in education to address the above-mentioned challenge. MM arranges large amounts of information visually and demonstrates the relationship between the separate topics of information. A mind map is usually formed about a single idea or broad topic, sketched as an image in the middle of a blank paper, to which related ideas – through words or images - are added. Main ideas are linked straight to the center, and extra ideas branch out from those main ideas (Hopper, 2016).

The human brain works in an associative way and has the ability to connect thousands of ideas (Anokhin, 1973). Mind mapping is radiant structured in a way that stimulates the different parts of the brain to interact (Buzan & Buzan, 1994). The use of color is one of the most effective aspects of MM. Psychologists have stated that color helps learners remember more compared to use colorless (i.e. black and white) imagery. Pictures, drawings, symbols, and other visual imagery are also important key elements of MM that serve as more effective memory aids than words (Anglin et al., 2004). Many studies highlight the advantages of using MM in education, specifically its effectiveness in learning, teaching research and solving problems. MM's spatial layout assists in making the new associations more obvious for the learner (Al-Jarf & others, 2009).

Most of the medical students who use MM, find it to be more efficient for information memorizing compared to other methods of self-study ways (Wickramasinghe et al., 2011). Using MM for lesson preparation might help teachers for recalling subject materials and boost teaching confidence (Boyson, 2009). The first study conducted on using MM in medical education (Farrand et al., 2002) found that MM significantly enhanced a learner's long-term memory. According to a study done on physical therapy students, 10 out of 14 stated that using MM results in organizing and understanding their courses more effectively (D'Antoni & Zipp, 2006).

Another study (Spencer et al., 2013) stated that MM improves the connection between thoughts, which assists in data holding, information gaining and broad comprehension. Yet another study (Holland et al., 2004) states that MM is an influential method used in designing projects and assignments. Using MM in writing improves the students' working as they turn out to be more creative in generating and joining thoughts. MM facilitates thinking with better clarity to realize associations between ideas to find problems' keys and analyze alternatives in patient care (Al-Jarf & others, 2009). In medical education, the advantage of using MM may be valuable for different students' specialties as it found to be beneficial tool for innovative thinking and cooperating with others.

In conclusion, further, to serving as a useful guide for health providers in the scope of GI disorders in their practice, this clinical education book could also be used as a practical guide for academic staff who are involved with dietetic clinical education. Registered dietitians in the practice, dietetic interns and students will also benefit from case scenarios that focuses on the MNT and applied NCP for disorders of the digestive system.

At last, the editors of this book would like to thank all the reviewers who participated in the improvement of this work for their thoughtful comments, valuable suggestions, and considerable efforts.

REFERENCES

Al-Jarf, R., & ... (2009). Enhancing freshman students' writing skills with a mind-mapping software. *Conference Proceedings of eLearning and Software for Education (ELSE), 1*, 375–382.

Aljaaly, E. A. (2019). Challenges and Reflections on the Experience and Development of the Profession of Nutrition and Dietetics: A Starting Point With the First Indigenous Dietitian in Saudi Arabia. In Handbook of Research on Indigenous Knowledge and Bi-Culturalism in a Global Context (pp. 95–119). IGI Global. doi:10.4018/978-1-5225-6061-6.ch006

Anglin, G. J., Vaez, H., & Cunningham, K. L. (2004). Visual representations and learning: The role of static and animated graphics. Handbook of Research on Educational Communications and Technology, 2, 865–916.

Anokhin, P. K. (1973). The Forming of Natural and Artificial Intelligence. *Impact of Science on Society*, *23*(3), 195–212.

Boyson, G. (2009). The use of mind mapping in teaching and learning. *The Learning Institute. Assignment*, *3*(8), 123–145.

Buzan, T., & Buzan, B. (1994). *The Mind Map Book*. Dutton.

Charney, P. (2010). *The Nutrition Care Process*. Academic Press.

D'Antoni, A. V., & Zipp, G. P. (2006). Applications of the mind map learning technique in chiropractic education: A pilot study and literature review. *Journal of Chiropractic Humanities*, *13*, 2–11. doi:10.1016/S1556-3499(13)60153-9

Farrand, P., Hussain, F., & Hennessy, E. (2002). The efficacy of themind map'study technique. *Medical Education*, *36*(5), 426–431. doi:10.1046/j.1365-2923.2002.01205.x PMID:12028392

Fkub, J. G. (2013). *NCP Step 1 : Nutrition Assessment*. Academy of Nutrition and Dietetics. https://www.ncpro.org/nutrition-assessment-snapshot

Hakel-Smith, N., Lewis, N. M., & Eskridge, K. M. (2005). Orientation to nutrition care process standards improves nutrition care documentation by nutrition practitioners. *Journal of the American Dietetic Association*, *105*(10), 1582–1589. doi:10.1016/j.jada.2005.07.004 PMID:16183359

Holland, B., Holland, L., & Davies, J. (2004). *An investigation into the concept of mind mapping and the use of mind mapping software to support and improve student academic performance*. Academic Press.

Hopper, C. H. (2016). *Practicing college learning strategies* (7th ed.). Cengage Learning.

Howe, M. J. A. (1970). Using students' notes to examine the role of the individual learner in acquiring meaningful subject matter. *The Journal of Educational Research*, *64*(2), 61–63. doi:10.1080/00220671.1970.10884094

Kris-Etherton, P. M., Akabas, S. R., Bales, C. W., Bistrian, B., Braun, L., Edwards, M. S., Laur, C., Lenders, C. M., Levy, M. D., Palmer, C. A., Pratt, C. A., Ray, S., Rock, C. L., Saltzman, E., Seidner, D. L., & Van Horn, L. (2014). The need to advance nutrition education in the training of health care professionals and recommended research to evaluate implementation and effectiveness. *The American Journal of Clinical Nutrition*, *99*(5), 1153S–1166S. doi:10.3945/ajcn.113.073502 PMID:24717343

Lacey, K., & Pritchett, E. (2003). Nutrition care process and model: ADA adopts road map to quality care and outcomes management. *Journal of the Academy of Nutrition and Dietetics*, *103*(8), 1061–1072. PMID:12891159

Litchford, M. D. (2015). *Nutrition Focused Physical Assessment: Making Clinical Connections*. Case Software & Books.

Madden, A., & Hoffman, R. (2019). Assessment of nutritional status. In *Manual of Dietetic Practice*. John Wiley & Sons.

Mahan, L. K., Escott-Stump, S., Raymond, J. L., & Krause, M. V. (2012). *Krause's food & the nutrition care process*. Elsevier Health Sciences.

Mathieu, J., Foust, M., & Ouellette, P. (2005). Implementing nutrition diagnosis, step two in the nutrition care process and model: Challenges and lessons learned in two health care facilities. *Journal of the Academy of Nutrition and Dietetics*, *105*(10), 1636–1640. PMID:16183367

Pudelko, B., Young, M., Vincent-Lamarre, P., & Charlin, B. (2012). Mapping as a learning strategy in health professions education: A critical analysis. *Medical Education*, *46*(12), 1215–1225. doi:10.1111/medu.12032 PMID:23171264

Shao, A., Drewnowski, A., Willcox, D. C., Krämer, L., Lausted, C., Eggersdorfer, M., Mathers, J., Bell, J. D., Randolph, R. K., Witkamp, R., & Griffiths, J. C. (2017). Optimal nutrition and the ever-changing dietary landscape: A conference report. *European Journal of Nutrition*, *56*(1), 1–21. doi:10.100700394-017-1460-9 PMID:28474121

Shaterjalali, M., Yamani, N., & Changiz, T. (2018). Who are the right teachers for medical clinical students? investigating stakeholders' opinions using modified Delphi approach. *Advances in Medical Education and Practice*, *9*, 801–809. doi:10.2147/AMEP.S176480 PMID:30519136

Skipper, A. (2008). Nutrition care process and model part I: The 2008 update. *Journal of the American Dietetic Association*. PMID:18589014

Spencer, J. R., Anderson, K. M., & Ellis, K. K. (2013). Radiant thinking and the use of the mind map in nurse practitioner education. *The Journal of Nursing Education*, *52*(5), 291–293. doi:10.3928/01484834-20130328-03 PMID:23550549

Swan, W. I., Pertel, D. G., Hotson, B., Lloyd, L., Orrevall, Y., Trostler, N., Vivanti, A., Howarter, K. B., & Papoutsakis, C. (2019). Nutrition Care Process (NCP) update part 2: Developing and using the NCP terminology to demonstrate efficacy of nutrition care and related outcomes. *Journal of the Academy of Nutrition and Dietetics*, *119*(5), 840–855. doi:10.1016/j.jand.2018.10.025 PMID:30660633

Swan, W. I., Vivanti, A., Hakel-Smith, N. A., Hotson, B., Orrevall, Y., Trostler, N., Howarter, K. B., & Papoutsakis, C. (2017). Nutrition Care Process and Model update: Toward realizing people-centered care and outcomes management. *Journal of the Academy of Nutrition and Dietetics*, *117*(12), 2003–2014. doi:10.1016/j.jand.2017.07.015 PMID:28988837

Wickramasinghe, A., Widanapathirana, N., Kuruppu, O., Liyanage, I., & Karunathilake, I. M. K. (2011). *Effectiveness of mind maps as a learning tool for medical students*. South East Asian Journal of Medical Education.

Yusoff, M. S. B., Rahim, A. F. A., Baba, A. A., Ismail, S. B., Pa, M. N. M., & ... (2013). Prevalence and associated factors of stress, anxiety and depression among prospective medical students. *Asian Journal of Psychiatry*, *6*(2), 128–133. doi:10.1016/j.ajp.2012.09.012 PMID:23466109

Section 1

Cases on Medical Nutrition Therapy for Upper Gastrointestinal Tract Disorders

Chapter 1
Dysphagia and Considerations for Nutritional Intervention

Maryanne Weatherill
https://orcid.org/0000-0002-2818-3676
University of West Georgia, USA

EXECUTIVE SUMMARY

This chapter discusses a clinical case from the interdisciplinary practice of dysphagia and the collaboration between speech-language pathology clinicians and dietetics professionals from the perspective of the speech-language pathologist. The discussion begins with an introduction to the normal swallowing process to better understand disordered swallowing and the role of therapeutic and compensatory interventions. Changes in swallowing that occur with normal aging and their impact are identified and reviewed. Common interventions and considerations in the clinical management of dysphagia from the perspective of the speech-language pathologist are included with rationale based on the current literature. Swallowing motor functions and factors in dysphagia decision making are discussed in relationship to clinical problem solving with a sample case and nutritional interventions. The chapter closes with general recommendations and conclusions to assist in learning and understanding of the concepts discussed.

INTRODUCTION

In healthcare settings, an interdisciplinary approach is applied to management of swallowing disorders (dysphagia) and this collaboration may include a dietetic professional and a speech-language pathologist (SLP), along with the patient, their family, and other members of the healthcare team. Speech-language pathologists

DOI: 10.4018/978-1-7998-3802-9.ch001

are professionals who assess, diagnose and treat dysphagia, as well as a variety of communication and cognitive disorders (ASHA, 2016). This case study chapter discusses the clinical problem of dysphagia from the perspective of a speech-language pathologist practicing in the United States. Dysphagia is identified as a risk factor for malnutrition, (Chen, Li, Fang, Lu, & He, 2019). This supports the need for close collaboration between the SLPs, who address the motor and sensory complications of dysphagia and the dietetic professionals who address the nutritional concerns. Insight into different perspectives on dysphagia and dysphagia management is important to understand the influences of dysphagia on clinical decision-making and patient outcomes.

Dysphagia is a disorder of swallowing that may affect a person's ability to safely and effectively meet their nutritional needs. A variety of medical conditions may result in dysphagia, including neurological conditions affecting a person's motor skills, or diagnoses or procedures that can affect function of the swallowing structures. For example, anterior cervical disc fusion (ACDF) procedures may result in a two-week post-surgical dysphagia incidence of up to 71%, with declining incidence over time (Cho, Lu, & Lee, 2013). Dysphagia has been identified through videofluoroscopic evaluation in 64% of patients assessed after acute stroke (Mann, Hankey, & Cameron, 2000). In addition to the effects of dysphagia on one's ability to adequately obtain nutrition and hydration, presence of dysphagia can influence morbidity, mortality, and quality of life (Gonzales-Fernandez, Ottenstein, Atanelov, & Christian, 2013). Based on an understanding of dysphagia as a disorder with multiple influences, perhaps a better working definition of dysphagia would encompass a broader perspective, such as: dysphagia is a multifactorial swallowing disorder that can affect a person's overall health and psychosocial well-being. Regardless of the reason for the dysphagia, each case is unique and intervention is dependent upon multiple factors that influence the overall management approach.

For discussion purposes, this chapter introduces a composite clinical case of a 75-year-old male who suffers from dysphagia as a result of a stroke. The American Heart Association reports that in the United States, over 795,000 people have a stroke annually (Go, et al., 2012). The incidence of dysphagia after stroke varies by location and severity of infarct but this diagnosis was selected for the case study due to documented high rates of resulting dysphagia. Research indicates that 64-78% of people post stroke demonstrated dysphagia when they were evaluated with instrumental studies in the acute hospital setting (Martino et al., 2005). Presence of a previous stroke is cited as a risk factor related to higher rates of malnutrition (Chen et al., 2019) with up to 62% of people suffering from malnutrition post stroke (Foley, Salter, Robertson, Teasell, & Woodbury, 2009). To better understand the case study, a basic review of normal swallowing, age-related changes in swallowing, disordered swallowing, swallowing assessments, and dysphagia management are presented.

Normal Swallowing Process

The act of swallowing is known as deglutition. Normal swallowing is a complex motor and sensory process involving the structures and functions of the head and neck based on signals received from and transmitted to the nervous system. Efforts of over 30 muscles and six cranial nerves coordinate to produce a normal swallow (Gonzales-Fernandez et al., 2013). Swallowing occurs in three main phases: oral phase, pharyngeal phase, and the esophageal phase. The oral phase has two sub-components: the oral preparatory phase and the oral propulsive stage.

A very simplified description of this process is as follows: 1) The oral preparatory phase encompasses the processing of the food or liquid bolus in the oral cavity, "preparing" the items to be swallowed. This preparation includes the action of the lips to prevent anterior leakage of the bolus from oral cavity, as well as teeth for mastication (chewing) and the use of the other oral structures including the tongue, cheeks, and palate to control, mash and form the bolus before moving it through the oral cavity for swallowing. 2) Once the bolus is prepared for swallowing, it is propelled through the oral cavity. This is primarily accomplished through tongue movement and control, in which the bolus is contained and moved posteriorly between the dorsum of the tongue, inferiorly, and the hard palate, superiorly. 3) The bolus transitions over the back of the tongue and enters the pharyngeal phase. During the pharyngeal phase, the soft palate is elevated to seal off the nasal cavity and the bolus is driven downward due to a variety of simultaneous, coordinated movements and pressure changes. At this time the larynx elevates and protective functions of the larynx are engaged to prevent aspiration and protect the airway. The pharyngeal phase ends when the upper esophageal sphincter (UES) relaxes and allows the bolus to pass into the esophagus. 4) The esophageal phase is bound by the UES and the lower esophageal sphincter (LES) that leads to the stomach. When the bolus has moved through the esophagus, the LES relaxes and the bolus moves into the stomach and the swallowing process is complete.

Effects of Aging on Swallowing

Normal swallowing is a dynamic and synchronized process that occurs with small variations from person to person. Normal variability is present between individuals and swallowing functions can change during the natural aging process. Presbyphagia is age related swallowing change and is considered normal and not a disorder. Age does not specifically cause dysphagia but changes related to aging can contribute to it (Groher & Crary, 2015). As a person ages, some common changes include decreased frequency of swallowing with research describing from 2-19 swallows per hour in healthy elderly people with a mean age of 82.4 years, and 16-76 times per hour for healthy adults with a mean age of 26.5 years (Tanaka, Nohara, Kotani, Matsumura, & Sakai, 2013). As people age, swallowing initiation may be slower and duration for UES opening may be longer (Namasivayam-MacDonald, Barbon, & Steele, 2018).

Age related changes can contribute to complications such as malnutrition in frail elderly people (Cichero, 2018). As people age, they may demonstrate decreased ability to regulate intake of nutrition resulting in a physiologic response known as "anorexia of aging" (Morely, 1997). As the aging process occurs, a person may experience changes in sensation or perception of food taste (Schiffman & Graham, 2000). Additionally, medications used for management of medical conditions may have side effects which affect intake due to alterations in taste or smell (Cichero, 2018), or a reduction in production of saliva and oral/pharyngeal moistness, influencing the overall condition of the oral environment (Cichero, 2017). When a neurological infarct such as stroke occurs, normal changes in taste sensation may be affected by damage to the cortical sensory areas, or the cranial nerves responsible for innervating the taste receptors. This damage can reduce function in an already limited system.

People may demonstrate difference in oral phase processing of boluses due to tooth loss and/or presence or absence of dentures. Presence or absence of partial dentures or complete dentures and their use may influence food choice and diet quality (Su, Yuki, Hirayama, Sato, & Han, 2020). In a study of denture use and nutritional status, denture use increased with age, and a relationship was found between denture use and increased complaints of chewing, biting, or swallowing difficulty (Papas, Palmer, Rounds, & Russell, 1998). In the same study, the researchers found that denture wearers also had lower protein intake than their dentate peers (Papas et al, 1998).

Disordered Swallowing

Two major possible consequences of dysphagia include malnutrition and aspiration, both of which can lead to further medical complications. Dysphagia can contribute to poor oral intake, with subsequent malnutrition and dehydration (Chen et al., 2019).

Dysphagia is closely associated with malnutrition risk and patients with dysphagia have a higher number of medical diagnoses (Blanař, Hödl, Lohrmann, Amir, & Eglseer, 2019). Crary et al., (2013) discuss higher BUN/Cr levels in acute stroke patients who had dysphagia, though 32% of the patients studied had malnutrition upon admission and could only theorize on the cause. The findings of Blanař et al., (2019) further support dysphagia screenings for patients at risk for malnutrition.

Aspiration occurs when the food, liquid, or other material enters the laryngeal vestibule and proceeds below the vocal folds into the trachea. Penetration is the term used when the food, liquid, or other material enters the laryngeal vestibule but does not progress below the level of the vocal folds. Aspiration can lead to pulmonary complications including aspiration pneumonia. There are many factors that determine whether a person will develop aspiration pneumonia or not. These can include the severity of the illness, along with other co-occurring factors including nil per os (NPO) status and the presence of bacteria in the oral cavity. In stroke patients, the relative levels of *Streptococcus spp.* and *Strep pneumoniae* bacteria increased significantly on saliva samples taken one-month post, and patients with suspected pneumonia during hospitalization demonstrated an association between presence of *Strep pneumoniae* development of aspiration pneumonia (Perry, Huckabee, Tomkins, & Milne, 2019).

Swallowing Assessment

Clinical Assessment

Swallowing assessments can be either clinical or instrumental. Clinical assessments can include "bedside" evaluation with a variety of screening or non-instrumental assessment tools. Clinical assessments are often more readily available to the patient than instrumental assessments. Drawbacks of clinical assessments include limitations in ability to detect and/or rule out aspiration, and the inability to clearly visualize all aspects of the swallow (McCullough et al., 2005).

Instrumental Assessment

Instrumental assessments are used to assess the structures and functions involved in swallowing and to determine a course of treatment. Videofluoroscopic swallowing evaluations are a type of moving x-ray study, conducted while administering different consistencies of barium, using a fluoroscope to visualize swallowing functions. Use of the fluoroscope for a swallowing evaluation is known by several names; videofluoroscopic swallowing study (VFSS), modified barium swallow (MBS) or modified barium swallow study (MBSS). The swallowing structures and functions are assessed in the lateral and anterior-posterior (AP) views. A benefit of the MBSS procedure is the ability to view all phases of the swallow, while a drawback includes exposure to radiation. Another instrumental evaluation common to the clinical setting is known as a fiberoptic endoscopic evaluation of swallowing (FEES). It includes directly viewing the structures involved in swallowing through the use of a flexible fiberoptic endoscope inserted through the nose, passed through the nasal cavity to view the pharyngeal cavity and the larynx. Benefits of the FEES assessment include direct visualization of the structures and no exposure to radiation, while drawbacks include inability to view all phases of the swallow.

Dysphagia Management

Ideally, dysphagia management will incorporate a multidisciplinary, collaborative approach. Use of a multidisciplinary approach is beneficial for identifying and treating patients with dysphagia and reducing pneumonia. In a study conducted by Aoki et al. (2016), 132 acute stroke patient admissions were examined pre- incorporation of a multidisciplinary team approach and compared to 173 acute stroke patient admissions post- incorporation of a multidisciplinary team approach. The patients in both groups exhibited similar rates of fever, but the pre- incorporation group demonstrated a significantly higher onset and diagnosis of pneumonia at 15.9% than the post- incorporation patients at 6.9% (Aoki et al., 2016). Formal team organization for dysphagia management in the Aoki et al. (2016) study also resulted in increased professional oral care with a dentist or dental hygienist from 12.9% to 51.7%; increase in instrumental swallowing assessments from 12.1% to 26%; individualized nutritional management; and implementation of mealtime patient body positioning by physical therapy and occupational therapy. All of which were felt to have contributed to an overall decrease in incidence of pneumonia.

From the perspective of the SLP, after the patient completes a swallowing evaluation, the SLP considers the patient's swallowing structures and functions, information about the patient's historical level of functioning, nutritional needs, medical status, personal goals and beliefs. This information is used to formulate a plan to address the identified motor or sensory issue(s), and physical intake and management of the prescribed nutritional source. The resulting plan may include direct rehabilitation approaches or compensatory management designed to compensate for the disorder.

Compensatory Approaches

Compensatory approaches address how the problem can be managed in the current situation in the present time. Compensatory approaches are not rehabilitative because they do not target skills to improve function. These approaches are only used to manage the current functional level of intake; to help the patient maximize his or her potential to obtain adequate nutrition to meet their needs; and minimize the risk of aspiration or other complications. Compensations can be direct approaches, giving the patient specific actions to compensate for, or overcome a deficit. One example is the patient who can drink thin liquids from a cup without difficulty, but demonstrates aspiration when using a straw. The approach for this patient would be to instruct in cup drinking only. The use of postural strategies including asking the person to turn their head or tuck their chin when swallowing would be considered a postural compensation.

Another compensatory approach for dysphagia management includes use of modified food and liquid textures. Modifying a food texture can include using a blender to create a pureed food texture, or using food thickeners to change the texture from a thin liquid as in water, to a thicker liquid similar to a blended yoghurt drink. An item can start out as one texture and become another. For example, one common misperception is that ice cream based milkshakes are considered a "thick" liquid, when they are not due to the melting and texture thinning that occurs. In an effort to standardize the food and liquid textures the International Dysphagia Diet Standardisation Initiative (IDDSI) was developed. This global initiative is an attempt to develop an understanding of food and liquids that could be applied across the continuum of care and from country to country. The classification system categorizes liquids from thinnest consistency (Level 0) to thickest (Level 4) and foods from most restrictive (Level 3) to least restrictive at Level 7 (IDDSI, 2016)

While modified diet textures have a role in dysphagia management they have been associated with negative consequences including dehydration and malnutrition (Gonzales-Fernandez et al., 2013) and should be used with caution. Diet texture modifications are common in practice, but should be incorporated only when deemed necessary after a visualization study as they do not always reduce aspiration and can increase risk for other medical complications including dehydration and malnutrition due to patient refusal. At that point, the potential complications of dehydration and malnutrition must be weighed against the risk for complications from aspiration during the decision making process.

Swallowing compensations including postural or positional strategies, as well as food and liquid texture modifications, must be visualized through an instrumental swallowing study prior to use. Their effectiveness cannot be fully evaluated without visualization. Clinicians can only see what is really happening as a result of these compensations if they are using imaging equipment such as with MBSS or FEES. Each of these compensatory strategies may help a person to manage their dysphagia, but it will not rehabilitate it.

Rehabilitative Approaches

Rehabilitative approaches to remediate the swallowing function are direct interventions performed by the SLP. They may involve use of therapeutic techniques, exercises, or modalities. These approaches are designed to directly influence the movement rate, range, accuracy, or strength of the swallow. Ideally, a person who demonstrates dysphagia and requires compensatory approaches initially will improve through rehabilitation and normalize the swallow to the point where the compensations, including diet texture restrictions can be discontinued.

SETTING THE STAGE

This case study is presented in medical chart form and is a composite representation of a typical patient admitted to the Emergency Department (ED) of a hospital in the U.S. In this setting, the patient will proceed through several phases of evaluation and treatment. Initially, they will receive a medical evaluation in the ED. The initial medical evaluation includes clinical assessments as well as relevant laboratory tests and imaging evaluations. The patient in this case discussion was admitted with symptoms that, through evaluation, lead to the diagnosis of cerebrovascular accident (CVA) or stroke.

When a person receives a CVA diagnosis in the ED, a specific treatment plan is initiated. This plan includes evaluations by other medical and rehabilitation professionals that typically occur after the patient leaves the ED and are transferred to the inpatient medical unit. These referrals include evaluations by speech-language pathologists, dietetics practitioners, physical therapists, occupational therapists, and may include other professionals as well as lab tests and imaging studies.

Often the patients may remain nil per os (NPO), or nothing by mouth, prior to screening by nursing staff or evaluation by the SLP. Each hospital may have their own screening protocol for identifying patients at risk for dysphagia. The speech-language pathologist's evaluation includes a clinical, or bedside swallowing assessment, and may include additional instrumental diagnostics including a modified barium swallow study/videofluoroscopic swallowing study (MBSS/VFSS), or a flexible fiberoptic endoscopic evaluation of swallowing (FEES).

CASE DESCRIPTION

Patient's Details

- Age: 75 years
- Gender: Male

Case History

Case description: The patient is a 75-year-old Caucasian male who presented to the Emergency Department at 13:30 on hospital admission day, with sudden-onset, generalized right-sided weakness affecting motor functions for his face, arm, and leg. He demonstrates slurred speech and word finding difficulties. Nursing staff administered a swallow screening, which the patient failed. Due to the symptoms he was displaying, he was made NPO until he received a clinical swallowing evaluation.

- Medical history: Includes hypertension, hyperlipidemia, and type II diabetes.
- Surgical history: Unremarkable.
- Smoking: 10-year 1 pack per day smoking history. Quit 30 years ago.
- Family history: Father with diabetes, cardiovascular disease, ischemic CVA, hypertension.

Main Medical Diagnosis

Left middle cerebral artery ischemic CVA

Demographics

- Marital status: The patient is married and lives with his wife in a one story home.
- Education: Master's degree in history.
- Occupation: Retired teacher.
- Ethnicity and religion: Caucasian, Non-denominational

Anthropometry

- Current weight: 113 kg
- Admission weight: 115 kg
- Height: 182 cm

Nutritionally Focused Physical Examination

- General appearance: No acute distress, drowsy but easily roused
- Heart: Regular rhythm and rate. S1, S2 present without S3, S4. No murmurs or gallops
- HEENT: R facial droop. R eye droop. Visual fields appear intact. Ears clear. No sinus drainage.
- Genitalia: Deferred
- Neurologic: Alert to voice, oriented to person, but not to place, or time. Unable to spell "world" forwards or backwards. Follows one-step commands 100%, 2 step commands 50%. 1/3 recall at approx. 5 minutes. Speech: low volume, slow rate, +word finding difficulty, difficulty naming objects (able to name pen but not purpose). Unable to do serial 7s.
- Extremities: No peripheral edema noted.
- Skin: Skin is warm, dry, and intact. No decubitus ulcers on initial exam

- Chest/lungs: Non-labored, no accessory muscle use. Symmetric breathing. CTAB. No rhonchi, egophony, or crackles on auscultation.
- Peripheral vascular: R arm and leg numbness, weakness
- Abdomen: Nontender, non-distended. BS+ normal. No organomegaly on palpation

Vital Signs

- Pulse: 85
- Temp: 37°C
- Blood pressure: 165/95
- Resp rate: 25

Food/Nutrition-Related History

The patient has been consuming a regular texture, 2 gram sodium, consistent carb diet prior to his hospitalization. Since admission, he has been NPO.

24-Hour Recall

Meal 1: NPO
Meal 2: NPO
Meal 3: 25% of pureed meal and 160cc moderately thick liquids

- Food allergies/intolerances: None
- Food purchase/preparations: The patient and his wife share in food purchase and preparation responsibilities
- Vitamin and mineral supplementation: None

Medications

- Spironolactone 100mg QD
- Atenolol 50mg QD
- Metformin 500ml BID

CHRONOLOGY OF KEY EVENTS

Clinical Evaluation of Swallowing

Time of evaluation: 14:00, 24.5 hours post admission
Reason for evaluation: The patient was admitted with a diagnosis of ischemic left middle cerebral artery cerebrovascular accident. Swallowing evaluation orders received as part of the stroke protocol.
Current diet texture: NPO, IV for hydration, no oral intake, no additional nutritional support

Clinical Assessment Procedure and Findings

The following food items were administered: applesauce and canned fruit. More challenging solid food items were deferred due to the patient's response to the items administered. Liquids in the following International Dysphagia Diet Standardization Initiative (IDDSI, 2016) consistencies were administered: Level 0 (thin), Level 2 (mildly thick) and Level 3 (moderately thick) liquids.

Oral Phase

The patient demonstrates right facial weakness at rest and in motion. He demonstrates poor lip seal on the right, with labial drooping and oral leakage of saliva. He is unable to complete lip rounding on the right and is unable to form lip seal against pressure or around spoon or straw.

Buccal strength impairment is evident in right facial drooping and accumulation of bolus trials in the right lateral sulcus, with residue present after swallowing. Buccal numbness is present and leads to the patient frequently biting his cheek due to this decreased oral sensation.

The patient retains natural teeth in well-maintained condition, serving as functional units for mastication. Oral bolus preparation is impacted through right-sided weakness of the muscles of mastication. This limitation results in ineffective mastication for solid food textures.

He demonstrates lingual weakness evident in inability to elevate tongue tip outside of oral cavity to lick lips and leaked material, with inability to fully lateralize tongue to clear food from the right lateral sulcus. In addition, food residue is present on the right dorsal tongue after swallowing.

Pharyngeal Phase

The patient demonstrates signs of decreased laryngeal function for airway protection. He exhibits a weak, breathy voice during speech tasks, and a volitional cough judged to be likely insufficient to fully expel any aspirated material from the airway. The patient demonstrates overt symptoms of pharyngeal dysphagia including multiple coughing episodes and expectoration, though the full extent of pharyngeal involvement cannot be determined without an instrumental assessment.

Recommendations from Clinical Assessment

During clinical evaluation, the patient demonstrates overt difficulty in the oral phase of the swallow with signs and symptoms that suggest pharyngeal involvement. Due to these findings and concerns for decreased airway protection and risk of aspiration, a modified barium swallow study was requested to further assess the patient's function and to assist in the therapeutic decision-making process.

Instrumental Swallowing Assessment

Time of evaluation: 12:30, 47 hours post admission
Reason for evaluation: To visualize swallowing, assess structures and functions, and assist in therapeutic decision-making including appropriate interventions and diet texture recommendations.
Current diet texture: NPO, IV for hydration, no oral intake, no additional nutritional support

Procedure

Videofluoroscopy included projections in the lateral and anterior-posterior views with the patient positioned in an upright sitting position. The following textures of barium following IDDSI standards were administered by cup, spoon, or straw or appropriate: Level 0 (thin), Level 2 (mildly thick), Level 3 (moderately thick) liquids, and Level 4 (puree), level 5 (minced and moist), and level 6 (soft and bite sized) food items mixed with barium. Boluses varied in size by mode of administration.

Results

In addition to supporting the clinical findings above the MBSS revealed oral phase deficits including poor lip seal with oral leakage; poor tongue coordination with decreased bolus formation; difficulty masticating solid food items; tongue rocking prior to propulsion to the back of tongue. During active mastication, some of the Level 5 and 6 food boluses escaped the oral cavity into the pharynx without being processed, then progressed over the back of the tongue into the vallecula with subsequent penetration to the level of the vocal folds prior to initiation of laryngeal elevation in the pharyngeal phase. For all textures, the patient demonstrated some degree of residue present in the vallecula after the swallow, decreased pharyngeal stripping, and decreased base of tongue retraction. Once the boluses passed the UES into the esophagus, they appeared to pass through to the distal esophagus without overt difficulty on a cursory esophageal sweep in the AP view. With liquid items, the boluses poured over the base of tongue into the vallecula and the pyriform sinuses with spillage into the airway prior to initiation of the pharyngeal swallow. The patient demonstrated insufficient airway protection with liquid items. Penetration was present with Levels 0, 2, 3 trials and aspiration present with Levels 0, and 2.

Results of the assessment based on the Penetration-Aspiration Scale (PENASP), (Rosenbek, Robbins, Roecker, Coyle, & Wood, 1996) as seen in Appendix, Table 1 are as follows:

IDDSI Level 0: PENASP 7 Material enters the airway, passes below the vocal folds, and is not ejected from the trachea despite effort

IDDSI Level 2: PENASP 7 Material enters the airway, passes below the vocal folds, and is not ejected from the trachea despite effort

IDDSI Level 3: PENASP 2 Material enters the airway, remains above the vocal folds, and is ejected from the airway

IDDSI Level 4: PENASP 1 Material does not enter the airway

IDDSI Level 5: PENASP 5 Material enters the airway, contacts the vocal folds, and is not ejected from the airway.

IDDSI Level 6: PENASP 5 Material enters the airway, contacts the vocal folds, and is not ejected from the airway

Impressions

The patient demonstrates oropharyngeal dysphagia characterized by difficulties in oral preparation of all consistencies, with inability to fully masticate level 6 food items, and poor ability to form a cohesive bolus with level 5 food items. These items did not maintain bolus cohesion as the items transitioned into and through the pharyngeal phase increasing risk for aspiration. The best oral and pharyngeal management occurred with the level 4 texture, and resulted in the least amount of oral and pharyngeal residue after completing the swallow. The patient demonstrated consistent aspiration during the swallow with coughing present on each trial of the aspirated level 1 liquid.

Recommendations

The patient demonstrates significant motor impairment of the oral and pharyngeal swallowing phases. He would benefit from a swallowing rehabilitation program based on the principles of neural plasticity and motor learning. Compensatory positioning strategies were not effective during the study and are therefore not recommended. Due to the deficits visualized on the MBSS study, diet modifications including level 3 (moderately thick) liquids and level 4 (puree) food items are recommended. Given the severity of the deficits seen on this study, there is concern that the patient may have difficulty consuming his modified diet in an efficient manner, thus putting him at risk for nutritional deficits.

DISCUSSION

The main aim of the nutrition therapy for this case is to integrate the patient's nutritional needs and functional limitations in a manner that best facilitates safe and adequate nutrition that supports quality of life while respecting the patient's personal and healthcare choices. As the patient was NPO for a minimum of 47 hours of his hospitalization without a source of nutritional intake, and before the instrumental swallowing assessment was conducted, the most immediate needs for this patient are his ability to obtain adequate nutrition and hydration as well as successful administration of medication. Though the standard for clinical evaluation is within the first 24 hours, it may not happen for a variety of reasons. These may include the patient not being alert and able to participate in a study, medically unstable, or the patient may need to be NPO for a different test, procedure, or surgery, thus delaying the assessment.

Just as there are many etiologies of dysphagia, there may be many correct solutions for addressing it. Management of patients with dysphagia requires a highly individualized problem-solving process and integrates consideration of a multitude of factors including the health status and projected course, current level of function, risk for complications, personal choices, and access to service issues. These factors must be considered within the interdisciplinary collaboration of the dietetic professional, SLP, physician, and others involved in the patient's care.

This case illustrates how the type and severity of dysphagia shapes the decision-making process for diet consistency recommendations made by the SLP after conducting an evaluation of swallowing. It highlights examples of clinical and instrumental swallowing evaluations and the different types of findings revealed by each. Findings are then translated into the recommendations that the SLP makes for the patient. These recommendations may include potential types of compensatory strategies, rehabilitation techniques, and diet texture recommendations. This is just one example of how dysphagia may present in a clinical case, as well as one interpretation of the results and recommended course. Two potential scenarios and courses of action are described below.

Scenario 1: The Patient Begins Oral Intake and Meets Nutrition and Hydration Needs

Ideally, the patient will be able to resume his oral intake and meet his nutrition and hydration needs. The dietetic professional and the SLP will collaborate to help assure the patient receives the diet texture recommended by the SLP that meets the recommendations for nutritional content identified by the dietetic professional. The patient will not experience any complications related to his swallowing deficits or health issues. The patient will begin the recovery process, receive recommended rehabilitation, and be able to normalize his diet texture. As he is able to manage more textures of food and liquid, he will still be relying on the dietetic professional to monitor his intake and make nutritional recommendations.

One consideration that warrants mention for a patient of this type who has not received substantial nutrition for 47 hours at the time of the instrumental assessment is refeeding syndrome. It consists of "a range of metabolic and electrolyte alterations occurring as a result of the reintroduction and/or increased provision of calories after a period of decreased or absent caloric intake" (daSilva et al., 2020). While the treatment of this syndrome is out of the scope of care for the speech-language pathologist and this paper, it is a consideration for the dietetic professional treating a patient in this type of scenario.

Scenario 2: The Patient Begins Oral Intake but Does Not Meet Nutrition and Hydration Needs

If the patient begins oral intake but does not meet his nutrition and hydration needs, then the SLP and dietetic professional will need to examine the underlying factors that are limiting the patient's ability to meet his needs and make recommendations for modifications or interventions. In the case of this patient, several factors place him at potential risk for malnutrition and dehydration including use of pureed foods and thickened liquids. He may find that these items have poor palatability and may refuse them. He may be experiencing decreased interest in participation related to depression related to his stroke. The patient in the presented case had a left middle cerebral artery CVA and as a result, is also struggling with communication issues that may limit his ability to understand recommendations or participate in his care. He may have social or economic factors that limit his access or participation in care.

Consider whether the patient is demonstrating poor intake related to aspects of his diet. The patient may not like the modified diet texture resulting in poor intake. Is the larger risk in this situation related to the risk for aspiration or the risk for malnutrition or dehydration? The patient may have sensory issues such as taste changes that limit his enjoyment of eating and influence his intake. If he recently began diet restrictions related to his health conditions this may also limit options for meals, and the combination of restrictions imposed by the new diet and the dysphagia diet may result in more limited meal options. He may not like the food at the facility and, due to his dietary or texture restrictions, may not be able to eat food his family brings him from home. How do the current diet restrictions affect the patient's quality of life and is this resulting in limited intake? A question to ask at this point is "is there any way to liberalize the diet and reduce the restrictions that may be contributing to the problem?"

Collaboration between the professionals involved in the patient's care while including the desires of the patient and his family may be an effective approach to the problem of poor oral intake. During the course of this collaboration, the patient and family can be instructed in foods that they can bring for the patient that meet the nutritional needs and are appropriate for the dysphagia diet. Relating to the dysphagia diet specifically, instructing the family in simple strategies to modify the food items at home to meet the textural requirements can potentially give the patient more food options and help improve intake.

The patient's communication limitations may influence his care. In our case study, the patient has dysarthria and aphasia. Dysarthria is commonly referred to as "slurred speech." Dysarthrias are a group of neurologically based motor speech disorders characterized by abnormalities in the fundamental control or execution of the target motor speech task (Duffy, 2013). He may have specific requests that he is unable to convey. Dysarthria is a speech sound production problem, while aphasia is a language content problem. Functionally, aphasia may have both expressive and receptive components, meaning that the person may have difficulty expressing language content to others or understanding the content of messages they receive. Aphasia is a multidimensional, acquired language impairment with a neurological basis, which can affect any or all language components (Papathanasiou & Coppens, 2017). Due to the presence of aphasia, he may not be following directions or participating in his care because he has difficulty understanding the information he is receiving.

Psychological factors such as depression can influence a person's engagement in their recovery process. Depression after stroke is a common issue for people in nursing facilities (Kowalska et al., 2015) and adjustment after stroke can be a barrier to achieving intrinsic regulation and progress in therapy. A general prevalence of depression after stroke has been reported as 30% to 36%, with 34%-36% prevalence during stroke rehabilitation (Visser et al., 2015). Depression may be present as an influencing factor in rehabilitation progress. In addition, depression may persist, with 40% of patients suffering post-stroke depression at 30-months (Shi et al., 2015). When specifically related to malnutrition, depression is considered a "major determinant" (Chen et al., 2019). The probability of depression after stroke is influenced by stroke severity and level of disability present after stroke (Shi et al., 2015). Often, some dysphagia treatment is available, but it is frequently not sufficient for the person to fully regain their lost function. Depression compounds these issues. Patients that demonstrate poor levels of intake and poor engagement in their own care post stroke may be experiencing depression and may benefit from appropriate medical referrals and intervention.

Management of swallowing disorders is influenced by the patient's motor functions and assessment findings, but it is critical to remember that a number of other factors warrant consideration. Patient factors including individual culture, beliefs, wants, needs, emotional state, as well as functional communication, cognition and motor functions can influence ability to engage and participate in the recovery process. Family influences such as familial and community support have a role in recovery. Factors such as socioeconomic status may limit access to treatments or interventions the patient needs to facilitate recovery. Not all of these factors may exist in every situation, but must be considered when outlining interventional approaches for each patient.

CONCLUSION

This chapter discusses swallowing and dysphagia from the standpoint of the speech-language pathologist as an interdisciplinary partner with the dietetic professional. An effective collaboration between the dietetic professional and the speech-language pathologist is critical to effectively address dysphagia. The normal swallowing process is complex. Knowledge of normal swallowing anatomy and physiology is essential for understanding the appropriate management of dysphagia and to address potential complications. This case study illustrates common features of dysphagia that may occur as a result of a stroke to demonstrate the need for interdisciplinary understanding as the basis for effective management of the individual with this disorder.

Dysphagia treatment provided by the SLP can be both rehabilitative and compensatory. A person's needs may change as they move through their medical intervention process. Recommendations for rehabilitation and/or compensations are usually made by the SLP, but they can have a significant impact on the problem solving process and interventions identified by the dietetic professional. A patient's therapeutic plan may be influenced by additional factors including ethical issues, and patient and family preferences. In addition, appropriateness of various nutritional and hydration sources, including enteral and parenteral means must be considered. A discussion of the ethical considerations surrounding dysphagia and nutritional sources and diet modifications is a critical component in the decision-making process.

Dysphagia is a disorder of deglutition and the potential complications of dysphagia vary widely. Dysphagia can result in mild issues such slow oral processing to the most severe consequences such as aspiration pneumonia or other respiratory issues, requiring the patient to receive enteral or parenteral nutrition. Patients with dysphagia also have the potential for nutritional and hydration deficits which can be complicated by other medical factors, or result in complication of their own, and can be particularly challenging for the dietitian and SLP. Medical factors can result in dietary restrictions from a nutritional standpoint, which may be further impacted by effects of dysphagia. Depression or other psychosocial factors may be challenges that limit a person's engagement in swallowing rehabilitation or desire to eat. Continued collaboration between the medical professionals, the patient, and the patient's family is necessary to successfully address dysphagia as well as the nutrition and hydration concerns that accompany it. Each case must be carefully considered from all aspects to account for and address the individual variability and multiple, ongoing decisions that must occur for dysphagia management to be effective.

DISCLOSURE

The author has no financial or non-financial conflicts of interest.

REFERENCES

American Speech-Language Hearing Association (ASHA). (n.d.). *About the CSD Professions*. Retrieved July 15, 2016, from https://www.asha.org/Students/Learn-About-the-CSDProfessions/

Aoki, S., Hosomi, N., Hirayama, J., Nakamori, M., Yoshikawa, M., Nezu, T., Kubo, S., Nagano, Y., Nagao, A., Yamane, N., Nishikawa, Y., Takamoto, M., Ueno, H., Ochi, K., Maruyama, H., Yamamoto, H., & Matsumoto, M. (2016). The multidisciplinary swallowing team approach decreases pneumonia onset in acute stroke patients. *Public Library of Science One*, *11*(5), e0154608. doi:10.1371/journal.pone.0154608 PMID:27138162

Blanař, V., Hödl, M., Lohrmann, C., Amir, Y., & Eglseer, D. (2019). Dysphagia and factors associated with malnutrition risk: A 5-year multicentre study. *Journal of Advanced Nursing*, *75*(12), 3566–3576. doi:10.1111/jan.14188 PMID:31452231

Chen, N., Li, Y., Fang, J., Lu, Q., & He, L. (2019). Risk factors for malnutrition in stroke patients: A meta-analysis. *Clinical Nutrition (Edinburgh, Lothian)*, *38*(1), 127–135. doi:10.1016/j.clnu.2017.12.014 PMID:29310894

Cho, S., Lu, Y., & Lee, D.-H. (2013). Dysphagia following anterior cervical spinal surgery: A systematic review. *The Bone & Joint Journal*, *95B*(7), 868–873. doi:10.1302/0301-620X.95B7.31029 PMID:23814234

Cichero, J. A. Y. (2017). Unlocking opportunities in food design for infants, children, and the elderly: Understanding milestones in chewing and swallowing across the lifespan for new innovations. *Journal of Texture Studies*, *48*(4), 271–279. doi:10.1111/jtxs.12236 PMID:28766752

Cichero, J. A. Y. (2018). Age related changes to eating and swallowing impact frailty: Aspiration, choking risk, modified food texture and autonomy of choice. *Geriatrics*, *3*(4), 69. doi:10.3390/geriatrics3040069 PMID:31011104

Crary, M., Humphrey, J. L., Carnaby-Mann, G., Sambandam, R., Miller, L., & Silliman, S. (2013). Dysphagia, nutrition, and hydration in ischemic stroke patients at admission and discharge from acute care. *Dysphagia*, *28*(1), 69–76. doi:10.100700455-012-9414-0 PMID:22684924

daSilva, J. S. V., Seres, D. S., Sabino, K., Adams, S. C., Berdahl, G. J., Wolfe Citty, S., ... Ayers, P. (2020). ASPEN consensus recommendations for refeeding syndrome. *Nutrition in Clinical Practice*, *35*(2), 178–195. doi:10.1002/ncp.10474 PMID:32115791

Duffy, J. (2013). *Motor speech disorders: Substrates, differential diagnosis, and management*. Elsevier.

Foley, N. C., Salter, K. L., Robertson, J., Teasell, R. W., & Woodbury, M. G. (2009). Which reported estimate of the prevalence of malnutrition after stroke is valid? *Stroke*, *40*(3), pe66–e74. doi:10.1161/STROKEAHA.108.518910 PMID:19164799

Go, A. S., Mozaffarian, D., Roger, V. L., Benjamin, E. J., Berry, J. D., Borden, W. B., ... Turner, M. B. (2012). Heart disease and stroke statistics—2013 update: A report from the American Heart Association. *Circulation*, 2–241. PMID:23239837

González-Fernández, M., Humbert, I., Winegrad, H., Cappola, A. R., & Fried, L. P. (2014). Dysphagia in old-old women: Prevalence as determined according to self-report and the 3-ounce Water Swallowing Test. *Journal of the American Geriatrics Society*, *62*(4), 716–720. doi:10.1111/jgs.12745 PMID:24635053

Groher, M. E., & Crary, M. A. (2015). *Dysphagia: Clinical management in adults and children* (2nd ed.). Elsevier.

Kowalska, J., Bojko, E., Szczepańska-Gieracha, J., Rymaszewska, J., & Rożek-Piechura, K. (2015). Occurrence of depressive symptoms among older adults after a stroke in the nursing home facility. *Rehabilitation Nursing*, *41*(2), 112–119. doi:10.1002/rnj.203 PMID:25772117

Mann, G., Hankey, G., & Cameron, D. (2000). Swallowing disorders following acute stroke: Prevalence and diagnostic accuracy. *Cerebrovascular Diseases (Basel, Switzerland)*, *10*(5), 380–386. doi:10.1159/000016094 PMID:10971024

Martino, R., Foley, N., Bhogal, S., Diamant, N., Speechley, M., & Teasell, R. (2005). Dysphagia after stroke: Incidence, diagnosis, and pulmonary complications. *Stroke*, *36*(12), 2756–2763. doi:10.1161/01.STR.0000190056.76543.eb PMID:16269630

McCullough, G. H., Rosenbeck, J. C., Wertz, R. T., McCoy, S., Mann, G., & McCullough, K. (2005). Utility of clinical swallowing examination measures for detecting aspiration post-stroke. *Journal of Speech, Language, and Hearing Research*, *48*, 1280-1293. doi: 1092-4388/05/4806-1280

Morely, J. E. (1997). Anorexia of aging: Physiologic and pathologic. *The American Journal of Clinical Nutrition*, *66*(4), 760–773. doi:10.1093/ajcn/66.4.760 PMID:9322549

Namasivayam-Macdonald, A. M., Barbon, C. E., & Steele, C. M. (2018). A review of swallow timing in the elderly. *Physiology & Behavior*, *184*, 12–26. doi:10.1016/j.physbeh.2017.10.023 PMID:29101012

Papas, A., Palmer, C., Rounds, M. C., & Russell, R. M. (1998). The effect of denture status on nutrition. *Special Care in Dentistry*, *18*(1), 17–25. doi:10.1111/j.1754-4505.1998.tb01354.x PMID:9791303

Papathanasiou, I., & Coppens, P. (2017). *Aphasia and related neurogenic communication disorders*. Jones & Bartlett Learning.

Perry, S. E., Huckabee, M. L., Tomkins, G., & Milne, T. (2020). The association between oral bacteria, the cough reflex and pneumonia in patients with acute stroke and suspected dysphagia. *Journal of Oral Rehabilitation*, *47*(3), 386–394. doi:10.1111/joor.12903 PMID:31698513

Rosenbek, J. C., Robbins, J. A., Roecker, E. B., Coyle, J. L., & Wood, J. L. (1996). A penetration-aspiration scale. *Dysphagia*, *11*(2), 93–98. doi:10.1007/BF00417897 PMID:8721066

Schiffman, S. S., & Graham, B. G. (2000). Taste and smell perception affect appetite and immunity in the elderly. *European Journal of Clinical Nutrition*, *54*(3), S54–S63. doi:10.1038j.ejcn.1601026 PMID:11041076

Shi, Y., Xiang, Y., Yang, Y., Zhang, N., Wang, S., Ungvari, G., ... Zhao, X. (2015). Depression after minor stroke: Prevalence and predictors. *Journal of Psychosomatic Research*, *79*(2), 143–147. doi:10.1016/j.jpsychores.2015.03.012 PMID:25868687

Su, Y., Yuki, M., Hirayama, K., Sato, M., & Han, T. (2020). Denture wearing and malnutrition risk among community-dwelling older adults. *Nutrients*, *12*(1), 151. doi:10.3390/nu12010151 PMID:31948104

Tanaka, N., Nohara, K., Kotani, Y., Matsumura, M., & Sakai, T. (2013). Swallowing frequency in elderly people during daily life. *Journal of Oral Rehabilitation*, *40*(10), n/a. Advance online publication. doi:10.1111/joor.12085 PMID:23855718

The International Dysphagia Diet Standardisation Initiative. (2016). *Complete IDDSI framework detailed definitions.* The International Dysphagia Diet Standardisation Initiative 2016. https://iddsi.org/framework/

Visser, M., Heijenbrok-Kal, M., van't Spijker, A., Oostra, K., Busschbach, J., & Ribbers, G. (2015). Coping, problem solving, depression, and health-related quality of life in patients receiving outpatient stroke rehabilitation. *Archives of Physical Medicine and Rehabilitation*, *96*(8), 1492–1498. doi:10.1016/j.apmr.2015.04.007 PMID:25921980

KEY TERMS AND DEFINITIONS

Aspiration: Aspiration occurs when the bolus enters the laryngeal vestibule and subsequently passes below the level of the vocal cords. The aspirated material may be expelled from the airway or remain in place.

Deglutition: The act of swallowing.

Dysphagia: Disorder of swallowing that may occur in the oral, pharyngeal, or esophageal phases. Dysphagia is a multifactorial swallowing disorder that can affect a person's overall health and psychosocial well-being. It may occur in the oral, pharyngeal, or esophageal phases.

Flexible Fiberoptic Endoscopic Evaluation of Swallowing: A type of instrumental swallowing assessment that uses a flexible fiberoptic endoscope passed through the nose to directly visualize the structures and dynamic process of deglutition. Also known as FEES.

Mastication: The act of chewing.

Penetration: Penetration occurs when the bolus enters the laryngeal vestibule and does not pass below the level of the vocal cords. The penetrated material may be expelled from the airway or remain in place.

Speech Pathologist: Also known as speech-language pathologist. A person who has specialized training and expertise in assessment and treatment of speech, language, voice, cognitive, and swallowing disorders. In the United States speech-language pathologists complete a certification process through the American Speech-Language-Hearing Association to receive the Certificate of Clinical Competence in speech-language pathology (CCC-SLP).

Videofluoroscopic Evaluation of Swallowing: A type of instrumental swallowing assessment that uses videofluoroscopic evaluation to view moving pictures of swallowing structures and functions through use of radiation and a contrast material such as barium. It allows assessment of the static and dynamic processes of deglutition. It is abbreviated as VFSS. This study is also known as a modified barium swallowing study (MBSS) or modified barium swallow (MBS).

APPENDIX

Table 1. The 8-Point Penetration-Aspiration Scale (PENASP)

1. Material does not enter the airway
2. Material enters the airway, remains above the vocal folds, and is ejected from the airway
3. Material enters the airway, remains above the vocal folds, and is not ejected from the airway
4. Material enters the airway, contacts the vocal folds, and is ejected from the airway
5. Material enters the airway, contacts the vocal folds, and is not ejected from the airway
6. Material enters the airway, passes below the vocal folds and is ejected into the larynx or out of the airway
7. Material enters the airway, passes below the vocal folds, and is not ejected from the trachea despite effort
8. Material enters the airway, passes below the vocal folds, and no effort is made to eject

From (Rosenbek et al., 1996)

Reprinted by permission from [Springer Nature Customer Service Centre GmbH]: [Springer Nature] [Dysphagia] [A Penetration-Aspiration Scale, Rosenbek, et al.], [1996]

Chapter 2
Gastroesophageal Reflux Disease

Rouba Khalil Naaman
King Abdulaziz University, Saudi Arabia

EXECUTIVE SUMMARY

This chapter discusses a gastroesophageal reflux disease (GERD) case. GERD is a common disorder affecting the gastrointestinal tract. It results from the relaxation of the lower esophageal sphincter, which leads to stomach acid reflux, which in turn causes heartburn and discomfort. Certain lifestyle factors and dietary choices aggravate this condition, leading to serious tissue damage. Management of GERD usually requires medications and lifestyle and dietary modifications. This case involves the symptoms and aggravating factors of GERD. It also shows the role of medical nutrition therapy in managing GERD symptoms. Moreover, it will allow dietetic professionals to assess GERD symptoms to plan for nutrition interventions and educate patients about the dietary manipulation required to reduce gastric acid secretions and relieve pain.

INTRODUCTION

Gastroesophageal reflux disease (GERD) is a chronic disorder characterized by the abnormal reflux of gastric acids into the esophagus, resulting in heartburn (Miwa et al., 2019). GERD affects up to 28% and 26% of the populations in North America and Europe, respectively. In the Middle East, approximately 33% of the population has GERD (El-Serag, Sweet, Winchester, & Dent, 2014).

DOI: 10.4018/978-1-7998-3802-9.ch002

The mechanism of GERD is mainly related to the relaxation of the lower esophageal sphincter (LES). When food is digested under normal conditions, the LES opens to allow the bolus to pass down into the stomach and then closes to prevent gastric content from going back to the esophagus. In GERD, the LES is relaxed, causing a backflow of gastric acids into the esophagus. If acid exposure is left untreated, it may result in severe complications, such as chronic esophagitis, esophageal ulcer, Barrett's esophagus, and esophageal cancer (Alshehri et al., 2020).

Obesity significantly increases the risk of GERD (Ayazi, Crookes, Peyre, Hagen, & Leers, 2007; El-Serag, Graham, Satia, & Rabeneck, 2005). Subjects with an increased abdominal circumference are at a significantly higher risk of having increased intra-abdominal pressure and therefore a relaxed LES. Hiatal hernia is another risk factor that is positively associated with the risk of GERD. It occurs when a part of the stomach is pulled into the diaphragm, resulting in gastric acid reflux and heartburn. Lifestyle risk factors, including poor sleep, excessive alcohol intake, large meals, late-night eating, and sedentarism, also trigger GERD symptoms.

The consumption of certain dietary factors contributes to LES relaxation and GERD. However, limited data are available on the association between certain foods and GERD symptoms. Studies have shown that peppermint, caffeine (coffee, tea, and soft drinks), acidic foods (citrus fruits and tomatoes), high-fat foods, and spicy foods are associated with increased esophageal irritation and heartburn (Meining & Classen, 2000).

Doctors diagnose GERD by asking patients about any experienced GERD symptom. Patients are asked whether they feel heartburn after meals and when lying down. When diagnosing GERD, other symptoms should be assessed, such as dental corrosion, dysphagia, cough, and chest pain.

The main aim of the medical management of GERD is to decrease gastric acid secretion. Proton-pump inhibitors (PPIs), histamine 2 (H_2) receptor antagonists, and antacids are the most common medications used to manage GERD. For patients who fail to respond to medications, surgical management maybe an option for managing GERD (Heidelbaugh, Nostrant, Kim, & Van Harrison, 2003).

Nutritional management for GERD involves dietary and lifestyle modifications. Patients should be advised to avoid food items that might aggravate GERD symptoms, maintain an ideal weight, and stop smoking. Moreover, patients need to avoid having large meals, eating late at night, and lying down after eating (Kaltenbach, Crockett, & Gerson, 2006).

To relief GERD symptoms and complications, it is important to understand risk factors of the disease and how it's diagnosed, assessed and managed. In this review, a brief about epidemiology, pathophysiology, etiology, diagnosis and management of GERD is provided.

EPIDEMIOLOGY

GERD is one of the most common gastrointestinal disorders seen by GI specialists. In North America, a high prevalence ranging from 18% to 29% has been reported. In Europe, GERD affects approximately 9% to 26% of the population. GERD prevalence in East Asia ranges from 9% to 33%. In Australia, up to 12% of the population is affected by the condition. In the Middle East, GERD prevalence ranges from 9% to 33% of the population (El-Serag et al., 2014).

PATHOPHYSIOLOGY

In order to manage GERD, the pathophysiology of the disease and how it develops should be understood. The esophagus is a 25 cm muscular tube that plays an essential role in food digestion; it receives and pushes food from the mouth to the stomach by contracting its muscles using esophageal peristalsis. It has a nonkeratinized stratified squamous epithelium lining in addition to submucosal glands, which protect the esophagus mucosa from gastric acid exposure by the release of bicarbonate, epidermal growth factor (EGF), prostaglandin E2 (PGE2) and mucin (Mahan & Raymond, 2017).

Sphincters are layers of muscles surrounding the esophagus that close and open to control foods' entrance to and exit from the esophagus. There are two sphincters located at the upper and lower parts of the esophagus: the upper esophageal sphincter (UES) and the LES. The esophagus closes and opens when the sphincters contract and relax, respectively. When food is digested, the LES opens to allow the bolus to pass down into the stomach and then closes to prevent gastric content from going back to the esophagus (Hershcovici, Mashimo, & Fass, 2011).

There are various mechanisms involved in GERD pathogenesis. These include motor abnormalities, anatomical abnormalities, and impaired resistance of the esophageal mucosa (De Giorgi, Palmiero, Esposito, Mosca, & Cuomo, 2006).

Motor Abnormalities

A normal esophagus can prevent itself from prolonged gastric acid exposure and protect its tissues from damage through LES contraction and esophagus closure. Most GERD patients (60%) have impaired LES function as their primary underlying mechanism of reflux (Zaninotto, DeMeester, Schwizer, Johansson, & Cheng, 1988). This causes a backflow of gastric acids into the esophagus, which increases esophageal mucosa acid exposure. This can be attributed to reduced LES pressure

(LESP), increased intra-abdominal pressure, or LES lengths shorter than 2 to 5 cm (Kahrilas, 2003).

Anatomical Abnormalities

Hiatal hernias occur when the upper portion of the stomach moves into the diaphragm, resulting in a lower LESP, prolonged gastric exposure, and heartburn. During the clearance of acid from the esophagus, hiatal hernia also permits gastric acids to accumulate in the hernia sac, hence increasing the chance of acid reflux with swallowing and when the LES is relaxed (De Giorgi et al., 2006; Mittal, Lange, & McCallum, 1987).

Impaired Resistance of the Esophageal Mucosa

The esophageal mucosa is a layer that protects the esophageal tissues against injuries resulting from gastric acid exposure. When the ability of the esophagus to resist mucosal injuries fails, the risk of GERD development increases (Chatila et al., 2020).

RISK FACTORS AND ETIOLOGY

GERD has a multifactorial etiology, and several factors are associated with the appearance of its symptoms. These include age, obesity, smoking, diet, excessive alcohol intake, consumption of large meals, late-night eating, and sleep disturbances (Almadi et al., 2014; Chatila et al., 2020; Nilsson, Johnsen, Ye, Hveem, & Lagergren, 2004).

Age and Gender

One study showed an association between GERD development and old age, but no other study has reported such an association (Diaz-Rubio, Moreno-Elola-Olaso, Rey, Locke, & Rodriguez-Artalejo, 2004; Wienbeck & Babnert, 1989).

Obesity

Obesity is another factor associated with GERD; it impairs the sphincter by increasing the intra-abdominal pressure and exerting pressure on the diaphragm, which might lead to hiatal hernia (Barak, Ehrenpreis, Harrison, & Sitrin, 2002; Wajed, Streets, Bremner, & DeMeester, 2001). A previous study that assessed the association between obesity and GERD showed that increased BMI is significantly associated with increased esophageal acid exposure and impaired LES (Ayazi et al., 2009).

Smoking

The strong association between tobacco smoking and GERD has been reported previously (Zheng, Nordenstedt, Pedersen, Lagergren, & Ye, 2007). There is evidence indicating the role of smoking in sphincter relaxation (Kahrilas & Gupta, 1990). It has been shown that when compared with non-smokers, chronic smokers have significantly lower LESP (Kahrilas & Gupta, 1990).

Dietary Factors

According to previous studies, the high consumption of fruits, sweets, and foods that are fatty, fried, sour, or spicy are significantly associated with heartburn and discomfort (Jarosz & Taraszewska, 2014). Some specific food items may exacerbate GERD symptoms. Previous evidence has reported an association between peppermint and chocolate and reduced LESP. (Newberry & Lynch, 2019). Acidic foods, such as citrus fruits, tomatoes, and spices, may result in esophageal mucosal irritation (Yeoh, Ho, Guan, & Kang, 1995). Fatty foods lower LESP and delay gastric emptying (Holloway, Lyrenas, Ireland, & Dent, 1997). According to Fox et al., (2007), a high-calorie diet is associated with a higher esophageal acid exposure compared with a low-calorie diet. The same study also showed that a high-fat diet is associated with a higher frequency of GERD symptoms.

Few studies assessed the association between beverages and GERD. Gomes & Dantas, (2014) reported that acidic beverages are associated with slower esophageal transit when compared with neutral beverages. Caffeine intake has also been linked to GERD, and it has been shown that caffeine reduces LESP, resulting in esophageal acid exposure (Lohsiriwat, Puengna, & Leelakusolvong, 2006). A positive relationship between excessive alcohol consumption and GERD was reported in a meta-analysis (Pan et al., 2019). It was shown that alcohol impairs esophageal motility in addition to reducing LESP (Castell, Murray, Tutuian, Orlando, & Arnold, 2004).

Lifestyle and Psychological Factors

Having a few meals a day or having large meals late at night are also associated with the development of GERD symptoms (Fujiwara et al., 2005; Surdea-Blaga, Negrutiu, Palage, & Dumitrascu, 2017). Limited studies have reported the association between sleep disturbances, psychological stress, and GERD (Jung, Choung, & Talley, 2010; Okuyama et al., 2017).

Hiatal Hernia

Hiatal hernia is another condition that is associated with GERD with an incidence range of 0.8% to 43% (Dent et al., 2012; Schlottmann et al., 2018). A positive association between hiatal hernia and the severity of GERD symptoms has been reported (Kahrilas, Lin, Chen, & Manka, 1999).

SIGNS, SYMPTOMS AND DIAGNOSIS

Typical Symptoms

Heartburn is a typical symptom occurring with reflux. It refers to the painful burning sensation caused by gastric acids flowing back up into the esophagus (Vakil et al., 2006). Regurgitation is another symptom that may occur with heartburn; abdominal muscles contract, leading to reflux of stomach contents into the mouth or throat (Vakil et al., 2006).

Atypical Symptoms

Atypical GERD symptoms that in most the cases they are caused by GERD include chronic cough, asthma, chest pain, nausea, dyspepsia, laryngitis, and bloating (Katz, Gerson, & Vela, 2013).

Alarm Symptoms

Additional symptoms that can be present in GERD patients include chest pain, dysphagia, anemia, weight loss, painful swallowing, and bleeding (Alzubaidi & Gabbard, 2015).

Diagnosis

To diagnose GERD, doctors ask patients about their experienced symptoms. According to the American College of Gastroenterology (2005), heartburn and regurgitation indicates the occurrence of GERD. In western countries, 4–10% and 10–30% of adult patients develop this symptom daily and weekly, respectively (El-Serag et al., 2004; El-Serag, Hill, & Jones, 2009) Patients should also be asked about experiencing other GERD symptoms, such as dental corrosion, dysphagia, cough, and chest pain.

MEDICAL AND SURGICAL MANAGEMENT

Medical Management

PPIs are commonly prescribed to manage GERD. PPIs help decrease the acid levels secreted by the parietal cells of the stomach. H2 receptor antagonists are used to treat mild cases of GERD. Antacids are used to neutralize gastric acids and relieve heartburn. Prokinetic agents, which enhance GI motility, are prescribed to cases with delayed gastric emptying.

Surgical Management

In some cases, surgical procedures are an effective approach to managing GERD. These situations include failure of medications to treat the disease, the inability of certain individuals to tolerate or afford medications for prolonged periods, those who develop GERD complications (such as Barrett's esophagus and esophageal stricture) (Stefanidis et al., 2010). Nissen fundoplication is a procedure that effectively manages GERD symptoms by preventing gastric acid from traveling in the wrong direction. Some studies have reported that gastric bypass surgery might also be effective in managing GERD (Chang & Friedenberg, 2014).

MEDICAL NUTRITION THERAPY

Lifestyle and dietary modifications are important in managing GERD symptoms. These modifications involve avoiding all factors that increase the development of the disease.

Lifestyle Modifications

Lifestyle modifications include avoiding the consumption of large meals (particularly late at night), reducing alcohol consumption, staying upright after meals for three hours, and quitting smoking (American College of Gastroenterology, 2005). A study showed that having one to two meals a day or having a big late meal instead of having dinner and supper might exacerbate the emergence of GERD symptoms (Jarosz & Taraszewska, 2014). Late-night eating has been found to exacerbate acid reflux compared with having meals at early times, in overweight patients in particular (Piesman, Hwang, Maydonovitch, & Wong, 2007). Weight loss is another factor that should be considered in overweight and obese individuals. A study showed that a decrease in the body mass index (BMI) by 3.5 kg/m^2 is associated with a 40%

reduction in symptom frequency (Jacobson, Somers, Fuchs, Kelly, & Camargo, 2006). The head elevation of the bed should also be considered for individuals who experience GERD symptoms at night.

Dietary Modifications

Regarding the dietary modifications, GERD-exacerbating food products, such as peppermint, chocolate, sweets, caffeine, spicy, fatty, sour, and acidic foods should be eliminated (Jarosz & Taraszewska, 2014). The elimination of carbonated drinks and caffeinated products should be considered, as they have also been linked to GERD symptoms (Song et al., 2011). Previous studies have shown that the Mediterranean diet and very low carbohydrate intake have a protective effect against GERD (Pointer, Rickstrew, Slaughter, Vaezi, & Silver, 2016; Surdea-Blaga et al., 2017). It has been found that a fiber-rich diet increases LESP and reduces heartburn symptoms (Morozov, Isakov, & Konovalova, 2018).

SETTING THE STAGE

The following case was obtained from a private gastrointestinal clinic in Jeddah, Saudi Arabia. A specialized gastroenterologist evaluated the case and prescribed certain medications to manage the disease. The patient was also referred to a dietitian for nutritional consultation, as lifestyle and dietary changes are recommended to manage heartburn and GERD symptoms. An approval for publication was obtained from the patient in this case. There was no conflict of interest, as the patient did not receive any financial support from the author to disclose the case in this chapter.

CASE DESCRIPTION

Patient's Details

- Age: 34 years old
- Gender: Female

Case History

Case description: The patient began experiencing heartburn and discomfort in high school. Her heartburn occurred about twice a week. However, the heartburn and discomfort have become more frequent this year, occurring almost every day.

This sensation worsens after she eats certain food products and after she goes to bed at night. She complains of symptoms that accompany heartburn, including dry cough and chest pain radiating to the back. She was referred to a dietitian to help her manage the heartburn.

- Medical history: Polycystic ovary syndrome
- Surgical history: None
- Smoking: Yes
- Family history: Mother and maternal grandmother-High blood pressure and asthma

Main Medical Diagnosis

Gastroesophageal Reflux Disease (GERD)

Demographics

- Marital status: Single-lives with mother, maternal grandmother; and aunt
- Education: Bachelor's degree in marketing
- Occupation: Previously, a secretary in a private clinic—now at home
- Ethnicity and religion: Arab, Muslim

Anthropometry

- Current weight: 86 kg
- Height: 162 cm

Table 1. Biochemical Data

Parameter	Reference	Patient's Results
Sodium	136-145	140
Potassium	3.5-5.5	4.0
Chloride	95-105	100
BUN (mg/dL)	8-18	10
Creatinine serum (mg/dL)	0.6-1.2	0.94
Glucose (mg/dL)	70-110	93
Magnesium (mg/dL)	1.8-3	2.0
Calcium (mg/dL)	9-11	10.90

continues on following page

Table 1. Continued

Parameter	Reference	Patient's Results
Bilirubin total (mg/dL)	≤1.5	1.1
Protein, total (g/dL)	6-8	6.9
Albumin (g/dL)	3.5-5	4.0
Prealbumin (mg/dL)	16-35	30
Ammonia (NH_3, µmol/L)	9-33	22
Alkaline phosphatase (U/L)	30-120	88
ALT (U/L)	4-36	5
AST (U/L)	0-35	15
CPK (U/L)	30-135 (Female) 55-170 (Male)	90
Lactate dehydrogenase (U/L)	208-378	220
Cholesterol (mg/dL)	120-199	226
LDL (mg/dL)	<130	138
HDL-C (mg/dL)	>55 (Female) >45 (Male)	50
Triglycerides (mg/dL)	35-135 (Female) 40-160 (Male)	131
WBC ($\times10^3/mm^3$)	4.8-11.8	9.2
RBC ($\times10^6/mm^3$)	4.2-5.4 (Female) 4.5-6.2 (Male)	4.2
Hemoglobin (g/dL)	12-15 (Female) 14-17 (Male)	13.4
Hematocrit (%)	37-47 (Female) 40-54 (Male)	37
Mean cell volume (µm3)	80-96	84.7
Mean cell Hgb (pg)	26-32	31
Mean cell Hgb content (g/dL)	31.5-36	36
RBC distribution (%)	11.6-16.5	11.9
Platelet count ($\times10^3/mm^3$)	140-440	436
Lymphocyte (%)	15-45	33.3
Monocyte (%)	3-10	8.0
Vitamin D (ng/ml)	30-100	12.0

Nutritional-Focused Physical Examination

- General appearance: Mild obese, 34 years old female, well-looking
- Heart: Regular heart rate and normal sound
- HEENT: Ear: itchy ear and sinusitis
- Genitalia: Normal
- Neurologic: Oriented and alert
- Extremities: No edema; normal strength and sensations
- Skin: Warm and smooth
- Chest/lungs: Lungs clear
- Peripheral vascular: Pulses full, no bruits
- Abdomen: No distention, no pain

Vital Signs

- Pulse: 73 BPM
- Temperature: 38 °C
- Blood pressure: 130/78 mm Hg
- Respiratory **rate:** 15 BPM

Food/Nutrition-Related History

The patient states that she has a very good appetite. She claims that most foods exacerbate her GERD symptoms. These include tomato sauce, cakes, jam, honey, and fresh fruits (such as bananas, strawberries, and citrus fruits). She usually skips breakfast and dinner. She drinks around three liters of water a day. She generally includes rice in her lunch and eats one bag of chips daily. She does one-hour aerobic workouts and a 30-minute treadmill exercise daily. Her weight is steady.

Table 2. 24-Hour Recall

6:00 pm:	1 bowl of salad (tabbouleh); 1 vanilla wafer
11:00 pm:	1 cup tea (with no added sugar); 1 small dates cookie (maamoul)
12:00 am:	Two oranges
3:00 am:	Half clementine; small piece of halloumi cheese

- Food allergies/intolerances: Self-reported kiwi allergy

- Food purchase/preparations: She purchases her food and meals are prepared by her aunt
- Vitamin and mineral supplementation: None

Medications

Ranitidine 150 mg daily, 500 mg Glucophage, Diane 35 daily.

NUTRITIONAL MANAGEMENT

Disease Pathophysiology and Management Mind Map

In order to plan for an effective nutrition intervention which will help to reduce the heartburn and relieve pain, it is important to understand the disease pathophysiology, etiology, symptoms. Figure 1 is a mind map which will help firstly to analyze the disease information with its all features and to construct the knowledge about the disease in a simplified way. Secondly, it will provide a list of medical and nutritional solutions which dietitians can think of when managing the disease.

Figure 1. A mind map of gastroesophageal reflux disease (GERD) etiology, pathophysiology and management
Developed by: Khalifa, N 2020

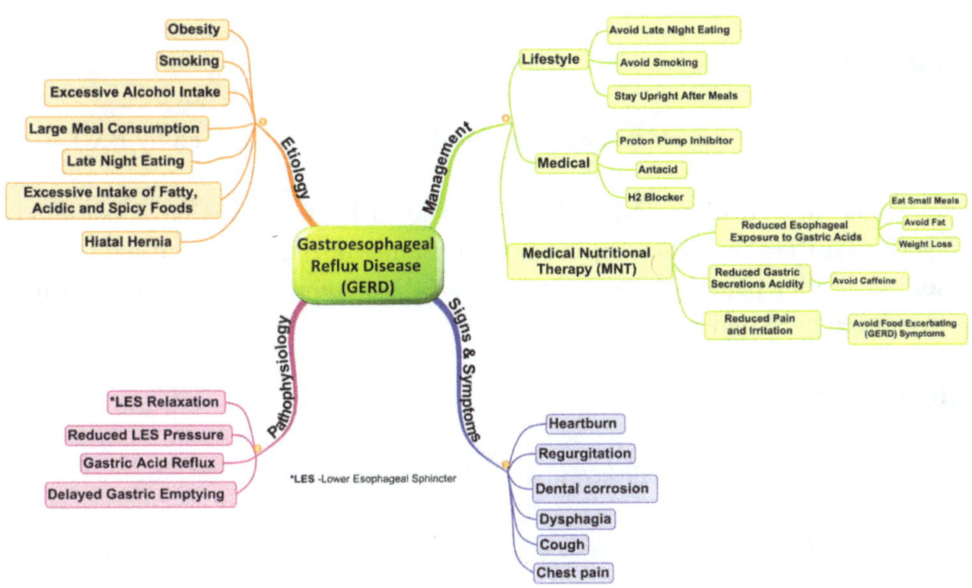

Main Aim of the Nutrition Therapy

- Decrease esophageal exposure to gastric acids.
- Decrease gastric secretion acidity.
- Prevent pain and irritation.

Adime Note

Assessment: The patient is a 34-year-old female with GERD who has been complaining of heartburn and gastric pain for years.

- **Anthropometry:**
  - BMI = 32.8 kg/m^2 (obese class 1)
  - Ideal body weight = 53.81 kg
- **Biochemical:**
  - Cholesterol (↑) 226 mg/dl, could be due to the high fat intake
  - LDL (↑) 138 mg/dl, could be due to the high fat intake
  - HDL-C (↓) 50 mg/dl, could be due to the low good-fat intake
  - Vitamin D (↓) 12.0 ng/ml, could be due to low sun exposure and lack of vitamin D supplement intake
- Clinical: Itchy ear, smooth skin, no abdominal pain or GI bleeding
- Dietary: No previous dietary restrictions, high carbohydrates and sugar intake, low vegetable and fiber intake, high fat intake, high intake of acidic foods, late-night eating

Diagnosis

Class 1 obesity (NC-3.3.3)[1] related to high calorie diet as evidenced by BMI, 32.8 kg/m2
Undesirable food choices (NB-1.7)[2] related to lack of knowledge about foods triggering GERD as evidenced by frequent consumption of high fat and acidic foods
Disordered eating pattern (NB-1.5)[2] related to lack of knowledge about healthy diet as evidenced by skipping of meals

Intervention

Diet prescription: 2300 kcal/day, low fat, low sugar, low salt

- Energy: Using Mifflin St. Jeor equation (Mifflin et al., 1990) for females;

(10×weight) + (6.25×height) – (5×age) – 161 = 1866.5×1.5(activity factor) = 2800kcal/day.

- For weight loss: 2800 – 500=2300kcal/day.
- Carbohydrates: (50%)
  1150/4 = 288 gm/day.
- Protein: (20%)
  460/4 = 115 gm/day.
- Fat: (30%)
  690/9 = 77 gm/day
- Fluids: 3 liters/day
  - Recommendations based on the National Institute of Diabetes and Digestive and Kidney Diseaes, 2014:
    - Avoid large meals; eat small frequent meals in order to prevent GERD symptoms.
    - Avoid late-night meals to reduce pain and irritation.
    - Avoid lying down after eating and stay upright after meals to relief GERD symptoms.
    - Avoid smoking to increase LES pressure.
    - Lose weight to prevent esophageal acid exposure, increase LES pressure and therefore reduce GERD symptoms frequency.
    - Avoid foods and beverages containing caffeine to increase LES pressure and therefore reduction in esophageal acid exposure.
    - Avoid GERD-exacerbating foods, including fatty, and acidic foods (such as citrus and tomatoes) to reduce esophageal mucosal irritation and increase LES pressure.
    - Consume a healthy, well-balanced diet with high fiber content to increase LES pressure and reduce the heartburn symptoms.
    - Consume multivitamin supplementation to overcome antacids' side effects.

Monitoring/Evaluation

- Monitor weight loss.
- Monitor biochemical tests (lipid profile in particular).
- Control gastric pain and heartburn.
- Adhere to prescribed diet.
- Eating pattern manipulation

CONCLUSION

This chapter presented a gastroesophageal case and provided a tool for dietetic professionals to assess GERD symptoms and plan for nutrition interventions required to reduce gastric acid secretions and relieve pain. The patient discussed in this chapter had been experiencing GERD symptoms for a long time. The analysis of the case showed the role of medical nutrition therapy in managing GERD symptoms and highlighted how the prescribed nutritional intervention should be individualized based on a patient's symptoms, habits, and preferences. Moreover, it showed the importance of critical thinking when making decisions and the need to use an evidence-based practice when planning for effective interventions.

REFERENCES

Almadi, M., Almousa, M., Althwainy, A., Altamimi, A., Alamoudi, H., Alshamrani, H., Alharbi, O. R., Azzam, N. A., Sadaf, N., & Aljebreen, A. (2014). Prevalence of symptoms of gastroesopahgeal reflux in a cohort of Saudi Arabians: A study of 1265 subjects. *Saudi Journal of Gastroenterology, 20*(4), 248–254. doi:10.4103/1319-3767.136982 PMID:25038211

Alshehri, S. S., Alzahrani, M. A. A., Jan, O. M., Aldughaither, A., Fahad, Alsalem, A. S., … Alghamdi, A. A. O. (2020). Prevalence, Causes, Risk Factors and Updates of Management of GERD. *EC Microbiology, 16*(2), 1–8.

Alzubaidi, M., & Gabbard, S. (2015). GERD: Diagnosing and treating the burn. *Cleveland Clinic Journal of Medicine, 82*(10), 685–692. doi:10.3949/ccjm.82a.14138 PMID:26469826

American College of Gastroenterology. (2005). *Updated ACG guidelines for diagnosis and treatment of GERD*. Retrieved April 21, 2020, from https://www.aafp.org/afp/2005/0615/p2376.html

Ayazi, S., Crookes, P. F., Peyre, C. G., Hagen, J. A., & Leers, J. M. (2007). Objective documentation of the link between GERD and obesity. *The American Journal of Gastroenterology, 102*, 138–139. doi:10.14309/00000434-200709002-00059

Ayazi, S., Hagen, J. A., Chan, L. S., DeMeester, S. R., Lin, M. W., Ayazi, A., Leers, J. M., Oezcelik, A., Banki, F., Lipham, J. C., DeMeester, T. R., & Crookes, P. F. (2009). Obesity and gastroesophageal reflux: Quantifying the association between body mass index, esophageal acid exposure, and lower esophageal sphincter status in a large series of patients with reflux symptoms. *Journal of Gastrointestinal Surgery*, *13*(8), 1440–1447. doi:10.100711605-009-0930-7 PMID:19475461

Barak, N., Ehrenpreis, E. D., Harrison, J. R., & Sitrin, M. D. (2002). Gastro-oesophageal reflux disease in obesity: Pathophysiological and therapeutic considerations. *Obesity Reviews*, *3*(1), 9–15. doi:10.1046/j.1467-789X.2002.00049.x PMID:12119661

Chang, P., & Friedenberg, F. (2014). Obesity and GERD. *Gastroenterology Clinics of North America*, *43*(1), 161–173. doi:10.1016/j.gtc.2013.11.009 PMID:24503366

Chatila, A. T., Nguyen, M. T. T., Krill, T., Roark, R., Bilal, M., & Reep, G. (2020). Natural history, pathophysiology and evaluation of gastroesophageal reflux disease. *Disease-a-Month*, *66*(1), 100848. doi:10.1016/j.disamonth.2019.02.001 PMID:30803725

De Giorgi, F., Palmiero, M., Esposito, I., Mosca, F., & Cuomo, R. (2006). Pathophysiology of gastro-oesophageal reflux disease. *Acta Otorhinolaryngologica Italica*, *26*(5), 241–246. PMID:17345925

Dent, J., Becher, A., Sung, J., Zou, D., Agréus, L., & Bazzoli, F. (2012). Systematic Review: Patterns of Reflux-Induced Symptoms and Esophageal Endoscopic Findings in Large-Scale Surveys. *Clinical Gastroenterology and Hepatology*, *10*(8), 863–873. e3. doi:10.1016/j.cgh.2012.02.028 PMID:22401904

Diaz-Rubio, M., Moreno-Elola-Olaso, C., Rey, E., Locke, G. R., & Rodriguez-Artalejo, F. (2004). Symptoms of gastro-oesophageal reflux: Prevalence, severity, duration and associated factors in a Spanish population. *Alimentary Pharmacology & Therapeutics*, *19*(1), 95–105. doi:10.1046/j.1365-2036.2003.01769.x PMID:14687171

El-Serag, H. B., Graham, D. Y., Satia, J. A., & Rabeneck, L. (2005). Obesity is an independent risk factor for GERD symptoms and erosive esophagitis. *The American Journal of Gastroenterology*, *100*(6), 1243–1250. doi:10.1111/j.1572-0241.2005.41703.x PMID:15929752

El-Serag, H. B., Hill, C., & Jones, R. (2009). Systematic review: The epidemiology of gastro-oesophageal reflux disease in primary care, using the UK General Practice Research Database. *Alimentary Pharmacology & Therapeutics*, *29*(5), 470–480. doi:10.1111/j.1365-2036.2008.03901.x PMID:19035977

El-Serag, H. B., Petersen, N. J., Carter, J., Graham, D. Y., Richardson, P., Genta, R. M., & Rabeneck, L. (2004). Gastroesophageal reflux among different racial groups in the United States. *Gastroenterology*, *126*(7), 1692–1699. doi:10.1053/j.gastro.2004.03.077 PMID:15188164

El-Serag, H. B., Sweet, S., Winchester, C. C., & Dent, J. (2014). Update on the epidemiology of gastro-oesophageal reflux disease: A systematic review. *Gut*.

Fox, M., Barr, C., Nolan, S., Lomer, M., Anggiansah, A., & Wong, T. (2007). The Effects of Dietary Fat and Calorie Density on Esophageal Acid Exposure and Reflux Symptoms. *Clinical Gastroenterology and Hepatology*, *5*(4), 439–444.e1. doi:10.1016/j.cgh.2006.12.013 PMID:17363334

Fujiwara, Y., Machida, A., Watanabe, Y., Shiba, M., Tominaga, K., Watanabe, T., Oshitani, N., Higuchi, K., & Arakawa, T. (2005). Association between dinner-to-bed time and gastroesophageal reflux disease. *The American Journal of Gastroenterology*, *100*(12), 2633–2636. doi:10.1111/j.1572-0241.2005.00354.x PMID:16393212

Gomes, D. C., & Dantas, R. O. (2014). Acidic and neutral liquid ingestion in patients with gastroesophageal reflux disease. *Arquivos de Gastroenterologia*, *51*(3), 217–220. doi:10.1590/S0004-28032014000300010 PMID:25296082

Heidelbaugh, J. J., Nostrant, T. T., Kim, C., & Van Harrison, R. (2003). Management of gastroesophageal reflux disease. *American Family Physician*, *68*(7), 1311–1318. PMID:14567485

Hershcovici, T., Mashimo, H., & Fass, R. (2011). The lower esophageal sphincter. *Neurogastroenterology and Motility*, *23*(9), 819–830. doi:10.1111/j.1365-2982.2011.01738.x PMID:21711416

Holloway, R. H., Lyrenas, E., Ireland, A., & Dent, J. (1997). Effect of intraduodenal fat on lower oesophageal sphincter function and gastro-oesophageal reflux. *Gut*, *40*(4), 449–453. doi:10.1136/gut.40.4.449 PMID:9176069

Jacobson, B. C., Somers, S. C., Fuchs, C. S., Kelly, C. P., & Camargo, C. A. Jr. (2006). Body-Mass Index and Symptoms of Gastroesophageal Reflux in Women. *The New England Journal of Medicine*, *354*(22), 2340–2348. doi:10.1056/NEJMoa054391 PMID:16738270

Jarosz, M., & Taraszewska, A. (2014). Risk factors for gastroesophageal reflux disease: The role of diet. *Przegląd Gastroenterologiczny*, *9*(5), 297–301. doi:10.5114/pg.2014.46166 PMID:25396005

Jung, H., Choung, R. S., & Talley, N. J. (2010). Gastroesophageal Reflux Disease and Sleep Disorders: Evidence for a Causal Link and Therapeutic Implications. *Journal of Neurogastroenterology and Motility*, *16*(1), 22–29. doi:10.5056/jnm.2010.16.1.22 PMID:20535322

Kahrilas, P. J. (2003). GERD pathogenesis, pathophysiology, and clinical manifestations. *Cleveland Clinic Journal of Medicine*, *70*(SUPPL. 5), S4–S19. doi:10.3949/ccjm.70.Suppl_5.S4 PMID:14705378

Kahrilas, P. J., & Gupta, R. R. (1990). Mechanisms of acid reflux associated with cigarette smoking. *Gut*, *31*(1), 4–10. doi:10.1136/gut.31.1.4 PMID:2318431

Kahrilas, P. J., Lin, S., Chen, J., & Manka, M. (1999). The effect of hiatus hernia on gastro-oesophageal junction pressure. *Gut*, *44*(4), 476–482. doi:10.1136/gut.44.4.476 PMID:10075953

Kaltenbach, T., Crockett, S., & Gerson, L. B. (2006). Are lifestyle measures effective in patients with gastroesophageal reflux disease? An evidence-based approach. *Archives of Internal Medicine*, *166*(9), 965–971. doi:10.1001/archinte.166.9.965 PMID:16682569

Katz, P. O., Gerson, L. B., & Vela, M. F. (2013). Guidelines for the Diagnosis and Management of Gastroesophageal Reflux Disease. *The American Journal of Gastroenterology*, *108*(3), 308–328. doi:10.1038/ajg.2012.444 PMID:23419381

Lohsiriwat, S., Puengna, N., & Leelakusolvong, S. (2006). Effect of caffeine on lower esophageal sphincter pressure in Thai healthy volunteers. *Diseases of the Esophagus*, *19*(3), 183–188. doi:10.1111/j.1442-2050.2006.00562.x PMID:16722996

Mahan, L. K., & Raymond, J. L. (2017). *Krause's food & the nutrition care process*. Elsevier.

Meining, A., & Classen, M. (2000). The role of diet and lifestyle measures in the pathogenesis and treatment of gastroesophageal reflux disease. *The American Journal of Gastroenterology*, *95*(10), 2692–2697. doi:10.1111/j.1572-0241.2000.03175.x PMID:11051337

Mifflin, M. D., St Jeor, S. T., Hill, L. A., Scott, B. J., Daugherty, S. A., & Koh, Y. O. (1990). new predictive equation for resting energy expenditure in healthy individuals. *The American Journal of Clinical Nutrition*, *51*(2), 241–247. doi:10.1093/ajcn/51.2.241 PMID:2305711

Mittal, R. K., Lange, R. C., & McCallum, R. W. (1987). Identification and mechanism of delayed esophageal acid clearance in subjects with hiatus hernia. *Gastroenterology*, *92*(1), 130–135. doi:10.1016/0016-5085(87)90849-3 PMID:3781181

Miwa, H., Igarashi, A., Teng, L., Uda, A., Deguchi, H., & Tango, T. (2019). Systematic review with network meta-analysis: Indirect comparison of the efficacy of vonoprazan and proton-pump inhibitors for maintenance treatment of gastroesophageal reflux disease. *Journal of Gastroenterology*, *54*(8), 718–729. doi:10.100700535-019-01572-y PMID:30919071

Morozov, S., Isakov, V., & Konovalova, M. (2018). Fiber-enriched diet helps to control symptoms and improves esophageal motility in patients with non-erosive gastroesophageal reflux disease. *World Journal of Gastroenterology*, *24*(21), 2291–2299. doi:10.3748/wjg.v24.i21.2291 PMID:29881238

National Institute of Diabetes and Digestive and Kidney Diseaes. (2014). *Eating, Diet, & Nutrition for GER & GERD*. Retrieved April 17, 2020, from https://www.niddk.nih.gov/health-information/digestive-diseases/acid-reflux-ger-gerd-adults/eating-diet-nutrition

Newberry, C., & Lynch, K. (2019). The role of diet in the development and management of gastroesophageal reflux disease: Why we feel the burn. *Journal of Thoracic Disease*, *11*(S12), S1594–S1601. doi:10.21037/jtd.2019.06.42 PMID:31489226

Nilsson, M., Johnsen, R., Ye, W., Hveem, K., & Lagergren, J. (2004). Lifestyle related risk factors in the aetiology of gastrooesophageal reflux. *Gut*, *53*(12), 1730–1735. doi:10.1136/gut.2004.043265 PMID:15542505

Okuyama, M., Takaishi, O., Nakahara, K., Iwakura, N., Hasegawa, T., Oyama, M., Inoue, A., Ishizu, H., Satoh, H., & Fujiwara, Y. (2017). Associations among gastroesophageal reflux disease, psychological stress, and sleep disturbances in Japanese adults. *Scandinavian Journal of Gastroenterology*, *52*(1), 44–49. doi:10.1080/00365521.2016.1224383 PMID:27571846

Piesman, M., Hwang, I., Maydonovitch, C., & Wong, R. K. H. (2007). Nocturnal Reflux Episodes Following the Administration of a a standardized meal. Does timing matter? *The American Journal of Gastroenterology*, *102*(10), 2128–2134. doi:10.1111/j.1572-0241.2007.01348.x PMID:17573791

Pointer, S. D., Rickstrew, J., Slaughter, J. C., Vaezi, M. F., & Silver, H. J. (2016). Dietary carbohydrate intake, insulin resistance and gastro-oesophageal reflux disease: A pilot study in European- and African-American obese women. *Alimentary Pharmacology & Therapeutics*, *44*(9), 976–988. doi:10.1111/apt.13784 PMID:27582035

Schlottmann, F., Andolfi, C., Herbella, F. A., Rebecchi, F., Allaix, M. E., & Patti, M. G. (2018). GERD: Presence and Size of Hiatal Hernia Influence Clinical Presentation, Esophageal Function, Reflux Profile, and Degree of Mucosal Injury. *The American Surgeon*, *84*(6), 978–982. doi:10.1177/000313481808400651 PMID:29981634

Song, J. H., Chung, S. J., Lee, J. H., Kim, Y. H., Chang, D. K., Son, H. J., Kim, J. J., Rhee, J. C., & Rhee, P. L. (2011). Relationship between gastroesophageal reflux symptoms and dietary factors in Korea. *Journal of Neurogastroenterology and Motility*, *17*(1), 54–60. doi:10.5056/jnm.2011.17.1.54 PMID:21369492

Stefanidis, D., Hope, W. W., Kohn, G. P., Reardon, P. R., Richardson, W. S., & Fanelli, R. D.SAGES Guidelines Committee. (2010). Guidelines for surgical treatment of gastroesophageal reflux disease. *Surgical Endoscopy*, *24*(11), 2647–2669. doi:10.100700464-010-1267-8 PMID:20725747

Surdea-Blaga, T., Negrutiu, D. E., Palage, M., & Dumitrascu, D. L. (2017). Food and Gastroesophageal Reflux Disease. *Current Medicinal Chemistry*, *26*(19), 3497–3511. doi:10.2174/0929867324666170515123807 PMID:28521699

Vakil, N., Van Zanten, S. V., Kahrilas, P., Dent, J., Jones, R., Bianchi, L. K., & Cesario, K. B. (2006). The Montreal definition and classification of gastroesophageal reflux disease: A global evidence-based consensus. *American Journal of Gastroenterology, 101*(8), 1900–20.

Wajed, S. A., Streets, C. G., Bremner, C. G., & DeMeester, T. R. (2001). Elevated body mass disrupts the barrier to gastroesophageal reflux. *Archives of Surgery*, *136*(9), 1014–1019. doi:10.1001/archsurg.136.9.1014 PMID:11529823

Wienbeck, M., & Barnert, J. (1989). Epidemiology of reflux disease and reflux esophagitis. *Scandinavian Journal of Gastroenterology*, *24*(sup156, S156), 7–13. doi:10.3109/00365528909091032 PMID:2662390

Yeoh, K. G., Ho, K. Y., Guan, R., & Kang, J. Y. (1995). How Does Chili Cause Upper Gastrointestinal Symptoms? *Journal of Clinical Gastroenterology*, *21*(2), 87–90. doi:10.1097/00004836-199509000-00004 PMID:8583092

Zaninotto, G., DeMeester, T. R., Schwizer, W., Johansson, K. E., & Cheng, S. C. (1988). The lower esophageal sphincter in health and disease. *American Journal of Surgery*, *155*(1), 104–111. doi:10.1016/S0002-9610(88)80266-6 PMID:3341525

Zheng, Z., Nordenstedt, H., Pedersen, N. L., Lagergren, J., & Ye, W. (2007). Lifestyle Factors and Risk for Symptomatic Gastroesophageal Reflux in Monozygotic Twins. *Gastroenterology*, *132*(1), 87–95. doi:10.1053/j.gastro.2006.11.019 PMID:17241862

KEY TERMS AND DEFINITIONS

Barrett's Esophagus: Is a GERD complication characterized by a change in the lining of the lower part of the esophagus such that it resembles the lining of the small intestine.

Esophageal Peristalsis: Is a sequence of esophageal muscles contractions which helps in the movement of the bolus to the stomach.

Gastric Acid: Is a fluid secreted by the stomach to help in the digestion process. It mainly comprises hydrochloric acid, sodium chloride, and potassium chloride.

Heartburn: Is a condition characterized by a painful burning feeling in the chest. It happens as a result of the stomach acid traveling back up into the esophagus.

Hiatal Hernia: Is a condition that occurs when a part of the stomach is pulled into the diaphragm, resulting in gastric acid reflux and heartburn.

Itchy Ear: Is a condition resulting from an ear infection.

Lower Esophageal Sphincter: Is a muscular layer located at the lower end of the esophagus where it meets the stomach. It prevents the stomach acid from going back up to the esophagus.

Non-Steroidal Anti-Inflammatory Drugs: Are drugs used to reduce pain, fever, and inflammation.

Polycystic Ovary Syndrome: Is a hormonal condition affecting women's hormonal levels wherein they may have elevated male-hormone (androgen) levels.

Reflux: Is a condition wherein stomach acid travels back up into the esophagus.

ENDNOTES

1 Nutrition Care Process 2018, Nutrition Diagnostic Terminology. Clinical (NC)/ Weight (3).

2 Nutrition Care Process 2018, Nutrition Diagnostic Terminology. Behavioral-Environmental (NB)/ Knowledge and Beliefs (1).

APPENDIX: ABBREVIATIONS

ALT: alanine aminotransferase
AST: aspartate aminotransferase
BMI: body mass index
BPM: beat per minute
BUN: blood urea nitrogen
CPK: creatine phosphokinase
EGF: epidermal growth factor
GERD: gastroesophageal reflux disease
GI: gastrointestinal
H_2: histamine 2
HEENT: head, eyes, ears, nose, throat
HDL: high -density lipoprotein
Hgb: hemoglobin
LDL: low-density lipoprotein
LES: lower esophageal sphincter
LESP: lower esophageal sphincter pressure
PGE2: prostaglandin E2
PPIs: proton pump inhibitors
RBC: red blood cells
WBC: white blood cells

Chapter 3
Peptic Ulcer Disease

Albatool Abumunaser
King Abdulaziz University, Saudi Arabia

EXECUTIVE SUMMARY

This chapter will discuss a peptic ulcer disease (PUD) case. PUD is a common gastrointestinal tract disease (GIT) that affects the stomach and duodenum. It is characterized by deep lesions into the mucosal thickness. Various dietary and behavioral choices could aggravate the epigastric pain associated with PUD and interfere with the healing process leading to complications. Management of PUD includes medical treatment with medications along with behavioral and nutritional changes. This case presents a complication of PUD, and choices exacerbating the condition. It will also discuss the role of medical nutrition therapy in minimizing the symptoms and promoting ulcer healing. Additionally, it will allow the dietetic professional to methodically assess the elements in the case that are relevant for planning the nutrition intervention; in addition to, educating the patient about dietary modifications to improve the patient's quality of life.

INTRODUCTION

Peptic ulcer disease (PUD) is an erosion or break of the gastric or duodenal mucosa, mainly caused by gastric juices due to disruption of mucosal integrity (Jameson et al., 2018; Mahan & Raymond, 2017). In the United Kingdom, United States, and Europe, about 1–2 people out of 1,000 will develop PUD (Sverdén, Agréus, Dunn, & Lagergren, 2019). The pathogenesis of PUD involves one of two mechanisms: an increase in the secretion of gastric juices or a decline in the protective factors against the endogenous and exogenous hostile factors that attack the gastroduodenal mucosa (Hall, 2011). The primary etiology of PUD includes Helicobacter pylori (*H.pylori*)

DOI: 10.4018/978-1-7998-3802-9.ch003

infection and nonsteroidal anti-inflammatory drugs (NSAIDs). Additionally, there are several other risk factors, such as severe stress, other comorbid conditions, advanced age, African-American ethnicity, and lifestyle factors such as smoking and drinking alcohol (Jameson et al., 2018). The most typical symptom of PUD is gnawing or burning epigastric pain, although some patients may be asymptomatic; it is essential to watch for alarming signs and symptoms because they may indicate complications (Ramakrishnan & Salinas, 2007; Sverdén et al., 2019). Because the epigastric pain is not specific to PUD, a radiographic or endoscopic diagnosis may be necessary to document a PUD diagnosis (Jameson et al., 2018). The medical management includes the usage of various medications, an endoscopic approach, and surgery; meanwhile, the nutritional intervention involves dietary adjustments according to the patient's overall profile and improvement of the overall nutrition to promote ulcer healing (Jameson et al., 2018; Mahan & Raymond, 2017).

EPIDEMIOLOGY AND PREVALENCE

Annually, PUD affects around 1–2 per 1,000 people in the United States, United Kingdom, and Europe, but incidence has been dropping over the years due to the reduction in *H.pylori* infections (Sverdén et al., 2019). Duodenal ulcers are estimated to affect 6–15% of the Western population, whereas gastric ulcers are less common. The prevalence of *H.pylori* infection in developing countries is about 80% (people usually get it by age 20), whereas it affects about 20–50% of the population in developed countries. NSAIDs-induced and endoscopy-documented PUD incidence is estimated to be around 15–30% among regular NSAIDs users (Jameson et al., 2018).

PATHOPHYSIOLOGY

To understand the pathogenesis of PUD, it is essential to explain the defense mechanism of the gastroduodenal mucosa and gastric secretion process. First, it is crucial to acknowledge that the innermost layer surrounding the lumen of the gastrointestinal (GI) tract, which is the GI mucosa, is always under attack by aggressive factors. These hostile factors can be either endogenous factors, such as hydrochloric acid (HCL), pepsin, and bile salts, or exogenous factors including medications, ethanol, and bacteria. Fortunately, the mucosal barrier is protected from those agents by a three-level defense mechanism: preepithelial, epithelial, and subepithelial (Jameson et al., 2018; Li et al., 2014). These levels maintain the mucosal integrity through: (a) the production of prostaglandins (PGs); (b) the secretion of mucus and bicarbonate (HCO_3-); (c) removal of excess acid by uninterrupted blood flow; (c) and the rapid regeneration of epithelial cells. The PGs are vital for the regulation of the release of HCO_3- and mucus, inhibition of the HCL acid secretion from parietal cells, and maintenance of mucosal blood flow (Jameson et al., 2018).

The process of PG synthesis involves the conversion of cell membrane's phospholipids into arachidonic acid through phospholipase A2 enzyme. Arachidonic acid will eventually either produce leukotrienes by lipoxygenase or PGs via enzyme cyclooxygenase (COX). Enzyme COX is further expressed differently in two isoforms: COX-1 and COX-2—in the host tissue and the tissue activated by an inflammatory stimulus, respectively. The COX-1 isoform is expressed in different tissues such as the gastric, kidney, platelets, and endothelial cells and is essential for the maintenance of renal function, platelet aggregation, and the integrity of the mucosal barrier. In contrast, the COX-2 isoform acts on any tissue by being expressed in macrophages, white blood cells, fibroblasts, and endothelial cells due to the release of cytokines in response to injury or inflammation (Gupta, n.d.; Jameson et al., 2018; Sylvester, 2019). As mentioned above, the mucus is an essential agent in maintaining the integrity of the mucosal barrier due to its composition (mucin and water), which allows it to form an alkaline and thick gel layer protecting it from the highly acidic environment and facilitating food movements. Typically, the mucous cells tend to secrete additional amounts of mucus in response to contact with food or irritants (Hall, 2011; Jameson et al., 2018). The HCO_3- is secreted by the epithelial cells of the pancreatic ducts as part of the pancreatic juices to form an alkali medium at the duodenum luminal surface; hence, it neutralizes the acidity of the chyme coming from the stomach (Hall, 2011). Another essential defense agent is nitric oxide (NO), which influences the vascular muscle tone and protects the gastric mucosal barrier by enhancing regular blood flow, mucus production, and the integrity of the epithelial cell barrier (Chaudhary & Singh, 2014; Jameson et al., 2018). NO also protects the mucosa by diminishing neutrophil infiltration and inhibiting the secretion of histamine (Amandeep, Robin, Ramica, & Sunil, 2012).

As previously stated, it is necessary to understand the mechanism and stimulants of gastric secretions (HCL and pepsin) to understand the development of PUD. HCL and pepsinogen/pepsin can be destructive in case of a disruption in the protective mechanisms. However, they play an essential physiological role in the digestion of protein into peptides, the absorption of several micronutrients—such as vitamin B12, calcium, and magnesium—and the destruction of bacteria ingested with food (Jameson et al., 2018). The body of the stomach has a group of cells called parietal cells that are responsible for the secretion of HCL acid and the intrinsic factor. An essential mechanism of HCL secretion includes pumping hydrogen ions (H+) via active transport through a hydrogen-potassium pump (H+/K+ ATPase), an acid-secreting pump; this process also enables the formation of HCO_3- from carbon dioxide and hydroxyl (Hall, 2011) . The process of gastric acid secretion involves three phases: (a) Cephalic phase; vagus nerve initiates this phase in response to the sight, smell, taste of food, or any sensory stimulus; (b) Gastric phase; the presence of food in the stomach and the distention of the stomach stimulates this phase; (c) Intestinal phase; the presence of nutrients in the duodenum of the small intestine continues the stimulation of a small amount of gastric acid secretion (Hall, 2011; Jameson et al., 2018). The process of acid secretion mentioned in the previous phases involves the release of acetylcholine, gastrin, and histamine (H_2), which are stimulants that parietal cells have receptors for, and the eventually activation of the pathways regulating H+/K+ ATPase. Acetylcholine is a neurotransmitter secreted by the vagus nerve endings or enteric nerves in response to sensory stimuli or gastric stretch that either stimulates the release of HCL through the parietal receptors or the release of gastrin from G-cells. Gastrin hormone is secreted by the gastric G-cells and is stimulated by the presence of protein, stomach distention, or acetylcholine. Once gastrin enters circulation, it either directly stimulates the release of HCL or stimulates the stomach's enterochromaffin-like cells to release H_2. Histamine diffuses into the parietal cells to activate the release of HCL because HCL secretion rate is directly proportional to the secretion of H_2 (Feher, 2017; Hall, 2011; Jameson et al., 2018). The parietal cells also express receptors for somatostatin, which is a hormone released from the gastric endocrine cells that inhibits gastric, biliary, and pancreatic secretions. The somatostatin inhibits HCL either directly or indirectly through the reduction of the secretion of several stimulants, including H_2 and gastrin (Feher, 2017; Jameson et al., 2018).

Furthermore, the chief cells of the stomach synthesize pepsinogen—the inactive form and precursor of the enzyme pepsin—where it is packaged and stored until gastric release in response to the presence of food. The secretion of pepsinogen is stimulated by acetylcholine and gastric acidity. The pepsinogen is activated by the acidic environment (PH < 2) into the proteolytic enzyme pepsin. Ultimately, the pathogenesis of PUD is caused by an imbalance between the gastric factors and the gastroduodenal defense mechanism mentioned above, resulting from either a reduction in the mucosal barrier's ability to protect itself or excessive secretion of HCL and pepsin caused by various factors, which will be discussed later (Hall, 2011; Jameson et al., 2018). The weakening of the mucosal barrier makes it easier to excavate through the epithelial cell of the mucosa and into muscularis mucosa through the submucosa, muscularis propria, or both; consequently, this results in the formation of inflammation and lesions/ulcers (Jameson et al., 2018; Mahan & Raymond, 2017).

RISK FACTORS AND ETIOLOGY

The primary risk factors or etiology to PUD are *H.pylori* infection and NSAIDs, but other factors may contribute to the development of PUD. *H.pylori* is a gram-negative, microaerophilic bacillus, spiral-shaped, and flagellated (motile) bacterium that colonizes the stomach and is characterized by its ability to survive harsh conditions (Amandeep et al., 2012; Jameson et al., 2018). *H.pylori* bacteria are found either deep inside the mucus gel of the gastric mucosa or attached between the epithelium and the mucus layer. The consequences of *H.pylori* infection vary from chronic gastritis to PUD, mucosa-associated lymphoid tissue (MALT) lymphoma, or gastric cancer, depending on interactions between the host's immune response and bacterial factors. Thus, only 10–15% of patients infected with *H.pylori* develop PUD, and it tends to be more common in duodenal ulcer patients, with a percentage of 50–70% compared to 30–60% in gastric ulcer patients—although the etiology of how it causes duodenal ulcer is still unclear. The pathogenesis and virulence of *H.pylori* depend on specific encoded proteins such as vacuolating toxin (VacA) and cytotoxin-associated gene A (CagA), which are part of 1,500 encoded genes in the *H.pylori* genome; hence, different consequences are based on the different strains and their ability to express the virulent factors. The pathogenic virulence allows the *H.pylori* infection to colonize the stomach, injure the mucosal barrier, and avoid the host's defense through the host immune cells. The process by which *H.pylori* infection induces PUD involves various mechanisms, including the translocation of CagA into the host cell and triggering a sequence of cellular events such as reducing HCL acid secretion. These events are accomplished by directly inhibiting the H+/K+ ATPase pump and producing the enzyme urease that breaks down urea into ammonia (NH_3); thus, protecting the bacteria from the harsh gastric conditions as the NH_3 alkalinizes the environment, facilitating epithelial cell damage (Jameson et al., 2018). VacA may also contribute to the destruction of the mucosal barrier by interfering with the function of the immune cells and inducing apoptosis of mucosal epithelial cells, thus disrupting the healthy balance between cell death and proliferation (Amandeep et al., 2012; Rassow, 2011). Other mechanisms include the inhibition of somatostatin and activation of gastrin, and the production of enzymes such as proteases and phospholipases to break down the glycoprotein of the mucin to weaken the mucus's defenses. Furthermore, expressing adhesion factors and attachment to the epithelial cells facilitate mucosal damage through the production of reactive oxygen species (ROS) and reducing the production of glutathione, leading to oxidative damage of the cellular components, such as DNA, proteins, and polyunsaturated fatty acids, and activation of proinflammatory cytokines, which may increase acid secretion (Chaudhary & Singh, 2014; Jameson et al., 2018).

NSAIDs is a term used to describe a group of medications that are characterized by their anti-inflammatory and antipyretic properties (Gupta, n.d.). Therefore, they are used to manage conditions such as headaches, chronic joint or arthritis pain, and musculoskeletal and menstrual pain; they also tend to be used in perioperative periods (Gupta, n.d.; Sylvester, 2019).The use of NSAIDs has been dramatically increasing over the years; the increased prescription and over-the-counter usage means more than 30 million people consume them daily (Bjarnason et al., 2018).The desired therapeutic effect is accomplished through their interference with the COX enzyme pathway, specifically the COX-2 isoform. Most conventional NSAIDs function by comprehensively hindering both isoforms; thus, the undesired side effects affect the cardiovascular, renal, hepatic, and GI systems (Bjarnason et al., 2018; Gupta, n.d.). Consequently, different types of NSAIDs would have different side effects based on the extent of COX-1 and COX-2 inhibition (Sylvester, 2019). About 25% of NSAIDs users are prone to develop gastric ulcers. Studies have shown that the rates range from 5% to 80% and 15% to 40% in short- and long-term usage, respectively (Bjarnason et al., 2018; Jameson et al., 2018). The pathogenesis of NSAIDs-induced ulcers and erosions involves two main mechanisms: topical actions and the inhibition of the COX-1 enzyme. Because NSAIDs are lipid-soluble weak acids, they can come into contact with the mucosal phospholipid layer, compromising its effectiveness and facilitating mitochondrial oxidative phosphorylation uncoupling, leading to the generation of ROS, the reduction of glutathione, and induction of apoptosis (Bjarnason et al., 2018). Hence, the increased permeability of the mucosal barrier and exposure to aggressive factors initiate gastric damage. Eventually, inhibition of the COX-1 enzyme is followed, which leads to gastroduodenal ulcers through the interference with the synthesis of PGs, reduction in the secretion of mucus and HCO_3^-, and reduction in mucosal blood flow and cell proliferation (Bjarnason et al., 2018; Jameson et al., 2018).

A rare etiology of PUD includes acid hypersecretory conditions such as Zollinger-Ellison syndrome or gastrinoma. Zollinger-Ellison syndrome is a tumor in the pancreas that leads to an unregulated release of the gastrin hormone, stimulating HCL acid production via the parietal cells (Jameson et al., 2018). Furthermore, stress ulcer or stress-induced ulcer, is a type of ulcer seen in critically ill patients or those with severe physiological stress such as severe illness or trauma, including hypotension, burns, surgery, sepsis, respiratory failure, multiple traumatic injuries, and brain trauma (Anand, 2020). The mechanism behind stress-induced ulcer involves the reduced mucosal blood flow due to the hypoperfusion associated with the illness or trauma, which leads to the breakdown of the mucosal defense barrier (Clarke, 2020; Plummer, Blaser, & Deane, 2014).

Additional factors that increase the risk of PUD development include first-degree relatives because children of patients with duodenal ulcers are three times more likely to develop an ulcer. Additionally, it seems that the risk increases with advanced age, being African-American, and having a prior chronic condition such as diabetes, coronary heart disease, chronic renal failure, chronic pulmonary disease, and liver cirrhosis (Jameson et al., 2018). Furthermore, the excessive use of corticosteroids in conjunction with NSAIDs increases the risk of PUD (Anand, 2020). There are also some lifestyle factors linked to the pathogenesis of PUD because they interfere with regular gastroduodenal defense mechanisms—though not independent factors. These include chronic alcohol consumption, which diminishes the gastric barrier through inhibiting the COX-1 receptor, thus reducing the secretion of PGs, mucus, and HCO_3-; inducing microvascular injury in the mucosa; and stimulating the release of ROS, which damages the cellular membrane through lipid peroxidation (Amandeep et al., 2012; Asali et al., 2018). Furthermore, cigarette or tobacco smoking is a significant risk factor that reduces the release of HCO_3- and mucus and synthesis of antioxidants, permitting the reflux of toxic duodenal contents and stimulating gastric acid secretion, thus causing necrotic lesions on the gastric mucosa (Amandeep et al., 2012; Li et al., 2014; Vomero & Colpo, 2014). According to several studies, smoking activates epithelial cell apoptosis of the mucosa and inhibits cell renewal, thus interfering with ulcer healing (Li et al., 2014).

CLINICAL PRESENTATION

The most common clinical presentation of PUD patients is an episodic gnawing or burning right upper quadrant (RUQ) epigastric pain that may or may not radiate to the back. However, it is not diagnostic because it is seen with conditions such as functional dyspepsia and gastritis as well. The pain can manifest when the stomach is empty, within 2–5 hours postprandial, or at night. The epigastric pain associated with duodenal ulcers can be relieved with antacids and food consumption; however, gastric ulcers can only be relieved by antacids because food intake tends to aggravate the pain. Nevertheless, in both types, the pain or discomfort tends to last for minutes or hours and can reappear for several days, weeks, or months. Furthermore, other symptoms include heartburn, dyspepsia, bloating, burping, nausea, vomiting, poor appetite, and weight loss (Mahan & Raymond, 2017; Ramakrishnan & Salinas, 2007). However, some patients can be asymptomatic until they suffer from a complication: in fact, 30% of older adults do not complain of abdominal pain (Ramakrishnan & Salinas, 2007; Sverdén et al., 2019).

Some emergency symptoms usually indicate a complication of PUD, including sharp, sudden, persistent, and severe abdominal pain, melena, hematemesis, or vomit that looks like coffee grounds. The severe complications associated with PUD include GI bleeding, perforation, and obstruction. Bleeding is the most common complication, which is the result of a blood vessel break and manifested by hematemesis or coffee-ground vomit, melena, and fatigue due to anemia, orthostasis, or syncope (Fashner & Gitu, 2015; Mahan & Raymond, 2017). Perforation occurs in 1 of 10,000 people per year due to excavation of the ulcer into the gastric or duodenal wall, possibly penetrating an adjoining organ, which is manifested by peritonitis from the release of contents and sudden, rapid, severe RUQ abdominal pain exacerbated by movement. Finally, a gastric obstruction can result from the restriction associated with scarring and inflammation of the ulcer; thus blocking the pathway of food leading to recurrent episodes of vomiting with large volumes containing undigested food, persistent bloating after eating, and early satiety (Fashner & Gitu, 2015; Mahan & Raymond, 2017; Ramakrishnan & Salinas, 2007).

DIAGNOSIS

Because the symptoms of PUD are similar to other conditions, such as functional dyspepsia, it is necessary to perform either an esophagogastroduodenoscopy (EGD) or a radiographic barium study procedure for the documentation of PUD. An EGD is more sensitive and specific for PUD diagnoses, compared to radiography, which its sensitivity decreases with small ulcers (<0.5 cm), previous scarring, or in postoperative patients. Additionally, an EGD allows for tissue biopsies to differentiate benign gastric ulcers from malignant ones and detect *H. Pylori* infection (Jameson et al., 2018). Other studies used for the detection of *H.pylori* include the stool antigen test, urea breath test, and serologic enzyme-linked immunosorbent assay (Jameson et al., 2018; Ramakrishnan & Salinas, 2007). Patients with symptoms suggesting a PUD diagnosis should be under observation for emergency symptoms. Referral to an immediate EGD is necessary for patients who are older than 55 years and those with emergency symptoms. In contrast, patients younger than 55 years with no emergency symptoms should only be tested for *H. pylori* infection and advised to discontinue NSAIDs, smoking, and alcohol usage (Ramakrishnan & Salinas, 2007).

MEDICAL MANAGEMENT

The medical approach to PUD involves various interventions. It includes the usage of medications such as antacids, sucralfate, proton-pump inhibitors (PPIs), and a histamine 2 receptor antagonist (H_2RA). Antacids act as buffering agents by neutralizing the gastric acid in the upper GI (Hall, 2011). Sucralfate provides a protective barrier by enhancing the release of PGs, mucus, and HCO_3-. Likewise, the ulcer drugs PPI and H_2RA interfere with the process of acid secretion through replacing histamine receptors and inhibiting the H+/K+ ATPase pump, respectively. Initially, it is essential to determine whether NSAIDs or *H.pylori* are involved to provide the appropriate therapeutic plan (Jameson et al., 2018). However, the long-term use of these medications could increase some micronutrient deficiencies due to their interference with the absorption of specific vitamins and minerals. For instance, use of PPIs and H_2RA may decrease the absorption of iron and vitamin B12, whereas PPIs alone could also reduce the absorption of calcium. Furthermore, some types of antacids can decrease the absorption of folate, iron, and phosphate (Pronsky, Elbe, & Ayoob, 2015).

To eradicate the *H.pylori* infection, the American College of Gastroenterology recommends a triple or quadruple therapy regimen for 10–14 days, followed by 4–6 weeks of PPIs or H_2RA. The triple therapy consists of a PPI with two types of antibiotics (amoxicillin or metronidazole + clarithromycin). The quadruple therapy is either a combination of a PPI or H_2RA with a bactericidal salt called bismuth, and two antibiotics (tetracycline and metronidazole) or concomitant PPI with three antibiotics (clarithromycin, amoxicillin, and metronidazole; (Jameson et al., 2018; Ramakrishnan & Salinas, 2007). However, in the case of NSAIDs-related PUD, COX-2-selective NSAIDs could be used instead, but primarily there will be one of two treatments: either discontinuing the use of NSAIDs and starting on PPIs or H_2RA or continuing the use of NSAIDs, in which case only PPIs are still feasible (Jameson et al., 2018). Other treatments involve EGD therapy in case of a bleeding ulcer through hemostatic therapy, injection therapy, thermal coagulation, hemostatic clips, or a combination, as well as surgical interventions in case of perforated ulcers or recurrent bleeding (Anand, 2020; Sverdén et al., 2019). Guidelines recommend the continuation of PPIs for 6–8 weeks after an EGD treatment of a bleeding ulcer (Tarasconi et al., 2020).

NUTRITIONAL MANAGEMENT

Nutritional therapy plays an essential role in the management of PUD because its primary goal is to enhance the repair and maintenance of the gastrointestinal mucosa, relieve pain and symptoms, and optimize nutritional status. In the past, drinking milk was considered part of the therapy due to the belief of its coating effect, but this has changed nowadays because it is known to increase gastric acid secretion (Mahan & Raymond, 2017). To promote wound healing, following a diet rich in protein and antioxidants such as zinc, selenium, vitamin A (beta-carotene), vitamin E, and vitamin C is recommended. Antioxidants help with ulcer healing by promoting regeneration of the damaged mucosal lining and protecting it from further damage. Food sources for these nutrients include carrots, kiwi, apple, cabbage, avocado, and hazelnuts (Kulshreshtha, Srivastava, & Singh, 2017). Likewise, following a diet rich in fiber is also advised because it aids in buffering the concentrated bile acids, the formation of mucin (a component of mucus), and the reduction of intestinal transit time and abdominal bloating because feces are quickly evacuated; this results in a reduction in pain and discomfort (Kulshreshtha et al., 2017; Vomero & Colpo, 2014).

Moreover, studies regarding the effect of probiotics on *H.pylori* show that it does not eradicate it but can decrease the bacterial load and improve symptoms (Vomero & Colpo, 2014). It is advisable to limit fat and specifically fatty foods because they stimulate the overproduction of gastric acids and enzymes (Kulshreshtha et al., 2017). Some studies show that cruciferous vegetables and broccoli, curcumin, green tea, black currant oil, and kimchi can help with *H.pylori* eradication by enhancing the gastric mucosal barrier. Although it might be ineffective, increasing the consumption of omega-3 and omega-6 is still advocated due to their potential mucosal protective effects (Escott-Stump, 2012; Mahan & Raymond, 2017). Nonetheless, avoiding the factors that would aggravate the symptoms and interfere with ulcer healing such as smoking, alcohol, and caffeine, is recommended due to their involvement in damaging the mucosal defenses (Mahan & Raymond, 2017; Vomero & Colpo, 2014). It is also better to limit spices, such as black pepper and chili, because they tend to increase gastric acid secretion, although it is individualized (Mahan & Raymond, 2017). Advising patients on increasing the consumption of vitamin B12, folic acid, and iron food sources might be necessary; besides, considering the need for supplements in case of prolonged use of antacids, PPIs, and H_2 blockers may also be necessary. Ultimately, patients must follow overall proper nutrition that is high in protein from up to 1.2 gm/kg/kg/day in the acute stage to 1.5 gm/kg/day in the recovery phase, eat antioxidant-rich food, and avoid any irritants because they may differ from person to person (Vomero & Colpo, 2014).

SETTING THE STAGE

The data for the following case study was collected from a hospital's Emergency Department. The patient was admitted to the hospital by a gastroenterologist for evaluation and management. The patient was prescribed medications for PUD management, and he was referred to a registered dietitian for nutritional consultation and education. No financial support for disclosing the case; thus, no conflict of interest.

CASE DESCRIPTION

Patient's Details

- Age: 56 years old
- Gender: Male

Case History

Case description: The patient came to the emergency department complaining of sharp, severe RUQ epigastric pain, nonradiating to the back, hematemesis, and melena, which started 5 days ago but is more persistent and not alleviated by medications. He has been diagnosed with gastritis that is usually controlled by Mylanta. For the past 2 months, he has been having a difficult time at work and getting little sleep. Because of his increasing migraine episodes, he started taking Advil almost twice a day. Furthermore, he started having occasional intermittent episodes of abdominal pain lasting for 15 min and sometimes associated with vomiting. He says that his appetite has decreased over the past month, and sometimes food exacerbates his pain. An upper EGD was performed, identifying a bleeding 1-cm gastric ulcer. After stopping the bleeding, the physician conducted a biopsy for *H.pylori* and gastric malignancy, but it came back negative.

- Medical history: Gastritis diagnosed 3 years ago and migraines since adolescence but increased over the past few years.
- Surgical history: n/a
- Smoking: Yes, cigarettes for the past 30 years (2–3 packs/day)
- Family history: Father and grandfather both suffered from peptic ulcers.

Main Medical Diagnosis

Peptic ulcer disease (PUD)

Demographics

- Marital status: Married with three children
- Education: Master's degree in business management
- Occupation: Chief financial officer at an international bank (10 hours/day for 6 days/week)
- Ethnicity and religion: African-American and Muslim

Anthropometry

- Current weight: 68 kg
- Usual weight: 76 kg
- Height: 178 cm

Table 1. Biochemical Data

Parameter	Patients Results	Reference
Albumin	30 g/L	35–50 g/L
Prealbumin	130 mg/L	150–360 mg/L
Total Protein	6.5 gm/dL	6.8–8.2 gm/dL
Alanine Amino Transferase	30 U/L	4–40 U/L
Aspartate Amino Transferase	25 U/L	10–37 U/L
Creatinine	100 μmol/L	Male: 53–106 μmol/L Female: 44–97 μmol/L
BUN	8 mmol/L	3.6–7.1 mmol/L
Sodium	146 mmol/L	136–145 mmol/L
Potassium	3.3 mmol/L	3.5–5.0 mmol/L
Chloride	108 mmol/L	98–106 mmol/L
Magnesium	0.99 mmol/L	0.65–1.05 mmol/L
Corrected Calcium	2.0 mmol/L	2.25–2.75 mmol/L
Iron	8 μmol/L	14–32 μmol/L
Serum Vitamin B12	220 pg/mL	210–911 pg/mL
Folate	20 ng/mL	2.8–40 ng/mL
Hemoglobin	8 mmol/L	Male: 8.7–11.2 mmol/L Female: 7.4–9.9 mmol/L
Hematocrit	39%	Male: 42–52% Female: 37–47%
Gastrin	110 pg/mL	0–100 pg/mL

Nutritional-Focused Physical Examination

- General appearance: Pale, mildly distressed
- Heart: Regular rate and rhythm and normal heart sounds
- HEENT: Eyes: pallor conjunctiva
- Genitalia: Normal
- Neurologic: Oriented and alert

- Extremities: Normal strength and sensations, no edema
- Skin: Pallor and dry
- Chest/lungs: Rapid breath, clear lung
- Peripheral vascular: Pulses full, no bruits
- Abdomen: Mild epigastric tenderness, severe right upper quadrant pain radiating to the back

Vital Signs

- Pulse: 87 bpm
- Temp: 36.9°C
- Blood pressure: 110/78 mm Hg
- Respiratory rate**:** 22 bpm

Medical Treatment Plan

- Patient was given 1.5 liters normal saline.
- Patient was administered with 80 mg bolus intravenous omeprazole, followed by a continuous 8-mg/h infusion for 72 hours.
- Patient was instructed to limit the intake of NSAIDs and stop smoking.
- Patient was prescribed Omeprazole 20 mg BID for home.
- Patient was referred to the registered dietitian for consultation.

Food/Nutrition-Related History

The patient states he has a poor appetite. He says that, when the pain strikes, eating exacerbates it. He eats the three main courses but does not tend to finish them, drinks more than three cups of coffee per day, and sometimes eats one to two snacks with his coffee. He is interested to know whether he should follow a specific diet to feel better. He jogs at the beach three times a week.

Table 2. 24-Hour Recall

Meal	Food Items and Quantities
Breakfast	American coffee with ½ cup milk + 1 slice of toast with butter
Snack	2 American coffees
Lunch	1 can of diet cola + ½ spicy chicken burger
Snack	2 American coffees + 1 bag of chips
Dinner	½ cup salad + 3 oz fried chicken + 1 small baked potato with chili sauce

- Food allergies/intolerances: None
- Food purchase/preparations: His wife buys and prepares the food, and he also order takeaway while at work.
- Vitamin and mineral supplementation: None

Medications

- Advil (Ibuprofen) for migraines (2–3 times/day for the past 2 months)
- Aspirin for migraines (once every 2 days for the past 2 weeks)
- Mylanta for gastritis (twice/day for the past month)

Nutritional Management

Disease Pathophysiology and Management Mind Map

Figure 1. A mind map of the presented case study (Khalifa, 2020)

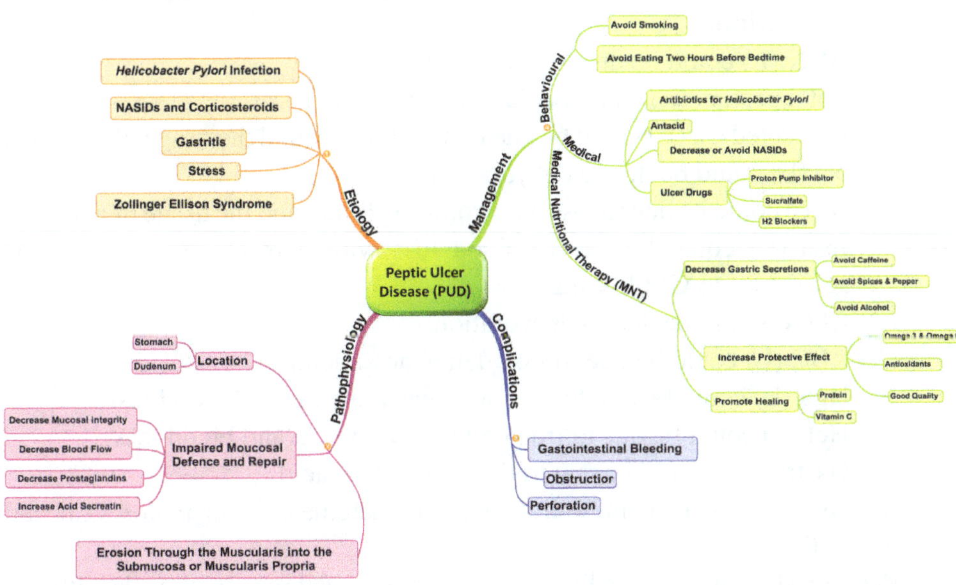

Main Aim of the Nutrition Therapy

- Promote wound healing (Antioxidants and protein) and anti-inflammatory protection (omega-3 and omega-6)

- Normalize nutritional status to prevent weight loss and micronutrient deficiencies (Vitamin B12, iron, and calcium)
- Minimize symptoms and aggravating pain through appropriate food choices

ADIME Note

Assessment: The patient is a 56-year-old male diagnosed with PUD complaining of epigastric pain, hematemesis, and melena.

- **Anthropometry:**
  - Ht: 178 cm, Wt: 70 kg, BMI: 21.4 kg/m2 (normal)
  - % Wt change: 7.9% in 1-month (severe weight loss)
  - UBW: 76 kg, % UBW: 92% (mild nutritional risk)
  - IBW: 78 kg, % IBW: 89% (mild nutritional risk)
- **Biochemical:**
  - Ab (L) could be due to inflammation secondary to the ulcer.
  - Prealbumin (L) could be due to inflammation secondary to ulcer and malnutrition
  - BUN (L) could be due to malnutrition.
  - Total protein (L) could be due to malnutrition.
  - Corrected Ca (L) could be due to malnutrition and the usage of antacids.
  - Na (L) could be due to dehydration.
  - K (L) could be due to loss with vomiting blood and the usage of antacids.
  - Iron (L) could be due to blood loss with hematemesis and melena secondary to GI bleeding.
  - Cl (H) could be due to dehydration.
  - RBC (L) could be due to iron deficiency anemia.
  - Hgb (L) could be due to iron deficiency anemia and blood loss.
  - Hct (L) could be due to iron deficiency anemia and blood loss.
  - Gastrin (H) could be due to the usage of antacids.
- **Clinical:** Epigastric pain, weight loss, hematemesis, and pallor skin and conjunctiva
- **Dietary:** The patient has a low appetite, consumes three main meals with one to two snacks per day, and complains of vomiting. According to his 24-hour recall, he consumed around 700 kCal, with 34.5 gm protein. Additionally, his diet is low in fiber and antioxidants and high in caffeinated beverages.

Diagnosis

Inadequate oral intake [NI-2.1][1] related to decreased appetite secondary to abdominal pain associated with peptic ulcer, as evidenced by PO < 50% of caloric and protein requirements.

Unintended weight loss [NC-3.2][2] related to decreased appetite secondary to fear of pain associated with peptic ulcer, as evidenced by 7.9% in 1 month.

Undesirable food choices [NB-1.7][3] related to food-and nutrition-related knowledge deficit, as evidenced by diet history (high intake of caffeine and spices and low consumption of fiber and protein).

Intervention

- **Prescription:**
  - Good quality nutrition: 2,000 kCal/day, 90 gm/day CHON
  - Energy: Using Mifflin-St. Jeor equation for men
    = (10 x weight) + (6.25 x height) – (5 x age) + 5
    = (10 x 70) + (6.25 x 178) – (5 x 56) + 5 = 1,538 x 1.3 (activity factor)
    = 2,000 kCal/day
  - Protein: (1.2–1.5 gm/kg) = 1.3 x 70 = 91 gm/day (18%)
  - Carbohydrates: (50–60%) = 2,000 x 55% = 1,100/4 = 275 gm/day
  - Fat: (25–30%) = 2,000 x 27% = 540/9 = 60 gm/day
  - Fluids: 30mL/kg = 30 x 70 = 2,100 mL/day

Recommendations

- Include an assortment of vegetables, fruits, and whole grains to increase fiber and antioxidant intake.
- Ensure adequate protein intake for wound healing, moderate consumption of fat with a focus on omega-3 and omega-6 sources, and iron-rich sources (lean meats).
- Decrease the intake of caffeine-containing beverages (coffee, tea, cola, and chocolates).
- Limit the consumption of certain spices (chili, peppermint, garlic, and black pepper), fried, and citric food and juices (orange and lemon).
- Eat smaller and more frequent meals, which may be better tolerated.
- Avoid eating 2–3 hours before bedtime.
- Avoid or decrease smoking.
- Consider iron, vitamin B12, and calcium supplementation with long-term use of medication.

Monitoring/Evaluation

- Nutritional status
  - Weight changes (prevent further weight loss)
  - Dietary intake (meets the requirements and appetite)
- Lab values (iron, B12, calcium, and albumin)
- GI symptoms (nausea, vomiting, and epigastric pain)

REFERENCES

Amandeep, K., Robin, S., Ramica, S., & Sunil, K. (2012). Peptic ulcer: A review on etiology and pathogenesis. *IRJP, 3*, 34-38. Retrieved from https://irjponline.com/admin/php/uploads/1161_pdf.pdf

American Dietetic Association. (2011). *International Dietetics and Nutrition Terminology (IDNT) Reference Manual, Standardized Language for the Nutrition Care Process* (3rd ed.). American Dietetic Association.

Anand, B. (2020). Peptic Ulcer Disease. *Medscape.* Retrieved from https://emedicine.medscape.com/article/181753-overview

Asali, A. M., Alghamdi, M. A., Fallatah, S. A., Alholaily, W. A., Aldandan, R. G., Alnosair, A. H., ... Alharbi, R. A. (2018). Risk factors leading to peptic ulcer disease: Systematic review in literature. *International Journal Of Community Medicine And Public Health, 5*(10), 4617–4624. doi:10.18203/2394-6040.ijcmph20183869

Bjarnason, I., Scarpignato, C., Holmgren, E., Olszewski, M., Rainsford, K. D., & Lanas, A. (2018). Mechanisms of Damage to the Gastrointestinal Tract From Nonsteroidal Anti-Inflammatory Drugs. *Gastroenterology, 154*(3), 500–514. doi:10.1053/j.gastro.2017.10.049 PMID:29221664

Chaudhary, A., & Singh, A. (2014). Peptic Ulcer: A Review on Epidemiology, Molecular Mechanism of Pathogenesis and Management. *International Journal of Chemistry and Pharmaceutical Sciences, 2*, 788–796. http://www.pharmaresearchlibrary.com/wp-content/uploads/2014/04/IJCPS2012.pdf

Clarke, R. C. (2020). Stress-Induced Gastritis. *Medscape.* Retrieved from https://emedicine.medscape.com/article/176319-overview

Escott-Stump, S. (2012). *Nutrition and diagnosis-related care* (7th ed.). Lippinocott Williams & Wilkins, Wolters Kluwer.

Fashner, J., & Gitu, A. C. (2015). Diagnosis and Treatment of Peptic Ulcer Disease and H. pylori Infection. *American Family Physician*, *91*(4), 236–242. https://www.aafp.org/afp/2015/0215/p236.html PMID:25955624

Feher, J. (2017). 8.2 - The Stomach. In J. Feher (Ed.), *Quantitative Human Physiology* (2nd ed., pp. 785–795). Academic Press. doi:10.1016/B978-0-12-800883-6.00078-1

Gupta, B. (n.d.). Non-steroidal Anti-inflammatory Drugs. *World Federation of Societies of Anaesthesiologists* Retrieved from https://www.wfsahq.org/components/com_virtual_library/media/8ea6b673c075492e525e15016eb2a6b1-Non-steroidal-Anti-inflammatory-Drugs--Update-24-2-2008-.pdf

Hall, J. E. (2011). *Guyton and Hall textbook of medical physiology* (12th ed.). Elsevier.

Jameson, J. L., Fauci, A. S., Kasper, D. L., Hauser, S. L., Longo, D. L., & Loscalzo, J. (2018). *Harrison's Principles of Internal Medicine* (20th ed., Vol. 2). McGraw-Hill Education.

Kulshreshtha, M., Srivastava, G., & Singh, M. (2017). Pathophysiological status and nutritional therapy of peptic ulcer: An update. *Environmental Disease*, *2*(3), 76–86. doi:10.4103/ed.ed_11_17

Li, L. F., Chan, R. L., Lu, L., Shen, J., Zhang, L., Wu, W. K., Wang, L., Hu, T., Li, M. X., & Cho, C. H. (2014). Cigarette smoking and gastrointestinal diseases: The causal relationship and underlying molecular mechanisms. *International Journal of Molecular Medicine*, *34*(2), 372–380. doi:10.3892/ijmm.2014.1786 PMID:24859303

Mahan, L. K., & Raymond, J. L. (2017). *Krause's Food & the Nutrition Care Process* (14th ed.). Elsevier.

Nahikian-Nelms, M., Sucher, K., & Lacey, K. (2016). *Nutrition therapy and pathophysiology* (3rd ed.). Cengage Learning.

Plummer, M. P., Blaser, A. R., & Deane, A. M. (2014). Stress ulceration: Prevalence, pathology and association with adverse outcomes. *Critical Care (London, England)*, *18*(2), 213–213. doi:10.1186/cc13780 PMID:25029573

Pronsky, Z. M., Elbe, D., & Ayoob, K. (2015). *Food-Medication Interactions* (18th ed.). Food-Medication Interactions.

Ramakrishnan, K., & Salinas, R. C. (2007). Peptic Ulcer Disease. *American Family Physician*, *76*(7), 1005–1012. https://www.aafp.org/afp/2007/1001/p1005.html PMID:17956071

Rassow, J. (2011). Helicobacter pylori vacuolating toxin A and apoptosis. *Cell Communication and Signaling*, *9*(1), 26. doi:10.1186/1478-811X-9-26 PMID:22044628

Sverdén, E., Agréus, L., Dunn, J. M., & Lagergren, J. (2019). Peptic ulcer disease. *BMJ (Clinical Research Ed.)*, *367*, l5495. doi:10.1136/bmj.l5495 PMID:31578179

Sylvester, J. (2019). Nonsteroidal Anti-inflammatory Drugs. *World Federation of Societies of Anaesthesiologists* Retrieved from https://www.wfsahq.org/components/com_virtual_library/media/a1363aaa0a41f691d0c5335673055a10-atow-405-00.pdf

Tarasconi, A., Coccolini, F., Biffl, W. L., Tomasoni, M., Ansaloni, L., Picetti, E., Molfino, S., Shelat, V., Cimbanassi, S., Weber, D. G., Abu-Zidan, F. M., Campanile, F. C., Di Saverio, S., Baiocchi, G. L., Casella, C., Kelly, M. D., Kirkpatrick, A. W., Leppaniemi, A., Moore, E. E., ... Catena, F. (2020). Perforated and bleeding peptic ulcer: WSES guidelines. *World Journal of Emergency Surgery; WJES*, *15*(1), 3–3. doi:10.118613017-019-0283-9 PMID:31921329

Vomero, N. D., & Colpo, E. (2014). Nutritional care in peptic ulcer. *Arquivos brasileiros de cirurgia digestiva: ABCD =. Arquivos Brasileiros de Cirurgia Digestiva*, *27*(4), 298–302. doi:10.1590/S0102-67202014000400017 PMID:25626944

Width, M., & Reinhard, T. (2018). *The Essential Pocket Guide for Clinical Nutrition* (2nd ed.). Wolters Kluwer Health.

KEY TERMS AND DEFINITIONS

Acetylcholine: A neurotransmitter that is released from the vagus nerve and other cholinergic nerves and acts in the GI by stimulating its activity.

Antacids: A group of medications used to provide relief by neutralizing the acidic environment in the stomach.

Chyme: The mixture of food and gastric secretion that passes down from the stomach.

Dyspepsia: Indigestion, which refers to a group of nonspecific symptoms, including upper abdominal pain or discomfort, fullness, gas, bloating, belching, or nausea.

Epigastric Pain: The discomfort or pain that is felt in the upper area of the abdomen, which could be because of acid reflux, gastritis, a peptic ulcer, or others.

Esophagogastroduodenoscopy: A procedure involving the passage of a long flexible tube with a light that examines the esophagus, stomach, and upper small intestine.

Gastritis: A term that describes inflammation of the stomach.

H2 Antagonist Receptors: A group of ulcer healing drugs used for inhibiting stomach acid by blocking the release of histamines, which are involved in the production of HCL (cimetidine, ranitidine, famotidine, and nizatidine).

Helicobacter Pylori: Gram-negative bacteria that are resistant to stomach acid and could result in various conditions, including gastritis, PUD, and gastric carcinoma.

Hematemesis: The condition of vomiting blood that is associated with upper gastrointestinal bleeding.

Intrinsic Factor: A glycoprotein that is secreted by the parietal cells to bind to vitamin B12 to facilitate its absorption in the terminal ileum.

Migraines: A condition characterized by a throbbing or painful sensation often at one side of the head that might be accompanied by nausea, vomiting, and sensitivity to light and sound.

Melena: The condition of passing black tarry stools, which are associated with upper gastrointestinal bleeding.

Nonsteroidal Anti-Inflammatory Drugs: A category of medications indicated for the reduction of inflammation, fever, pain, and prevention of blood clots (Aspirin, ibuprofen, naproxen, diclofenac, celecoxib, and others).

Parietal Cell: A gastric gland cell at the basement membrane that is responsible for the secretion of HCL and intrinsic factor.

Prostaglandins: A group of fatty acids derived from esterified arachidonic acids that are critical for gastric defense due to regulating mucus and HCO_3 release, inhibiting parietal cell secretion of HCL, and maintaining mucosal blood flow.

Proton-Pump Inhibitors: A group of ulcer-healing drugs used for inhibiting stomach acids through blocking the H+/K+ ATPase enzyme that is involved in the HCL production and which are the most potent acid inhibitory agents (omeprazole, esomeprazole, lansoprazole, rabeprazole, and pantoprazole).

Serologic Enzyme-Linked Immunosorbent Assay: A test that measures antibodies in the blood that are specific to *H.pylori*, but which does not differentiate between an active or past infection.

ENDNOTES

1 NI: refers to the Intake domain, defined as "actual problems related to intake of energy, nutrients, fluids, bioactive substances through oral diet or nutrition support." (2): refers to Oral or Nutrition Support Intake, defined as "actual or estimated food and beverage intake from oral diet or nutrition support compared with patient goal" (American Dietetic Association, 2011).

2 NC: refers to the Clinical domain, defined as "nutritional findings/problems identified that relate to medical or physical conditions." (3): refers to Weight, defined as "chronic weight or changed weight status when compared with usual or desired body weight" (American Dietetic Association, 2011).

3 NB: refers to the Behavioral/Environmental domain, defined as "nutritional findings/problems identified that relate to knowledge, attitude/beliefs, physical environment, access to food, or food safety." (1): refers to Knowledge and Beliefs, defined as "actual knowledge and beliefs as related, observed, or documented" (American Dietetic Association, 2011).

APPENDIX: ABBREVIATIONS

Ab: Albumin
BMI: Body mass index
Bpm: Beats per minute, breath per minute
BUN: Blood urea nitrogen
Ca: Calcium
Cl: Chloride
CagA: cytotoxin-associated gene A
COX: Cyclooxygenase
EGD: Esophagogastroduodenoscopy
GI: Gastrointestinal
Gm: Gram
H_2: Histamine
H+/K+ ATPase: Hydrogen-potassium pump
H_2RA: Histamine 2 receptor antagonist
HEENT: Head, eyes, ears, nose, throat
HCL: Hydrochloric acid
HCO_3-: Bicarbonate
Hct: Hematocrit
Hgb: Hemoglobin
H.pylori: Helicobacter pylori
Ht: Height
IBW: Ideal body weight
K: Potassium
Kg: Kilogram
MALT: Mucosa-associated lymphoid tissue
Na: Sodium
NH_3: Ammonia
NO: Nitric oxide
NSAIDs: Nonsteroidal anti-inflammatory drugs
PGs: Prostaglandins
PPIs: Proton-pump inhibitors
PUD: Peptic ulcer disease
RBCs: Red blood cells
ROS: Reactive oxygen species
RUQ: Right upper quadrant
UBW: Usual body weight
VacA: Vacuolating toxin
Wt: Weight

Section 2

Cases on Medical Nutrition Therapy for Lower Gastrointestinal Tract Disorders

Chapter 4
Diarrhea/Constipation

Shoug Alashmali
https://orcid.org/0000-0001-5675-2832
King Abdulaziz University, Saudi Arabia

EXECUTIVE SUMMARY

This chapter will discuss a case of diarrhea/constipation. Diarrhea and constipation are functional bowel disorders (FBDs) of the mid or lower gastrointestinal (GI) tract. These FBDs result from intestinal motility dysfunction and/or changes in intestinal fluid absorption, which in turn leads to bloating, discomfort, and occasionally, abdominal pain. Certain dietary choices aggravate these conditions, leading to serious complications. Management of diarrhea/constipation usually requires the use of medications and/or lifestyle modifications. The presently discussed case involved factors that exacerbated the conditions of diarrhea/constipation. This case serves as an example of the role of medical nutrition therapy in managing FBDs (particularly diarrhea and constipation). Moreover, this case will allow the dietetic professional to assess the causes of diarrhea/constipation in order to plan for the nutrition intervention and educate the patient about the dietary manipulations required to reduce their symptoms.

INTRODUCTION

Diarrhea and constipation are considered functional bowel disorders (FBDs) of the mid or lower gastrointestinal (GI) tract (Ibrahim & Stribling, 2019). FBDs are defined as any problem to the stomach or bowel, thus, they can be identified by symptoms alone. Therefore, symptom-based classification is necessary for clinical diagnosis, evidence-based management, and research of these disorders. FBDs include irritable bowel syndrome (IBS), functional bloating, functional constipation, functional

DOI: 10.4018/978-1-7998-3802-9.ch004

diarrhea, and unspecified FBD. To distinguish these symptomatic conditions from transient gut symptoms, FBDs must have occurred for the first time 6 months prior and must have been present for 3 days per month over the last 3 months, indicating current activity (Longstreth et al., 2006). Previous diagnostic criteria for FBDs suggested an absence of any structural or biochemical disorders. However, previous research has confirmed that functional gut disorders can manifest as structural and biochemical disorders. Furthermore, IBS, functional bloating, functional constipation, and functional diarrhea can have multiple etiologies. The prevalence of FBDs among the general population ranges from 15% to 20% worldwide (Barnes et al., 2019). In the Middle East, it is estimated that the prevalence of FBDs has reached 18% of the population (Chang et al., 2010). Half of the adults who suffer from chronic abdominal pain and stool irregularity have FBDs (Häuser et al., 2012). The prevalence of FBDs within gender groups varies depending on the symptoms. For example, the prevalence of diarrhea tends to be greater in males than in females (Abuzerr et al., 2019), while constipation has a higher prevalence in females than in males (female-to-male ratio of 2.2; Lee et al., 2014).

Although FBDs are considered symptomatic disorders rather than serious diseases, the overall healthcare costs of these disorders are estimated to be in the range of several billion US dollars in the United States alone due to lost wages and disability (Peery et al., 2015). FBDs can interfere with everyday activities; for example, patients may repeatedly be absent from work or may find themselves giving up pleasurable activities, such as food-related gatherings, visits to restaurants, and vacations (Häuser et al., 2012). Thus, FBDs have a great impact on individuals by reducing their quality of life through social effects and the necessity of medical treatments (Neri & Iovino, 2016). The cost to society of an FBD is considerably raised by the necessity of diagnostic tests and treatments, especially when there is no specific indication. Frequent absences from work, even with medical excuses, could also place a load on medical care costs and on society.

Diarrhea/Constipation

Diarrhea is characterized by the passing of frequent and/or loose or watery stools. Other researchers have described diarrhea as an abnormality in stool production, reaching >200 g/day in adults or >20 g/kg in children (Said, 2009). Few studies have diagnosed functional diarrhea as specifically distinct from IBS, so it is impossible to provide a precise frequency. The World Health Organization (WHO) identifies diarrhea as the second leading cause of death worldwide. Each year, approximately 800,000 children under the age of five will die from the consequences of diarrhea. Therefore, the prevention and treatment of diarrhea is a primary focus of public health interventions throughout the world (WHO, 2017). Diarrhea has been reported to be as prevalent as 22.7% among all age groups in the Middle East versus 5–10% in developed countries (Abuzerr et al., 2019).

Unlike diarrhea, constipation is characterized by straining during bowel movements, hard stools, and a decrease in the frequency of bowel movements (fewer than three per week; Said, 2009; Choung et al., 2006). It is also accompanied by abdominal discomfort, headaches, backaches, and the passing of gas (Nelms, 2016). The cycle of waste elimination usually depends on the individual's health, the type of food eaten, when it was eaten, and when the individual takes time to defecate (Whitney & Rolfes, 2016). Constipation is also considered one of the most common GI complaints. Approximately 63 million individuals suffer from constipation. Symptoms of constipation result in more than 4 million physician visits and 5 million prescriptions each year (U.S. Department of Health and Human Services, 2013).

Pathophysiology

The mechanism of diarrhea/constipation is mainly related to intestinal motility dysfunction and changes in fluid absorption. Under normal conditions, contractions of the smooth muscle of the GI tract balance fluid absorption via the intestine and regulate the movement of food through the small intestine and colon.

Diarrhea

Diarrhea can be classified as either acute, persistent, or chronic. Acute diarrhea lasts less than two weeks, persistent diarrhea lasts two to four weeks, and chronic diarrhea lasts more than four weeks (Said, 2009). There are two unbalanced mechanisms, osmotic and secretory, that result in diarrhea. In osmotic diarrhea, fluid passively moves into the bowel lumen down the osmotic gradient as a result of an increase in intestinal osmolality to >300 mOsm/L, which leads the intestinal contents to move quickly through the intestines (Nelms, 2016). This type of diarrhea is mostly caused by maldigestion of nutrients, excessive intake of sorbitol or fructose, enteral feeding, and some laxatives. Once the causative factor is removed, the diarrhea will cease. In secretory diarrhea, the bowel mucosa secretes excessive amounts of fluid and electrolytes into the intestine, thus adding more fluid to the food residue (Whyte & Jenkins, 2012). The underlying cause of this type of diarrhea is disease rather than hyperosmolality. The pathophysiology of secretory diarrhea could be related to activation of a physiological pathway by a toxin or inherent abnormalities in the enterocytes (Whyte & Jenkins, 2012). Diarrhea can lead to considerable fluid and salt losses. However, the composition of the fluids produced by diarrhea is different from that of vomiting. Stomach fluids lost through vomiting are highly acidic, whereas the intestinal fluids lost through diarrhea are almost neutral. Therefore, medical attention and proper replacement of fluid loss are important in managing diarrhea (Surawicz, 2010).

Constipation

Constipation involves a net reabsorption of electrolytes and fluids back into the body via the colon (Sleisenger et al., 2006). Constipation also involves colonic motility dysfunction (Andrews & Storr, 2011), which causes drier and larger stool to pass through the anal canal.

Etiology and Risk Factors

The causes of diarrhea and constipation are varied and potentially multifactorial. The common approach to classification groups diarrhea and constipation under disease-related and/or lifestyle-related (i.e., medication and diet) causes (Table 1).

Diarrhea

Diarrhea is a symptom of many medical conditions and treatments. Diarrhea could occur as a result of infection (e.g., foodborne illness caused by bacteria, protozoa, or viruses) or as a side effect of antibiotics or other medications, such as laxatives and antacids containing magnesium hydroxide (Whyte & Jenkins, 2012). These medications generally cause diarrhea either by increasing GI motility or by altering the normal flora of the colon, such as anti-diarrheal agents (Johnston et al., 2011). Food ingredients, such as alternative types of sugar sorbitol and fat olestra, may also cause diarrhea in some people. If a food ingredient is the cause of diarrhea, it must be omitted from the diet, at least temporarily. If medication is responsible for diarrhea, a different medicine or different form (e.g., injectable versus oral) of the medicine may alleviate the problem (Whitney & Rolfes, 2016). Enteral feedings are often implicated as a cause of diarrhea. Although changing formula types or reducing the rate of feeding is often proposed as a solution to diarrhea caused by enteral feeding, evidence for the effectiveness of this strategy is limited (Delegge & Berry, 2009). Some studies have shown that enteral feeding can be continued in such cases unless there is abdominal pain, fever, distention, or fluid output greater than the fluid input (Delegge & Berry, 2009). Rapid transit and malabsorption could be indicated if the stool output appears visually similar to the taken formula.

Diarrhea may also occur as a result of disorders of the GI tract, such as IBS or colitis. The most common cause of these disorders is IBS, which is estimated to have a worldwide prevalence of approximately 11% (Canavan et al., 2014). IBS is also associated with the presence of recurrent abdominal pain related to alterations in bowel habits; further information regarding IBS is covered as a full chapter in this book (Lacy & Patel, 2017).

Constipation

Lifestyle risk factors, including compromised mobility and inadequate toileting facilities, can result in constipation (Said, 2009; Leung, 2007). Failure to respond to the defecation signal is a common complaint of constipation patients, and this signal may not return for several hours during defecation process (Whitney & Rolfes, 2016). As a result, fluids continue to be withdrawn from the fecal matter, resulting in hard and dry stool. The use of certain medications, such as calcium channel blockers, diuretics, antidepressants, and anticonvulsants, has also been found to trigger constipation (Schiller et al., 2017). Over-the-counter medications, such as iron, calcium, and even non-steroidal anti-inflammatory (NSAIDS) drugs, can also result in constipation.

Constipation can also be a side effect of a medical problem, such as slowed colonic transit, bowel obstruction, or other sources of obstruction (e.g., fecal impaction, adhesions, or even tumors). Other medical conditions that can cause constipation include pelvic floor dysfunction (i.e., storage of fecal contents in the rectum for long periods of time), IBS, scleroderma, amyloidosis, and neurological disorders (e.g., Parkinson's disease and multiple sclerosis; Nelms, 2016).

Another lifestyle risk factor for FBDs is diet. Dietary factors play a major role in the pathogenesis of diarrhea/constipation and are proposed to interact with our intestinal and colonic epithelia through immune-mediated reactions, stimulation of the enteric nervous system through chemical stimuli, luminal distention through mechanical forces, and other unknown mechanisms (Gibson & Shepherd, 2012). Some studies have shown that certain dietary factors, such as excessive sugar, alcohol and/or caffeine intake, have been linked to diarrhea (Whyte & Jenkins, 2012), while inadequate fiber and/or water intake have been linked to constipation (Madoff, 2012).

Clinical Manifestations

Diarrhea

The etiology of diarrhea can result in other stool characteristics. For example, the composition, volume, and foul smell of a diarrhea patient's stool are typically consistent with the etiology of their diarrhea. The color of the stool can also be an indication of the diarrhea's etiology. Hematochezia refers to bright-red blood on the surface of the stool, which indicates stool contamination with blood from the rectum or anus. Occult blood results from bleeding in the lower GI tract, while melena is a type of dark stool contaminated with blood from the upper GI tract. Mucus in the stool may also be indicative of secretory diarrhea and may be infectious in origin. High electrolyte levels are also consistent with secretory diarrhea (Said, 2009). The presence of leukocytes in the stool indicates a form of bowel inflammation, such as inflammatory bowel disease, which is discussed in a full chapter of this book. Other clinical manifestations of diarrhea include abdominal pain and cramping. Diarrhea generally originates from the distal colon if defecation relieves cramping. However, diarrhea generally originates from the small bowel if abdominal pain and cramping continue after defecation. Other clinical and biochemical symptoms, such as weight loss, dehydration, and electrolyte and acid-base imbalances, are dependent on the volume of stool lost and represent the most serious consequences of diarrhea.

Constipation

Symptoms of constipation include decreased frequency of bowel movements. Bowel movements associated with constipation are often hard and pellet-like. Abdominal pain, bloating, and gas are common accompanying symptoms. According to the Bristol Stool Form Scale (BSFS; Whitney & Rolfes, 2016), many types of stool can occur in response to the etiology of constipation. Types 1 and 2 on the BSFS represent separate, hard, and nut-like lumps of stool (difficult to pass), while Types 3, 4, and 5 resemble sausages, sausages or snakes, or soft blobs, respectively (easy to pass). However, Types 6 and 7 on the BSFS are used to describe diarrhea, as the stool represented by these types is fluffy and watery (Madoff, 2012).

Diagnosis

Diarrhea

The most important step in determining the proper form of treatment for diarrhea is diagnosing the underlying etiology of the diarrhea. Many factors should be considered in this process, including hydration status, the presence of blood in the stool, the age of the patient, and whether the patient has an immunological disease. Other factors that should be assessed include when the symptoms started, how long they have persisted, past medical procedures or surgeries, current medications, and the intake of food-symptoms relationship (Whitney & Rolfes, 2016). Diagnosis of diarrhea usually begins with stool cultures to examine for microorganisms (viral and/or bacterial), parasites, leukocytes, lactoferrin, and the presence of blood. More invasive procedures, such as flexible sigmoidoscopy, upper endoscopy, and colonoscopy, may also assist in diagnosis. Determination of the osmolality and electrolyte content of the stool can also assist in the diagnosis process by differentiating between osmotic and secretory diarrhea; however, this type of diagnosis is less commonly used in clinical practice (Hasler & Owyang, 2012). Other clinical tests to consider include blood tests for complete blood count, electrolyte, albumin, and thyroid stimulating hormone (TSH) levels. Some bacteria, such as *C. difficile* and toxic substances, require specific diagnostic tests, including stool sample cultures, tests of cytotoxicity, and toxin enzyme immunoassays (McDonald et al., 2018). Other symptoms, such as rectal bleeding, unexplained weight loss, nausea, and vomiting, should be assessed as well.

Constipation

As with diarrhea, the process of diagnosing constipation includes a complete assessment of patient history and laboratory tests of complete blood count, TSH, and other serum chemistries. Additional procedures may include colonoscopy or flexible sigmoidoscopy. Physical identification of constipation can be achieved using the Rome III criteria. The Rome III criteria were established to define constipation as a symptomatic condition under specific factors. For a case to meet these criteria, at least two of the following symptoms must have occurred for at least 12 non-consecutive weeks within the last year (Longstreth et al., 2006; Ternent et al., 2007): straining, lumpy or hard stools, sensation of incomplete evacuation, sensation of anorectal obstruction/blockage, and/or manual maneuvers to facilitate (e.g., digital evacuation and support of the pelvic floor) in at least 25% of defecations; and/or fewer than three defecations per week. Moreover, stool that cannot be made loose without the use of laxatives is not classified as a component of IBS (Drossman, 2006).

Management

Medical

The predominant therapies for FBDs include medical and nutritional management. These treatments vary depending on the cause and severity of the FBD. The main target of medical management for diarrhea/constipation is to decrease symptoms and prevent further progression.

Diarrhea

Antidiarrheal agents, such as diphenoxylate (Lomotil), are among the most common medications used to stop diarrhea. Loperamide (Imodium) is also often effective for the treatment of diarrhea.

Constipation

The most effective treatments for constipation include osmotic laxatives, which work by drawing water into the colon, and stimulant laxatives, such as bisacodyl (e.g., Dulcolax) and senna (e.g., Senecott), which work by signaling for the muscles and nerves of the intestine to contract. Moreover, newer prescription medications, such as lubiprostone (Amitiza), linaclotide (Linzess), and plecanatide (Trulance), have been prescribed to patients with idiopathic constipation (Madoff, 2012). For those who fail to respond to constipation medications, surgical management may be an option to manage this condition. One currently popular practice is colonic irrigation, which is the internal washing of the large intestine with a powerful enema machine. This kind of cleansing may be unnecessary and can be hazardous, especially for those with histories of digestive diseases. Side effects of this practice may present as minor (e.g., abdominal pain, bloating, nausea, and vomiting) or severe (e.g., kidney failure, pancreatitis, and infections), sometimes leading to death (Mishori et al., 2011). Other problems may arise from equipment contamination, intestinal perforation, or electrolyte imbalances.

Medical Nutrition Therapy

Dietary therapies are often implemented in place of medication due to the high association between symptom onset and the ingestion of certain foods (Tuck & Vanner, 2018). Thus, patients should be advised to avoid food items that might aggravate diarrhea/constipation conditions.

Nutrition therapy for diarrhea has many goals. The first goal is to restore normal fluid, electrolyte, and acid-base balance. The second is to decrease GI motility. Other goals of nutrition therapy are to thicken the consistency of the stool by rebalancing the GI tract with normal flora and to gradually introduce foods to return to a normal diet without worsening symptoms (Academy of Nutrition and Dietetics, 2014; Duro & Duggan, 2007).

Diarrhea

Nutrition therapy for diarrhea usually starts with making the patient NPO (nothing by mouth) or prescribing clear liquids. Recent evidence has emphasized the importance of stimulating the GI tract by feeding the patient rather than providing them with clear liquids. Feeding can speed the recovery process, while clear liquids, which are high in simple carbohydrates, can increase the osmolality of the GI tract and worsen diarrhea due to hyperosmolality. In adults and older children, the introduction of solid foods should begin with a low-residue diet, which involves adding refined starches, such as rice, and then slowly adding other foods to the diet (Nelms, 2016).

Rehydration is another important step in the nutritional management of diarrhea. Mild diarrhea can be managed with simple rest and avoidance of strenuous activity as well as increased liquid intake (e.g., through clear juices and soups) to replace fluid losses (Whitney & Rolfes, 2016), whereas chronic diarrhea may require more intensive care involving oral rehydration solutions. Examples of oral rehydration solutions are Pedialyte and Rehydralyte. Additionally, the WHO has a standard oral rehydration solution recipe, which includes the following ingredients: 1/3 to 2/3 tsp table salt, 3/4 tsp sodium bicarbonate, 1/3 tsp potassium chloride (a salt substitute), 1 1/3 Tbsp sugar or rice powder, and 1 L bottled or sterile water (Kelly & Nadeau, 2004; Khan et al., 2005).

Nutrition therapy should also focus on avoiding beverages and foods with high sugar contents, such as lactose, sucrose, and fructose; sugar alcohols (e.g., sorbitol, xylitol, and mannitol); caffeine; and alcoholic beverages. Gas-producing foods should be avoided as well. Sources of soluble fiber and resistant starch, such as banana flakes, apple powder, and other pectin sources, are the most typically used routes to thicken stool consistency.

The BRAT (bananas, rice, applesauce, and toast) eating pattern has been used to guide food choices in cases of acute diarrhea but does not provide a sufficient variety of nutrients for long periods of use (Duro & Duggan, 2007). Another step in the treatment of diarrhea is the use of probiotics and prebiotics (Johnston et al., 2011). These foods and supplements support the growth of healthy flora and/or help to rebalance the GI tract with healthy bacteria. Probiotics and prebiotics have many roles in diarrhea management. First, they increase short-chain fatty acid (SCFA) production, thus promoting water and electrolyte absorption in the colon and reducing the incidence of diarrhea (O'Keefe, 2008). Another role of probiotics and prebiotics is that of improving the mucosal defense system of the GI tract and reducing the growth of harmful bacteria. Therefore, probiotics and prebiotics can be useful parts of treatment for many types of diarrhea, including radiation-induced diarrhea, diarrhea secondary to rotavirus, and traveler's diarrhea (Nelms, 2016). However, dosages for probiotics and prebiotics have not yet been established due to a lack of information needed to make dosage recommendations as well as the difficulty of maintaining the viability of the probiotics (Quigley, 2012; Douglas & Sanders, 2008). Medical attention should be sought if diarrhea is bloody, worsens, or persists because severe diarrhea can be life threatening, especially in infants, young children, elderly people, and immunocompromised people.

Constipation

As with diarrhea, lifestyle modifications (e.g., increased fiber intake, fluid intake, probiotics and prebiotics, and exercise) are recommended for the treatment of constipation before medications are considered. Adequate fiber and fluid intake serve as the foundation of nutrition therapy for constipation treatment. One dietary measure recommended for adults by clinicians is to gradually increase dietary fiber intake to 25–35 g per day over the course of one or two weeks (one to two high-fiber foods each day; Slavin, 2008). Due to variations in individual tolerance, especially among older adults, some patients may not be able to achieve high levels of fiber intake via food alone; these patients may require fiber supplementation. Fiber helps to increase stool weight, which allows for more consistent bowel movements and a colonic transit time of two to four days (Slavin, 2008). Fibers found in fruits, vegetables, whole grains, and resistant starch can help to prevent constipation by increasing fecal mass. In the GI tract, fiber attracts water, creating soft, bulky stools that stimulate bowel contractions to push the contents along. These contractions strengthen the intestinal muscles. Further, the water content of stools can ease elimination, reduce pressure in the rectal veins, and help to prevent hemorrhoids. Fiber also plays a role in maintaining a healthy colon and reducing the risk of developing other diseases, such as colon cancer and diverticulosis. The increased bulk physically stimulates the upper GI tract, promoting peristalsis throughout GI tract. Drinking plenty of water, in conjunction with eating high-fiber foods, helps to prevent constipation. Adults should ingest a minimum of 2 L of water per day (approximately 8–10 glasses/day).

Probiotics and prebiotics have also been recommended for the treatment of constipation. For example, the intake of fructans or fructooligosaccharides (FOS) has been shown to soften feces and assist in treating constipation. Fructans are defined as chains of fructose molecules with glucose on their terminal ends. Common examples of fructans include inulin and levan, which are available in wheat-containing grain products, such as breads, cereals, and pastas. FOS are linear chains made up of only fructose units. FOS are naturally found in plants such as onion, chicory, garlic, asparagus, banana, and artichoke, among many others (Sabater-Molina et al., 2009).

Similarly, physical activity improves the muscle tone and motility of the digestive tract. As little as 30 minutes of physical activity per day can help prevent or alleviate constipation. Eating prunes (or dried plums, as some have renamed them) can also be helpful. Prunes are high in fiber and also contain a laxative substance.

A few dietary approaches have been utilized to address FBDs (including diarrhea/constipation), such as the low food chemical diet/elimination diet; the low amine/histamine diet; the low capsaicin diet; the gluten-free diet; and recently, the low fermentable oligo-, di-, mono-saccharides and polyols (FODMAP) diet (Tuck &

Vanner, 2018; Halmos, 2017). However, limited data are available on the efficacies of these diets, and previous dietary approaches have raised concerns regarding their complexity, restrictiveness, nutritional adequacy, and effectiveness. A recent study suggested a new dietary approach for the management of diarrhea/constipation conditions known as the 5Ad dietary protocol (Ibrahim & Stribling, 2019). This protocol depends on its simplicity of administration as a long-term regime for all forms and severities of FBDs. The 5Ad dietary protocol focuses on excluding foods with large amounts of components, such as oligosaccharides, resistant proteins, food additives, and highly processed/refined foods. This dietary protocol emphasizes foods from the five food groups (at least one item per group/day) as foods to be consumed, rather than foods to avoid, to ensure a balanced and complementary diet. Fruits and vegetables (~1 kg/day) are important components of this protocol, as they ensure adequate dietary fiber intake. Patients with FBDs are advised to include low-lactose dairy products in their diets to ensure adequate calcium intake. Further, the 5Ad dietary protocol encourages the consumption of whole foods to reduce the need to purchase unhealthy, costly, and commercial gluten-free FODMAP alternatives (Ibrahim & Stribling, 2019). This protocol has been shown to improve stool consistency and frequency in both those with diarrhea and those with constipation.

If lifestyle and diet changes do not succeed in correcting constipation, then clinicians might recommend the use of stool softeners (as mentioned above). These products are best used for brief periods of time, as frequent laxative use can lead to dependency and can upset the body's fluid, salt, and mineral balances. Other laxatives could interfere with the absorption of fat-soluble vitamins. Treatment of this complication may require hospitalization, antibiotics, and/or surgery.

SETTING THE STAGE

The following case was obtained from an outpatient clinic in a governmental hospital in Jeddah, Saudi Arabia. The patient was evaluated by a gastroenterologist who prescribed certain medications to manage the symptoms either diarrhea or constipation. Then, the dietitian has provided nutritional consultation related to lifestyle and dietary interventions to manage the conditions of diarrhea and/or constipation. There was no conflict of interest as the patient did not receive any financial support for reporting this case in this chapter.

CASE DESCRIPTION

Patient Details

- Age: 49 years old
- Gender: Female

Case History

Case description: Patient complained of episodes of diarrhea and chronic constipation that began 20 years ago, after normal child delivery via the vaginal route. She also suffered from abdominal pain in the central and left upper quadrant of the abdomen after eating specific foods. She mentioned other critical symptoms accompanying this abdominal pain, including bloating, nausea, and feelings of discomfort. The physician referred the patient to the dietitian in order to help her manage both her diarrhea and her constipation.

- Medical history: Acute sinusitis, dryness of eye, posterior tibial tendinitis, meniscal injury
- Surgical history: None
- Smoking: No
- Family history: Mother and father had type II diabetes mellitus

Main Medical Diagnosis

Diarrhea/Constipation

Demographics

- Marital status: Married with one son
- Education: Bachelor's degree in social sciences
- Occupation: Housewife
- Ethnicity and religion**:** Arab, Muslim

Anthropometry

- Current weight: 77.3 kg Height: 156 cm

Table 1. Biochemical Data

Parameter	Reference	Patient's Results
Sodium	136–145	142
Potassium	3.5–5.5	4.1
Chloride	95–105	104
BUN (mg/dL)	8–18	8.7
Creatinine serum (mg/dL)	0.6–1.2	0.52
Glucose (mg/dL)	70–110	82.8
Magnesium (mg/dL)	1.8-3	1.9
Calcium (mg/dL)	9-11	9.7
Bilirubin, total (mg/dL)	£1.5	0.5
Protein, total (g/dL)	6–8	7.8
Albumin (g/dL)	3.5–5	4.4
Prealbumin (mg/dL)	16–35	33
Ammonia (NH3, μmol/L)	9–33	25
Alkaline phosphatase (U/L)	30–120	51
ALT (U/L)	4–36	18
AST (U/L)	0–35	19
CPK (U/L)	30–135 (Female) 55–170 (Male)	100
Lactate dehydrogenase (U/L)	208–378	240
Cholesterol (mg/dL)	120–199	150.6
LDL (mg/dL)	<130	92.7
HDL-C (mg/dL)	>55 (Female) >45 (Male)	66.4
Triglycerides (mg/dL)	35–135 (Female) 40–160 (Male)	120
WBC (×103/mm3)	4.8–11.8	10.4
RBC (×106/mm3)	4.2–5.4 (Female) 4.5–6.2 (Male)	4.5
Hemoglobin (g/dL)	12–15 (Female) 14–17 (Male)	14
Hematocrit (%)	37–47 (Female) 40–54 (Male)	38
Mean cell volume (μm3)	80–96	85.6
Mean cell Hgb (pg)	26–32	30
Mean cell Hgb content (g/dL)	31.5–36	35
RBC distribution (%)	11.6–16.5	12.5

continues on following page

Table 1. Continued

Parameter	Reference	Patient's Results
Platelet count (×103/mm3)	140–440	430
Lymphocyte (%)	15–45	40
Monocyte (%)	3–10	7
Vitamin D (ng/ml)	30–100	78
Vitamin B6 (μg/ml)	5–50	7.7
Vitamin B12 (ng/ml)	200–900	212
TSH (mU/L)	0.4–4	1.15

Nutritional Focused Physical Examination

- General appearance: Mildly obese, 49-year-old female; healthy appearance
- Heart: Regular heartrate and normal heartbeat sound
- HEENT: Nose: Acute sinusitis
- Genitalia: Normal
- Neurologic: Oriented and alert
- Extremities: No edema; normal strength and sensations
- Skin: Warm and smooth
- Chest/lungs: Lungs clear with no chest pain
- Peripheral vascular: Full pulse with no bruits
- Abdomen: Distention and pain

Vital Signs

- Pulse: 84 BPM
- Temperature: 36.5 °C
- Blood pressure: 119/92 mmHg
- Respiratory rate: 20 BPM

Food/Nutrition-Related History

Patient mentioned that her appetite was very good. She mentioned that some foods worsened her diarrhea while others worsened her constipation. Specifically, cabbage, onion, coffee, and added sugar exacerbated her diarrhea, while dairy products and red meat aggravated her constipation. She reported a habit of skipping breakfast, and she drank approximately 1500 mL of water or less per day. Her lunches tended to include mainly rice. She also reported walking for 30 minutes some days of the week (2–3 days/week). Her body weight had fluctuated over the past four months (between 76, 79.3, 75.4, and 77.3 kg).

Table 2. 24-Hour Recall

2:00 pm:	1 bowl of green salad; 1 bowl of rice; a quarter of an entire chicken with tomato sauce
7:00 pm:	1 cup of orange juice (with added sugar); 30 g of canned tuna; half (60 g) of white bread
9:00 pm:	½ cup of coffee (Arabic coffee); 2 pieces of dates
12:00 am:	Half a slice (60 g) of white bread; 2 tablespoons of white cheese

- Food allergies/intolerances: None
- Food purchases/preparations: Patient's husband purchased food and the patient prepared meals
- Vitamin and mineral supplementation: None

Medications

Loperamide (for diarrhea, as needed) and laxatives or Bisacodyl (for constipation, as needed)

Figure 1. Diarrhea/constipation causes, pathophysiology, and medical nutrition therapy mind map
(Developed by: Khalifa, N 2020)

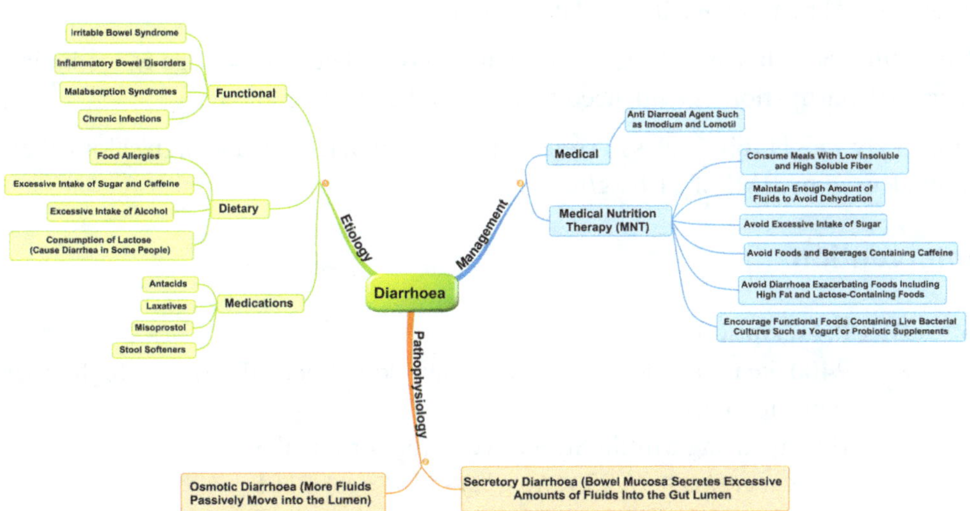

Nutritional Management

Disease Pathophysiology and Management Mind Map (Figure 1)

The Main Aims of Nutrition Therapy

- To decrease diarrhea and its consequences
- To decrease constipation and its consequences
- To prevent abdominal pain and bloating

ADIME Note

Assessment: The patient was a 49-year-old female who had complained of episodes of diarrhea/constipation lasting for years.

- **Anthropometry:**
  - BMI = 31.8 kg/m2 (obese class 1)
  - Ideal body weight = 53.54 kg
- **Biochemical:** Within normal range
- **Clinical:** Abdominal pain, bloating, smooth skin, no rectum bleeding
- **Dietary:** No previous dietary restrictions, high sugar and caffeine intake, low vegetable and fiber intake, high fat intake

Diagnosis

Diarrhea/constipation symptoms related to high sugar, high fat, and low fiber intake as evidenced by food/nutrition-related history

Unhealthy food choices related to a deficit of food-related knowledge exacerbating diarrhea/constipation as evidenced by high intake of sugar and fat

High body weight (obese class 1) related to physical inactivity and high calorie diet, as evidenced by BMI of 31.8 kg/m^2

Intervention

- **Diet Prescription:**
  - 2400 kcal/day, low fat, low sugar, low fiber (diarrhea), high fiber (constipation)
  - Energy, using Mifflin St. Jeor equation for females: $(10 \times weight) + (6.25 \times height) - (5 \times age) - 161$

= 1832 × 1.3 (*activity factor*) = 2381.6 *kcal/day*

- For weight loss: 2400 - 500 = 1900 *kcal/day*
- Carbohydrates: (50%) 950/4 = 238 *gm/day*
- Protein: (20%) 380/4 = 95 *gm/day*
- Fat: (30%) 570/9 = 63 gm/day
- Fluids: (as stated below)

Recommendations

- **Diarrhea**
  - Adequate fluid intake of 2–3 L/**day to a**void dehydration
  - Consume a healthy, well-balanced diet with low insoluble fiber and high soluble fiber intake
  - Avoid excessive sugar intake
  - Avoid foods and beverages containing caffeine
  - Avoid diarrhea-exacerbating foods, including high-fat and lactose-containing foods
  - Encourage functional foods containing live bacterial cultures, such as yogurt and probiotic supplements
- **Constipation**
  - Avoid sedentary lifestyle
  - Increase fluid intake by 3 L/day
  - Consume a healthy, well-balanced diet with high fiber intake (gradual increase up to 25–35 g/day)
  - Avoid constipation-exacerbating foods, such as red meat and dairy products

Monitoring/Evaluation

- Monitor body weight (losses or gains)
- Control stool consistency
- Adherence to prescribed diet

CONCLUSION

Constipation and diarrhea are FBDs of the lower GI tract. A comprehensive evaluation is necessary to determine the underlying cause of either diarrhea and/or constipation. The medical nutrition therapy for either condition is unique for each individual. Therefore, a dietitian should assess the causes of diarrhea/constipation carefully to identify the dietary and/or other factors that might be impacting these symptoms and furthermore providing the right nutritional intervention. Future studies should investigate more nutritional protocols to have an immediate effect to manage these conditions.

REFERENCES

Abuzerr, S., Nasseri, S., Yunesian, M., Hadi, M., Mahvi, A. H., Nabizadeh, R., & Abu Mustafa, A. (2019). Prevalence of diarrheal illness and healthcare-seeking behavior by age-group and sex among the population of Gaza strip: A community-based cross-sectional study. BMC Public Health, *19(1), 704. doi:1*0.*11*8612889-019-7070-0 PMID:31174512

Academy of Nutrition and Dietetics. (2014). Diarrhea. Nutrition care m*anual. Retrieved Apri*l 3, 2020 from www.nutritioncaremanual.org

Andrews, C. N., & Storr, M. (2011). The pathophysiology of chronic constipation. Canadian Jour*nal of Gastroenterology, 25(suppl b), B1*6–B21. doi:10.1155/2011/169319 PMID:22114753

Canavan, C., West, J., & Card, T. (2014). The epidemiology of irritable bowel syndrome. Clinical E*pidemiology, 6, 71–80. P*MID:24523597

Chang, J., Locke, G. III, McNally, M., Halder, S. L., Schleck, C. D., Zinsmeister, A. R., & Talley, N. J. (2010). Impact of functional gastrointestinal disorders on survival in the community. The Ame*rican Journal of Gastroenterology, 105(4*), *8*22–832. doi:10.1038/ajg.2010.40 PMID:20160713

Choung, R. S., Locke, G. R., Schleck, C. D., Zinsmeister, A. R., & Talley, N. J. (2006). Cumulative incidence of chronic constipation: A population-based study 1988–2003. Gast*roenterology, 13*0, *A*–508.

Delegge, M. H., & Berry, A. (2009). Enteral feeding: Should it be continued in the patient with C*lostridium difficile* enterocolitis? P*ractical Gastroenterology, 33(*3), 40–49.

Douglas, L. C., & Sanders, M. E. (2008). Probiotics and prebiotics in dietetics practice. *Journal of the American Dietetic Association*, *108*(3), 510–521. doi:10.1016/j.jada.2007.12.009 PMID:18313433

Drossman, D. A. (2006). The functional gastrointestinal disorders and the Rome III process. *Gastroenterology*, *130*(5), 1377–1390. doi:10.1053/j.gastro.2006.03.008 PMID:16678553

Duro, D., & Duggan, C. (2007). The BRAT diet for acute diarrhea in children: Should it be used? *Practical Gastroenterology*, *31*(6), 60–68.

Gibson, P. R., & Shepherd, S. J. (2012). Food choice as a key management strategy for functional gastrointestinal symptoms. *The American Journal of Gastroenterology*, *107*(5), 657–666. doi:10.1038/ajg.2012.49 PMID:22488077

Guo, Q., Goldenberg, J. Z., Humphrey, C., El Dib, R., & Johnston, B. C. (2019). Probiotics for the prevention of pediatric antibiotic-associated diarrhea. *Cochrane Database of Systematic Reviews*, *4*, CD00482.

Halmos, E. P. (2017). When the low FODMAP diet does not work. *Journal of Gastroenterology and Hepatology*, *32*, 69–72. doi:10.1111/jgh.13701 PMID:28244666

Hasler, W. L., & Owyang, C. (2012). Approach to the patient with gastrointestinal disease. In D. L. Longo, A. S. Fauci, D. L. Kasper, S. L. Hauser, J. Jameson, & J. Loscalzo (Eds.), *Harrison's principles of internal medicine* (18th ed.). McGraw-Hill.

Häuser, W., Layer, P., Henningsen, P., & Kruis, W. (2012). Functional bowel disorders in adults. *Deutsches Ärzteblatt International*, *109*(5), 83–94. PMID:22368721

Ibrahim, F., & Stribling, P. (2019). A 5Ad dietary protocol for functional bowel disorders. *Nutrients*, *11*(8), E1983.

Kelly, D. G., & Nadeau, J. (2004). Oral rehydration solution: A "low-tech" oft neglected therapy. *Practical Gastroenterology*, *28*(10), 51–62.

Khan, A. M., Sarker, S. A., Alam, N. H., Hossain, M. S., Fuchs, G. J., & Salam, M. A. (2005). Low osmolar oral rehydration salts solution in the treatment of acute watery diarrhea in neonates and young infants: A randomized, controlled clinical trial. *Journal of Health, Population and Nutrition*, *23*(1), 52. PMID:15884752

Lacy, B. E., & Patel, N. K. (2017). Rome criteria and a diagnostic approach to irritable bowel syndrome. *Journal of Clinical Medicine*, *6*(11), E99. doi:10.3390/jcm6110099 PMID:29072609

Lee, T. H., Choi, S. C., Park, M. I., Park, K. S., Shin, J. E., Kim, S. E., Jung, K. W., Koo, H. S., Kim, W. J., Cho, Y. K., Kim, Y. S., Lee, J. S., & and. (2014). Constipation misperception is associated with gender, marital status, treatment utilization and constipation symptoms experienced. *Journal of Neurogastroenterology and Motility*, *20*(3), 379–387. doi:10.5056/jnm14011 PMID:24935009

Leung, F. W. (2007). Etiologic factors of chronic constipation: Review of the scientific evidence. *Digestive Diseases and Sciences*, *52*(2), 313–316. doi:10.100710620-006-9298-7 PMID:17219073

Longstreth, G. F., Thompson, W. G., Chey, W. D., Houghton, L. A., Mearin, F., & Spiller, R. C. (2006). Functional bowel disorders. *Gastroenterology*, *130*(5), 1480–1491. doi:10.1053/j.gastro.2005.11.061 PMID:16678561

Madoff, R. D. (2012). Chronic constipation: From evaluation to treatment. *International Foundation for Functional Gastrointestinal Disorders*, *02*, G1075–G1084.

McDonald, L. C., Gerding, D. N., Johnson, S., Bakken, J. S., Carroll, K. C., Coffin, S. E., Dubberke, E. R., Garey, K. W., Gould, C. V., Kelly, C., Loo, V., Shaklee Sammons, J., Sandora, T. J., & Wilcox, M. H. (2018). Clinical Practice Guidelines for Clostridium difficile Infection in Adults and Children: 2017 Update by the Infectious Diseases Society of America (IDSA) and Society for Healthcare Epidemiology of America (SHEA). *Clinical Infectious Diseases*, *66*(7), e1–e48. doi:10.1093/cid/cix1085 PMID:29462280

Mishori, R., Otubu, A., & Jones, A. A. (2011). The dangers of colon cleansing. *The Journal of Family Practice*, *60*(8), 454–457. PMID:21814639

Nelms, M. (2016). *Nutrition therapy and pathophysiology* (3rd ed.). Cengage Learning.

Neri, L., & Iovino, P. (2016). Bloating is associated with worse quality of life, treatment satisfaction, and treatment responsiveness among patients with constipation-predominant irritable bowel syndrome and functional constipation. *Neurogastroenterology and Motility*, *28*(4), 581–591. doi:10.1111/nmo.12758 PMID:26867677

O'Keefe, S. J. (2008). Nutrition and colonic health: The critical role of the microbiota. *Current Opinion in Gastroenterology*, *24*(1), 51–58. doi:10.1097/MOG.0b013e3282f323f3 PMID:18043233

Peery, A. F., Crockett, S. D., Barritt, A. S., Dellon, E.S., Eluri, S., Gangarosa, L.M., Jensen, E.T., Lund, J.L., Pasricha, S,, Runge, T., Schmidt, M., Shaheen N.J., Sandler, R.S. (2015). Burden of gastrointestinal, liver, and pancreatic diseases in the United States. *Gastroenterology, 149*(7), 1731–1741.

Quigley, E. M. M. (2012). Prebiotics and probiotics: Their role in the management of gastrointestinal disorders in adults. *Nutrition in Clinical Practice*, *27*(2), 195–200. doi:10.1177/0884533611423926 PMID:22127952

Sabater-Molina, M., Larqué, E., Torrella, F., & Zamora, S. (2009). Dietary fructooligosaccharides and potential benefits on health. *Journal of Physiology and Biochemistry, 65*(3), 315–328. doi:10.1007/BF03180584 PMID:20119826

Said, H. (2009). Cell and molecular aspects of human intestinal biotin absorption. *The Journal ofNutrition, 139*(1), 158–162. doi:10.3945/jn.108.092023 PMID:19056639

Schiller, L. R., Pardi, D. S., & Sellin, J. H. (2017). Chronic diarrhea: Diagnosis and management. *Clinical Gastroenterology and Hepatology, 15*(2), 182–193.e3. doi:10.1016/j.cgh.2016.07.028 PMID:27496381

Slavin, J. L. (2008). Position of the American Dietetic Association: Health implications of dietary fiber. *Journal of the American Dietetic Association, 108*(10), 1716–1731. doi:10.1016/j.jada.2008.08.007 PMID:18953766

Sleisenger, M. H., Feldman, M., Friedman, L. S., & Brandt, L. J. (2006). *Sleisenger & Fordtran's gastrointestinal and liver disease: Pathophysiology, diagnosis, management* (8th ed.). Saunders.

Surawicz, C. M. (2010). Mechanisms of diarrhea. *Current Gastroenterology Reports, 12*(4), 236–241. doi:10.100711894-010-0113-4 PMID:20532705

Ternent, C. A., Bastawrous, A. L., Morin, N. A., Ellis, C. N., Hyman, N. H., & Buie, W. D. (2007). Standards practice task force of the American Society of Colon and Rectal Surgeons. Practice parameters for the evaluation and management of constipation. *Diseases of the Colon and Rectum, 50*(12), 2013–2022. doi:10.100710350-007-9000-y PMID:17665250

Tuck, C. J., & Vanner, S. J. (2018). Dietary therapies for functional bowel symptoms: Recent advances, challenges, and future directions. *Neurogastroenterology and Motility, 30*(1), e13238. doi:10.1111/nmo.13238 PMID:29094792

U.S. Department of Health and Human Services. (2013, September 10). *Digestive diseases statistics for the United States*. National Digestive Diseases Information Clearinghouse. Retrieved May 1, 2020 from http://digestive.niddk.nih.gov/statistics/statistics.aspx#specific

Whitney, E. N., & Rolfes, S. R. (2016). *Understanding nutrition*. Cengage Learning.

Whyte, L. A., & Jenkins, H. R. (2012). Pathophysiology of diarrhea. *Paediatrics & Child Health, 22*(10), 443–447. doi:10.1016/j.paed.2012.05.006

World Health Organization. (2017). *Diarrhoeal disease. Fact Sheet No. 330*. World Health Organization Website. Retrieved May 1, 2020 from http://www.who.int/mediacentre/factsheets/fs330/en/

KEY TERMS AND DEFINITIONS

Constipation: A functional bowel disorder that presents as infrequent evacuation (i.e., bowel movements), difficult evacuation, incomplete evacuation, or evacuation of small or hard stools but does not meet the criteria for IBS.

Diarrhea: A functional bowel disorder that presents as a continuous or recurrent syndrome characterized by the passage of loose (i.e., mushy) or watery stools without abdominal pain or discomfort.

Diverticulosis: A condition in which the intestinal walls develop bulges in weakened areas, most commonly in the colon. These bulging pockets, known as diverticula, can worsen constipation, entrap feces, and become painfully infected and inflamed (diverticulitis).

Functional Bowel Disorders: A term that describes problems with the functioning of the stomach and bowels. Examples include irritable bowel syndrome and functional dyspepsia.

Irritable Bowel Syndrome: A disorder in which intermittent abdominal pain is associated with a range of symptoms, such as diarrhea, constipation, or alternating episodes of both.

APPENDIX

Table 3. Pathophysiology of diarrhea/constipation.

Diarrhea	Constipation
Functional - Irritable bowel syndrome - Inflammatory bowel disorders - Malabsorption syndromes - Chronic infections Dietary - Food allergies - Excessive intake of sugar and caffeine - Excessive intake of alcohol - Consumption of lactose (cause diarrhea in some people) Medications - Laxatives - Antacids - Stool softeners - Misoprostol	Idiopathic (unexplained) Congenital - Hirschsprung's disease Functional - Irritable bowel syndrome - Normal or slow-transit constipation - Pelvic floor dysfunction Structural - Stricture - Intestinal pseudo-obstruction Medications - Antidepressants - Analgesics - Diuretics - Long-term laxatives use - Antihypertensives - Antiparkinsonian agents Myopathic - Systemic sclerosis Neurogenic - Multiple sclerosis - Parkinson's disease - Spinal cord injury Endocrine/metabolic - Diabetes mellitus - Hyperthyroidism - Pregnancy - Scleroderma Environmental Compromised immobility - Inadequate toileting facilities Dietary - Inadequate fiber intake - Inadequate calorie and fluid intakes

Abbreviations

ALT: alanine aminotransferase
AST: aspartate aminotransferase
BMI: body mass index
BPM: Beat per minute
BUN: blood urea nitrogen
CPK: creatine phosphokinase
FBDs: functional bowel disorders

FODMAP: fermentable oligo-, di-, mono-saccharides and polyols
GI: gastroesophageal
HEENT: head, eyes, ears, nose, throat
HDL: high -density lipoprotein
Hgb: hemoglobin
LDL: low-density lipoprotein
MNT: medical nutrition therapy
RBC: red blood cells
TSH: Thyroxine stimulating hormone
WBC: white blood cells

Chapter 5
Celiac Disease

Haalah M. Shaaker
King Abdulaziz University, Saudi Arabia

EXECUTIVE SUMMARY

This chapter reveals and discusses a case involving celiac disease (CD). CD is a common, lifelong, genetically-based autoimmune disorder that causes inflammation of the proximal small intestine. This disease is triggered by eating foods containing gluten, which causes intestinal discomfort. Gluten is a protein that is found naturally in wheat, barley, and rye and is common in foods such as bread, pasta, cookies, and cakes. Many pre-packaged foods, lip balms and lipsticks, hair and skin products, toothpaste and vitamin and nutrient supplements contain gluten, although it is rarely found in medicine. The key to living with CD is to follow a gluten-free diet. This case shows the role of medical nutrition therapy in managing and preventing the undesirable symptoms of CD. Moreover, it allows dietetic professionals to assess celiac patients' conditions and provide them with relief from undesirable symptoms, while also establishing an effective follow-up plan with each patient.

INTRODUCTION

Celiac disease (CD) is characterized by an immune response to the introduction of wheat gluten and proteins related to rye and barley that stimulate an inflammatory response, atrophy villous and crypt hyperplasia in the small intestine (Alaedini & Green, 2005). A systematic review and meta-analysis showed that the prevalence of CD is approximately 1.1% to 1.7% in a sample of 275,818 people (Singh et al., 2018). The true prevalence of CD in the Kingdom of Saudi Arabia (KSA) is not known since no national epidemiological studies have been carried out. However, regional data shows that it is a common disorder in this part of the world (Saeed et

DOI: 10.4018/978-1-7998-3802-9.ch005

al., 2017). In the Middle East, certain studies show that a high prevalence of CD has been found in Iran, in both the general population and at-risk groups, such as among patients with irritable bowel syndrome or type 1 diabetes (Rostami et al., 2004). CD results from an inappropriate T-cell-mediated immune response against ingested gluten in people that are genetically predisposed to react negatively to gluten (Africa, 2002). The disease is linked to genes that code for human leukocyte antigens DQ2 and DQ8, with transglutaminase 2 appearing to be an important element of CD (Alaedini & Green, 2005). CD involves mucosal malabsorption, whereby intestinal villi are decreased in number, with less absorptive surfaces, fewer enzymes in the damaged cells and markedly elongated crypts. Symptoms and signs include diarrhea, irritability, a distended abdomen, easy fatigue, pallor, weight loss, vomiting, anemia and frequent, strong-smelling stools that are pale and foamy.

Several risk factors are associated with developing CD. For example, Down syndrome is frequently associated with CD, which is related to the prevalence of IgA-antigliadin and IgA-antiendomysium antibodies in children with Down syndrome(Carlsson et al., 1998). Type 1 diabetes mellitus (T1DM) is another risk factor that is positively associated with the incidence of CD. Both T1DM and CD share the same genetic background and abnormal immune response in the small intestine, involving inflammation and a changeable grade of enteropathy (Volta & Villanacci, 2011). Moreover, possible risk factors include infant feeding practices, excluding children who were breastfed beyond the introduction of gluten into their diets. While the former may seemingly be at a lower risk of acquiring CD, it is notable that the consumption of significant amounts of gluten early in life may increase the risk of acquiring CD in the future. However, the data assessing the impact of feeding infants with gluten is inconsistent (Ludvigsson & Fasano, 2012) .

The only way to confirm a CD diagnosis is to have an intestinal biopsy (Fernández-Bañares et al., 2014). However, a simple blood test is also available to check for CD. Several different antibodies are produced by an immune system that views gluten as a threat, including the tTG-IgA test, IgA endomysial antibody (EMA), total serum IgA, deamidated gliadin peptide (DGP IgA and IgG) and the intestinal fatty acid-binding protein (I-FABP) (Leffler et al., 2007) .

Currently, the single treatment for CD is the elimination of all dietary sources of gluten. Gluten can be classified into four subclasses: albumins, globulins, gliadin and glutenins. In wheat, the injurious constituent is the prolamin fraction of a-gliadin, with the equivalent in rye and barley being secalin and hordein, respectively. Studies have shown through enzymatic degradation that the damaging fraction is an acidic polypeptide with a molecular weight of less than 1,500 Da (Shaw, 2014). Maintaining a gluten-free diet (GFD) concerns the real need to exclude all potential sources of wheat, rye and barley and to maintain a commitment to this rule for life, as shown in the below figure:

Figure 1. Celiac disease (CD) cases, The basic gluten-free diet adapted from (Macdonald, 2007)
**Oats are considered to be one of the complicating factors because they can be mixed and contaminated with gluten-containing wheat during different stages of the former's production, including when they are being packaged, stored, processed and transported. Thus, consumers should be aware of this contamination issue.*

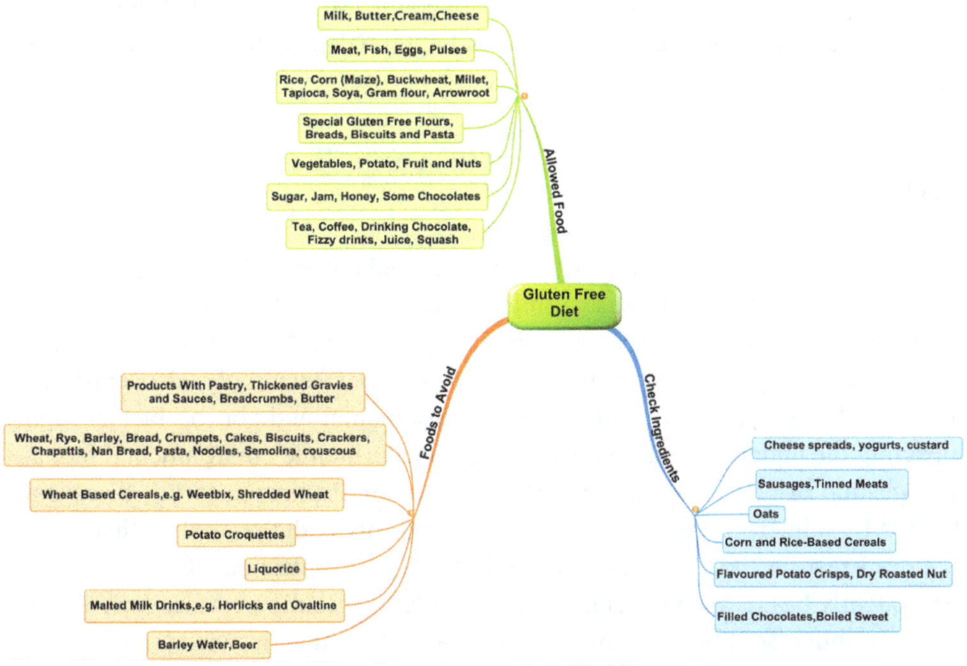

EPIDEMIOLOGY

In 2018, a study conducted a meta-analysis and review of many studies worldwide to estimate the global prevalence of CD and recognize variations in its pervasiveness within different countries and populations. In this case, the term "prevalence" refers to the percentage of people who have a disease at or during a specific period of time. The results found the current global prevalence of CD to be 1.4% based on blood tests and 0.7% based on biopsy results. The prevalence of CD was 0.4% in South America, 0.5% in Africa and North America, 0.6% in Asia and 0.8% in Europe and Oceania. The prevalence was higher in females than in males and was significantly more common in children than adults. The study indicated that the predominance of CD varies based on one's gender, age and origin (Singh et al., 2018).

CD is a common risk factor for type 1 diabetes in Saudi Arabia, Israel and Iran, with 2% to 8% of diagnosed patients having the latter (Rostami et al., 1999). It is also a comparatively common cause of constant diarrhea in Kuwait, Iraq, and Iran (Rostami et al., 1999). In fact, an analysis of wheat consumption within these states has illustrated that they have the highest global wheat consumption per capita, which is greater than 150 kg for each person annually (Cummins & Roberts-Thomson, 2009). Although few studies have been conducted concerning the scope of CD genetics, the existing ones have shown that citizens in countries such as Israel, Iran, Turkey and Saudi Arabia are prone to having HLA-DQB1*02, which is a CD-related gene (Gujral et al., 2012).

PATHOPHYSIOLOGY

CD is a condition that is characterized by intestinal enteropathy, especially among people that are genetically susceptible to it. This condition is induced by the consumption of gliadin or any other related prolamins. Moreover, wheat, barley and rye also trigger CD intestinal enteropathy. Oat sensitivity also exists at a minor level in the CD population, with environmental and genetic factors highly impacting the underlying mechanism of CD. The principle environmental factor is the ingestion of gluten and those with a genetic predisposition to this disease are affected by numerous genes. The reason behind this is the resistance that gliadin peptides exert on the enzymes produced in the gastrointestinal (GI) tract, which consequently has damaging effects. This is because gliadin peptides have distinct chains of amino acid that are specific to HLA-DQ2, which is considered a class II major histocompatibility complex that prefers glutamine residues as well for the tissue transglutaminase (tTG)-mediated deamidation, thereby ultimately altering intestinal permeability (Gujral et al., 2012) .

Moreover, Sams and Hawks explained the pathophysiology in their research in a similar way. They listed the factors causing CD as a union of four main factors: environmental factors, a genetic predisposition, gluten exposure and an autoimmune reaction. Gluten consists of a particular peptide division of proteins, such as prolamines, glutenin, gliadin, hordein, and secalin. These substances become more resistant to digestion by the internal enzyme, consequently reaching the body's intestine in their complex form. In normal cases, these peptides are tolerated by a healthy intestine as the intestinal wall is intact and blocks intestinal translocation. In a person with CD, these peptides can trigger an inflammatory response when moving across the intestinal epithelium from the lumen and traveling to the lamina propria, which results in the elongation of the crypt cells and the flattening of intestinal villi along with a further systemic immune response (Sams & Hawks, 2014).

RISK FACTORS AND ETIOLOGY

High-risk groups are people who may have higher CD prevalence rates within the general celiac population. The most common high-risk groups are first-degree relatives, individuals with osteopenia (bone disease), insulin-dependent diabetes types (particularly children) and people who are diagnosed with anemia, autoimmune hepatitis, primary biliary cirrhosis and other liver disorders. In addition, this group includes those with thyroid disease and other autoimmune endocrinopathies and dermatitis herpetiformis along with other skin disorders and neurological disorders, including those experiencing seizures and ataxia. Furthermore, those with genetic disorders, including Down syndrome and Turner's syndrome, are also at higher risk.

When analyzing all the factors that indicate that one has a higher risk for developing CD, having a family history of first-degree relatives with CD is considered to be the most relevant risk factor, with the likelihood of developing CD being equal to or greater than 20% (Freeman, 2010). Some studies observed a higher incidence of CD among siblings with the same parents. A study of Swedish teens and children below 20 years of age with known cases of insulin-dependent diabetes indicated that a minor proportion (0.7%) of those diagnosed with CD were symptomatic at the beginning of the clinical diagnosis. However, upon screening the percentage of silent CD cases during a follow-up assessment that took place five years later, a conclusive prevalence of 10% was found. Therefore, the prevalence of CD can grow over a period of time, especially in groups that are at high-risk of developing CD (Gujral et al., 2012).

Weaning from breastfeeding along with the timing of gluten introduction also plays a significant role that may contribute to the incidence of CD (Gujral et al., 2012). Aside from gluten exposure, infectious diseases are another dominant factor involved in the pathogenesis and disease development of CD in the first year of life. Remarkable studies have shown various types of infections that trigger the development of CD, such as Campylobacter jejuni, Adenovirus type 12, hepatitis C virus, enterovirus, rotavirus and the Giardia lamblia infection. Since an examination of genetically disposed individuals revealed that they have common viral sequences of 8 to 12 amino acids with the toxic fraction of gliadin, they are consequently susceptible to having the immunological responses associated with CD. Some initiating factors, such as the unmasking of gastric surgery, smoking cessation and gluten overload can also activate the disease, which can become possible in unexpected circumstances (Gujral et al., 2012).

SIGNS AND SYMPTOMS

There are typical symptoms of CD which are very common and well-known among many populations, including abdominal distention, chronic diarrhea, malabsorption, failure to thrive and weight loss. However, atypical symptoms include anemia, having a short stature, osteopenia, hepatic stenosis, dermatitis, ataxia, primary biliary cirrhosis, isolated hepertransamonasemia, recurrent aphthous stomatitis, alopecia, dental enamel, dermatitis herpetiformis, recurrent pericarditis, psoriasis, cardiomyopathy, dilatative polyneuropathy, epilepsy, vasculitis, myasthenia gravis, hypothyroidism and hyperthyroidism (Gujral et al., 2012).

The term "gluten intolerance" is used to describe a person who has symptoms regardless of whether she or he has CD. Gluten sensitivity terminology is commonly used to describe people who have reported unspecific symptoms, without having immunological reactions and subsequent intestinal damage. Both terminologies are usually used to define and specify overlapping symptoms like abdominal cramps, diarrhea or nausea after eating gluten. A GF diet should not be followed by patients who have experienced the previously mentioned symptoms without receiving a confirmed medical diagnosis of CD. There are many reasons for this, including the fact that symptoms could be attributed to other medical diagnoses for which prescribing a GF diet is not the exact treatment. Moreover, it is difficult to diagnose individuals with CD if they have been following a GF diet over a long period of time. Finally, a GF diet is considered to be expensive and restrictive if it were to be followed unnecessarily in the long run (Manhan & Janice, 2017).

MEDICAL MANAGEMENT

Considerable medical management in the first place is applied to manage comorbidities in CD patients. This is because the only effective treatment available for individuals with CD is a strict lifelong GFD.

MEDICAL NUTRITION THERAPY

Currently, all medical nutrition therapy (MNT) strategies for CD patients prioritizes omitting gluten from an individual's diet. This dietary approach excludes the intake of all barley, rye and wheat, which are considered the main sources of the prolamin fragments. Generally, nutritional deficiencies should be considered and regularly assessed to determine whether there is a need for any nutritional supplements.

Moreover, patients who are newly diagnosed or presented with severe symptoms involving nutrient deficiencies, such as prolonged prothrombin time, neuropathy and night-blindness, should be closely examined by clinicians to determine their vitamin B9, red blood cell ferritin and active vitamin D levels. If a patient suffers from GI symptoms, such as severe diarrhea or notable weight loss, the physician should consider checking the patient's vitamin levels, such as their fat-soluble vitamin (like vitamin A, vitamin E and vitamin K) and mineral (like zinc) levels. Furthermore, those who suffer from malabsorption may benefit from being provided with vitamin D and calcium after assessing bone health for osteopenia, osteoporosis or any other bone issues. Electrolytes and fluid maintenance and replacement are highly essential for those who are dehydrated due to severe diarrhea; thus, general vitamin-mineral supplements should be taken to at least cover their dietary reference intake (DRI) recommendations.

Most GF products are not fortified with essential nutrients like other grain products, with the former commonly lacking iron, folate, B12 and other B vitamins. Hence, the dietary intake of those who consume such products could be poor, incomplete and unbalanced unless they are provided with sufficient partial supplementation. Depending on the nature of the anemia that might be accrued, it should be treated with iron, vitamin B12 or vitamin B9. In addition, CD patients occasionally have lactose intolerance or fructose intolerance. A diet that is low in lactose or fructose may be beneficial in mitigating any undesirable symptoms associated with such intolerances. However, the lactase enzyme may return to function normally again during the remission period of the GI tract, which enables the person to tolerate foods containing lactose. The foods that CD patients can safely ingest without any concern include most fruits and vegetables (as they do not naturally contain gluten), unseasoned meats, non-gluten containing grains and plain dairy products. The effect of consuming oats on CD populations in particular is rather questionable as various studies have reported that oats are completely safe if they have not been contaminated by grains that contain gluten (Garsed and Scott, 2007). Nonetheless, some CD patients still experience intolerance and undesirable symptoms after ingesting oats. Thus, this group should avoid GF oats in their meal plans and substitutes in recipes can be recommended, such as substituting wheat flours which used to make various food items, with flours made from rice, corn, nuts, soybean, potatoes, buckwheat, quinoa, garbanzo beans, arrowroot or amaranth.

Patients who follow a well-balanced GFD will not need additional nutritional supplementation since nutrients' absorption becomes more efficient during the intestinal mucosal healing process.

The role of registered dietitian nutritionists (RDN) is extremely critical for CD patients. As soon as they are diagnosed, patients should be referred to the RDN so that they can be given individualized instructions on how to manage their dietary habits and prevent undesirable symptoms, along with receiving continuous guidance and support from reliable sources. Persons with CD commonly require frequent counseling sessions to be educated and follow-up on their dietary habits. Dietitians could also arrange to form a creative support group for CD patients (Vege et al., 2015).

Patients and their caregivers can expect many challenges when following GFDs. Such diets require a major lifestyle shift with regard to the consumption of traditional grains, which is a standard feature of Western diet since a majority of foods are made with wheat, like pasta, bread and other baked items. This is also due to the modification in the flavors and texture of many desired foods using substitute flours. On the other hand, these dramatic changes can be made easier by improving the taste of food so that it is palatable once the adjustment is made. In GF baked items, gums such as guar gum and cellulose can be used to provide the elasticity required to trap leavening gases in baked goods. Moreover, food makers can add some flavor-enhancing spices, such as cardamom, ginger, mint, lemon, and more, to improve the taste of GF foods. Reading every single food label for each product that is to be used is also a very common requirement so as to figure out whether there are any hidden gluten-containing ingredients in a product. An ideal GFD requires scrutinizing the food labels of all baked products and packaged foods. Consumers must be aware of the ingredients of all products that might be used during the preparation of a meal, other than the main gluten-containing products. Many items also use mixtures when preparing one ingredient, which may have already been contaminated through contact with any grains. Thus, providing the patient with handouts, educational videos, interactive counselling sessions or any other individualized counselling approach is highly recommended. A sufficient follow-up plan with CD patients will also have a positive outcome, making the lifestyle modification easier for patients and their care givers, by providing them with continuous educational sessions so as to overcome all challenges that may be faced (Manhan & Janice, 2017)

FUTURE THERAPUTIC APPROACHES FOR CD

Firstly, considerable medical management must be applied to manage comorbidities in CD patients. This is because the only effective treatment available for individuals with CD is a strict lifelong adherence to a GFD. On the other hand, promising future treatment approaches have been presented in many conducted studies, as is discussed further below.

The hydrolysis of the toxic gliadin peptide is one such further approach, which has four categories. The first category includes prolyl endopeptidases (PEPs), which are endoproteolytic enzymes that can be found in plants or numerous micro-organisms. These enzymes help break down a specific type of gluten (proline) into small particles (peptides), a form that enables digestion by the intestinal enzymes, which are called aminopeptidases and carboxypeptidases (Matysiak-Budnik et al., 2005). The second category is ALV003, which is a fusion of PEP with an endoprotease from barley germination, which has been treated with wheat flour and tested in CD cases. Surprisingly, the results showed that by using the ALV003 pre-treatment, there was no significant reduction in the incidence of the symptoms that were usually triggered when gluten was consumed. However, ALV003 succeeded in suppressing the immunological responses that were caused by CD patients' ingestion of gluten (Gujral et al., 2012).

The third therapeutic approach involves adding lactobacilli to sourdough for fermentation. This approach involves lysing the peptides that were found in proline and glutamine in order to minimize their immunotoxicity. A fusion of oats with fermented wheat flour, buckwheat and millet allows sourdough bread to retain standard baking features, with one study reporting that this kind of bread is generally well-tolerated by CD patients (Di Cagno et al., 2004).

The last therapeutic approach is VSL#3, referring to lyophilized bacteria that contain probiotics, including certain bifidobacterial, such as Bifidobacterium infantis, Bifidobacterium longum and Bifidobacterium breve. This also comprises lactobacilli like Lactobacillus delbrueckii subsp, Lactobacillus bulgaricus, Lactobacillus plantarum, Lactobacillus casei and Lactobacillus acidophilus. Lastly, this remedy also includes Streptococcus salivarius subsp. thermophiles. The main use of these probiotics is to break down the peptides found in gliadin with pretreated flour and then test their efficacy on a rat's GI system (Angelis et al., 2006).

A greater understanding of the pathogenesis of CD allows promising treatments to take place in the future, either through the hydrolysis of the toxic gliadin peptide, as has been explained above, or using other approaches. These could include restoration of the intestinal structure, restoration of the immune system's tolerance toward gluten, modulation of the immune-gliadin reaction, blockage of selective deamidation of specific glutamine residues by tissue and the prevention of toxic gliadin peptide absorption. Implementing each of these methods involves different mechanisms as each has its own validity.

SETTING THE STAGE

Patients' data were obtained from a pediatric gastroenterological clinic in a governmental hospital in Jeddah, Saudi Arabia. Medical team members involved were a pediatric gastroenterologist and a pediatric endocrinologist. There was no conflict of interest as the patient and his parents did not receive any financial support from the author to disclose the presented case.

CASE DESCRIPTIVE

Patient Details

- Patient name: AA Gender: Male
- Date of Birth: 24/01/2007 Age: 13 years
- Date of assessment: 02/03/2020

Case History

Medical History: AA is a 13 year-old boy with a known case of Down syndrome, hyperthyroidism and controlled insulin-dependent diabetes mellitus. He was diagnosed with CD two years ago, experiencing symptoms at that time including the severe weight loss of 3% in one week, bloating and loose diarrhea 5 to 7 times per day. The patient has recently regained 4 kgs of weight over the last 6 months.

- Chief complaint: The patient was presented as an out-patient at the celiac clinic for routine follow-up with no active complaints.
- Surgical history: None
- Smoker: No
- Family History: One younger sibling has Down syndrome, his maternal grandmother and father have diabetes mellitus and his maternal grandfather has CD.

Main Medical Diagnosis

Celiac Disease (CD)

Demographics

- Education: Intermediate degree (studying at a school for special needs)
- Occupation: None
- Household members: Mother, father and 2 sisters
- Ethnicity/ Religion: Saudi/ Muslim

Anthropometrics

- Height: 151cm
- Current weight: 35 kg
- Usual body weight: 31 kg

- History of weight loss: 3% in one week (two years ago)
- BMI: 15.3 kg/m2

Table 1. Biochemical Data

Test	Reference	Result	
TSH (mlU/L)	0.5-2	5.26	High
WBC (K/ul)	4.8-11.8	4.0	Low
RBC (M/ul)	4.2-5.4 (Females) 4.5-6.2 (Males)	5.46	Normal
Hb (g/dl)	12-15 (Females) 14-17 (Males)	10	Low
MCH (pg)	27-33	26.5	Low
Creatinine (umol/L)	20-110	75	Normal
Urea (mmol/L)	1.8-7.1	5	Normal
Total protein (g/L)	60-83	58	Low
Albumin (g/L)	35-55	31	Low
Calcium (mmol/L)	2.2-2.7	2.36	Normal
Magnesium (mmol/L)	0.85-1.10	0.95	Normal
Phosphate (mmol/L)	1.12-1.45	1.56	Normal
Potassium (mmol/L)	3.5-5.5	4.50	Normal
Sodium (mmol/L)	136-145	141	Normal
Chloride (mmol/L)	95-105	105	Normal
HbA1C (%)	4-5.7	6.0	High
Vitamin D (ng/ml)	30-100	116.2	High
Serum iron (umol/L)	10.7-30.4	8.5	Low
TIBC (umol/L)	42.9-80.5	59.2	Normal
Ferritin (ng/ml)	12-150 (Females) 12- 300 (Males)	20.7	Normal
Thyroid Peroxidase Antibody (IU/ml)	<35	> 1000	High
Tissue Transglutaminase – IgA (U/ml)	<3	1665.8	High

Nutrition-Focused Physical Examination

- General appearance: Patient looks pale, especially his face and the palms of both hands
- Heart: Regular rate and rhythm, heart sounds normal

- Genitalia: Not performed
- Rectal: Not performed
- Neurologic: Alert and oriented, although he has learning difficulties
- Extremities: Noncontributory
- Skin: Warm and no dryness
- Chest/lungs: Normal breathing sounds, lungs are clear
- Abdomen: Currently tender with normal bowel motion with current GFD: 1-2 times a day of a semi-soft consistency. However, when some gluten-containing food is introduced, the patient may experience one or more of these symptoms (loose diarrhea 4 to 6 times), bloating and abdominal discomfort
- Urologic: Normal urine output, light color, 6 times daily and no urination discomfort

Vital Signs

- Pulse rate: 76 BPM
- Temperature: 36.8 C degree
- Blood pressure 118/76 mm Hg
- Respiratory: 12 breaths/ minute

Food/Nutrition-Related History

A complete dietary history obtained from the mother**:**

Over the past three months, the patient's mother started to apply a GFD when feeding her child as ordered by a peer physician. She was also given educational materials about GFDs from the celiac clinic.

Table 2. Obtainment of 24-hour dietary recall: (United States Department of Agriculture, n.d.)

Meal	Content	Calories	Protein
Breakfast	½ slice of gluten free bread + 1 scrambled egg + 1 tbs of cream cheese	197 kcal	8.24 gm
School Snack	1 small croissant + whole milk (240ml)	291 kcal	11.8 gm
Lunch	15 tbs of rice cooked with 2 tbs of ready-to-use sauce + 1 tbs of tomato sauce and some spices + ¼ chicken + 1 cup of green salad with 1 tsp of salad sauce	546 kcal	34.23 gm
Snack	1 packet of buttered popcorn (known as Albatal chips)	72 kcal	1 gm
Dinner	¼ Tamees bread (bread with margarine) + 2 tbs of cooked fava beans with 2 tsp of olive oil and some salt	311 kcal	9.6gm
Total		1,417 kcal/day	75gm/day

- Usual intake: 3 main meals and 2 snacks daily
- Fluid intake: 1.5 to 2 L of water
- Food preferences: Likes: Juices, whole milk and cream cheese. Dislikes: GF flour and red meat
- Food allergies/intolerances/aversions: Only gluten-containing products. According to the mother, the child experiences discomfort only when he eats more than 1 meal containing gluten.
- Vitamin and mineral supplementation: Furros sulphate 325 mg/day as an iron supplement, on-and-off vitamin D supplement of 50,000 IU once a week (although this is currently on hold since his lab results are normal).
- Previous nutrition therapy: None; the mother had never previously consulted a dietitian and she is not well educated on GFDs and diabetic diets.
- Food purchase/preparation: Mother and grandmother
- Appetite: Good
- Chewing or swallowing difficulties: None

Medications

The patient was taking Thyroxine 150mcg/day for his thyroid condition and currently held based on the physician's order. To control his diabetes, he is only taking Lantus (long-acting insulin) 6 units once a day every 24 hours. The mother is also not aware of iron supplement interaction as she gives her child the iron supplement (Furros sulphate tablets 325 mg/day) with meals containing dairy products.

Nutritional Management

Disease Pathophysiology and Management Mind Map (Figure 2)

Main Aim of The Nutrition Therapy

- Provide nutritional education about GFD
- Ensure appropriate growth patterns
- Prevent nutrient malabsorption
- Prevent food-drug interactions
- Prevent undesirable gastrointestinal symptoms
- Maintain controlled blood glucose levels

Figure 2. Celiac disease (CD) cases, pathophysiology, and medical nutrition therapy mind map. Adopted from (Manhan & Janice, 2017), and developed by Khalifa, N 2020

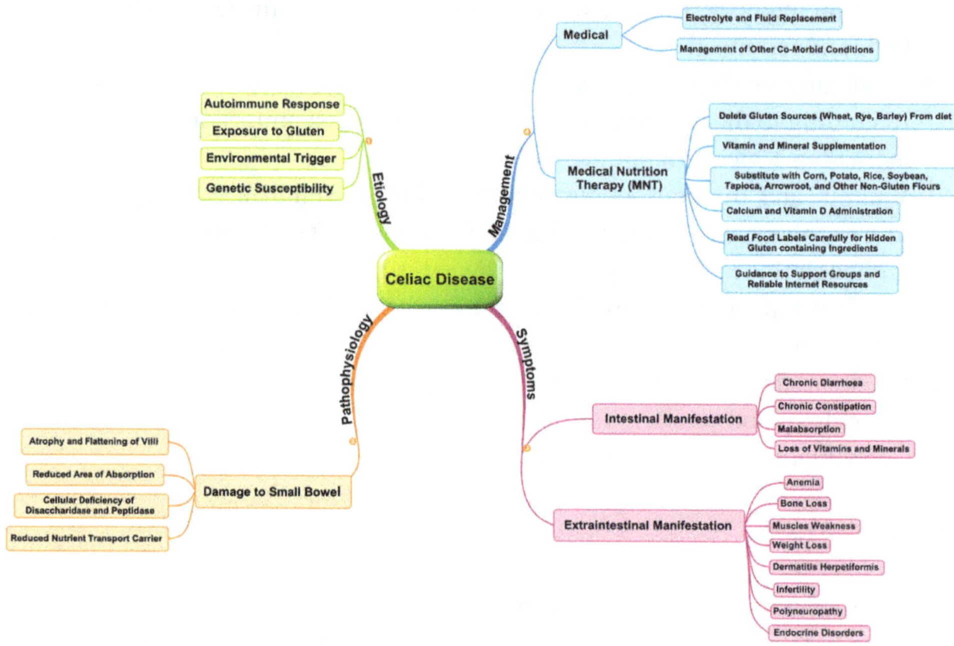

ADIME Note

Assessment

The patient is a 13 year-old boy with a known case of CD, Down syndrome, hyperthyroidism and controlled insulin-dependent diabetes mellitus. He usually complains of diarrhea and bloating whenever he ingests food containing gluten.

Anthropometric

- Current body weight: 35 kg
- Height: 151 cm
- BMI: 15.3 kg/m2
- Usual body weight: 31 kg
- History of weight loss: 3% in one week (two years ago)
- % weight change: he recently gained 4 kg over the past 6 months on his low-gluten diet
- Weight for age: 10th -25th Percentile (healthy for most pediatric patients)

- Ideal weight for age: 44 kg
- Height for age: 75th – 90th Percentile (healthy for most pediatric patients)
- Ideal height for age: 144 cm

Growth charts designed for children with Down Syndrome were used to assess the patient's growth and anthropometrics (Growth Charts for Children with Down Syndrome, n.d.) and an interpretation of the anthropometric measurements was adopted from the book *The Essential Pocket Guide for Clinical Nutrition* (Width & Reinhard, 2018).

Table 3. Biochemical: (Based on an interpretation of Width and Reinhard's (2018) abnormal lab values)(Width & Reinhard, 2018)

Test	Reference	Result		Interpretation
TSH (mIU/L)	0.2-2	5.26	H	Hyperthyroidism
WBC (K/ul)	4.8-11.8	4.0	L	May indicate dietary deficiency of iron or B12
Hb (g/ dl)	12-15 (Females) 14-17 (Males)	10	L	Anemia
MCH (pg)	27-33	26.5	L	Anemia
Total protein (g/L)	60-83	58	L	Decreased muscle mass
Albumin (g/L)	35-55	31	L	May indicate protein malabsorption
Serum Iron (umol/L)	10.7-30.4	8.5	L	Insufficient dietary iron intake or intestinal malabsorption of iron

Clinical

The patient looks pale which may indicate anemia. He currently experiences normal bowel motions during his GFD: 1-2 times a day of a semi-soft consistency. However, when some gluten-containing food is introduced, the patient may experience one or more of these symptoms: loose diarrhea 4 to 6 times, bloating and abdominal discomfort. All vital signs are normal.

Dietary

The patient is consuming 92% of the total caloric requirements and 98% of the total protein requirements. Thus, it is not an indication to start nutrition support. The patient is not complaint to his GFD and he is consuming high-fat foods.

Diagnoses

1. Undesirable food choices related to the nutrition-related knowledge deficit about GFD, as evidenced by uncomfortable symptoms when ingesting foods containing gluten.
2. Food-medication interaction related to the lack of food-drug interaction awareness, as evidenced by low laboratory results of hemoglobin, mean corpuscular hemoglobin and ferritin. He is also taking iron supplements with dairy products, as reported by the mother.

The problem, etiology, signs and symptoms (PES) statement was adopted from a nutrition diagnostic terminology form (Academy of Nutrition and Dietetics, 2014)

Intervention

1. **Calculating nutritional requirements:** (Width & Reinhard, 2018)
   a. *Calories: By estimating the energy requirements for pediatrics*:
   DRI (boys aged 12-13) × weight
   = 44 × 35 = 1,540 kcal /day
   b. *Protein: By estimating the protein requirements for pediatrics*:
   DRI (boys aged 12-13) × weight
   = 0.94 × 35 = 32.9 gm/day

   However, it counts only 8.5% of the total caloric needs.
   Thus, we will go to the macronutrient distribution of 20% of the protein of the total caloric needs, to compensate the protein malabsorption
   = 1,540 × 0.2 = 308 / 4 = 77 gm/day

   c. *Carbohydrates: 45% of the total caloric needs as recommended for diabetic patients*
   = 1,540 × 0.5 = 693 / 4 = 174 gm/day
   d. *Fat: 35% of the total caloric needs*
   = 1,540 × 0.35 = 540 / 9 = 60 gm/day
   e. *Fluids: By using baseline fluid requirements*
   1,500ml + (20ml/kg for each kg > 20kg) = 1,500 + 300 = 1,800 ml /day
2. **Nutrition prescription:**
   Diabetic GFD (1,540kcal/day, 77gm protein/day, 1,800 ml/day fluids)
3. **Goals and recommendations**:
   a. *Educate the caregiver about GFDs with handouts for instructions and recipes, including*:

i. A handout with a table reveals foods that do and do not contain gluten.
ii. A handout about GF products and how to read food labels to make sure that the purchased product does not contain gluten (Figure 1)
iii. Provide the mother with an overview of the autoimmune reaction toward gluten-containing food in a simple way. Thus, the mother can understand the reason behind the undesirable symptoms that come along with gluten ingestion.
iv. Recommend some handbooks for GF recipes

b. *Instruct the mother to provide a window of 4 hours before and after the consumption of iron supplementation pills and calcium-containing foods to avoid food-drug interaction, because calcium-containing food will decrease the bioavailability of the iron supplement*:
i. Provide the mother with a list of calcium-containing food items. For example, this includes milk, yogurt, cheese, other dairy products, leafy vegetables, nuts, tofu, soya drinks with added calcium, sardines and pilchards (where a person can eat the bones).
ii. Explain to the caregiver that the lowered iron bioavailability caused by the inappropriate calcium intake timing will not improve the serum iron status.

c. *Educate the patient about their diabetic diet and how to maintain blood glucose levels*:
i. Encourage the patient to consume complex carbohydrates, such as whole grains and brown rice, but to also be aware of gluten content.
ii. Stay away from simple sugars, such as sweets, chocolates, nectar, packaged juices with added sugar, carbonated beverages and soft drinks.
iii. Consume the recommended 4 to 5 servings of fruits a day
iv. Avoid foods that are high in sodium, such as table salt, chips, pickles, fast food and processed meat.

d. *Encourage the patient to avoid consuming high-fat foods, to minimize excessive weight gain and to control his or her blood glucose levels.*
i. Recommend foods are low in saturated fat, cholesterol and whole fat, such as lean meat, low-fat milk and yogurt and grilled meals (instead of fried items).

e. *Provide a detailed individualized diet plan to the patient and his mother along with a food exchange list so that they can have a variety of food alternatives*:

Table 4. Diabetic gluten-free diet (1,540kcal/day, 77gm protein/day, 1,800 ml/day fluids)

Meal	Content	Calories	Protein
Breakfast	2 scrambled eggs + 1 cup of low-fat yogurt + 1.5 cups of GF cereals + 2 cups of water	380 kcal	22 gm
School snack	1 cup of low-fat milk + 3 dates	160 kcal	8 gm
Lunch	90 gm of cooked chicken + 1 cup of rice + 2 cups of green salad with some seasonings that are low in sodium and lemon juice + 2 cups of water	435 kcal	21 gm
Snack	30 gm of nuts + 1 cup of low-fat yogurt + 1 cup of water	165 Kcal	15 gm
Dinner	60 gm of cooked fish or lean meat + 2 slices of GF bread + 2 cups of water	290 kcal	14 gm
Bedtime snack	3 cups of plain popcorn + 1 cup of water	70 kcal	0 gm
Total	Using the food exchange list (Ucsf, 2008)	1,500kcal/day	80gm/day

Monitoring and Evaluation

- Weight changes and growth patterns
- Nutritional plan adherence
- Lab values (iron, Hb, ferritin, vitamin D and calcium)
- Anemia and paleness of the skin
- Undesirable GI symptoms (diarrhea and bloating)

REFERENCES

Academy of Nutrition and Dietetics. (2014). eNCPT Reference Manual. Author.

Africa, N. (2002). a 1*501, B 1*02). *English Journal*, *346*(3), 180–188. doi:10.1056/NEJMra010852

Alaedini, A., & Green, P. (2005). Review Narrative Review : Celiac Disease : Understanding a Complex. [PubMed]. *Annals of Internal Medicine*, *142*, 289. doi:10.7326/0003-4819-142-4-200502150-00011

Angelis, M. De, Rizzello, C. G., Fasano, A., Clemente, M. G., Simone, C. De, Silano, M., Vincenzi, M. De, Losito, I., & Gobbetti, M. (2006). VSL#3 probiotic preparation has the capacity to hydrolyze gliadin polypeptides responsible for Celiac Sprue. Biochimica et Biophysica Acta - Molecular Basis of Disease, 1762(1), 80–93. https://doi.org/ doi:10.1016/j.bbadis.2005.09.008

Carlsson, A., Axelsson, I., Borulf, S., Bredberg, A., Forslund, M., Lindberg, B., Sjöberg, K., & Ivarsson, S.-A. (1998). Prevalence of IgA-Antigliadin Antibodies and IgA-Antiendomysium Antibodies Related to Celiac Disease in Children With Down Syndrome. *Pediatrics*, *101*(2), 272–275. doi:10.1542/peds.101.2.272

Cummins, A. G., & Roberts-Thomson, I. C. (2009). Prevalence of celiac disease in the Asia-Pacific region. *Journal of Gastroenterology and Hepatology*, *24*(8), 1347–1351. doi:10.1111/j.1440-1746.2009.05932.x

De Angelis, M., Rizzello, C. G., Fasano, A., Clemente, M. G., De Simone, C., Silano, M., De Vincenzi, M., Losito, I., & Gobbetti, M. (2006). VSL#3 probiotic preparation has the capacity to hydrolyze gliadin polypeptides responsible for Celiac Sprue. Biochimica et Biophysica Acta. [PubMed]. *Molecular Basis of Disease*, *1762*(1), 80–93. doi:10.1016/j.bbadis.2005.09.008

Di Cagno, R., De Angelis, M., Auricchio, S., Greco, L., Clarke, C., De Vincenzi, M., Giovannini, C., D'Archivio, M., Landolfo, F., Parrilli, G., Minervini, F., Arendt, E., & Gobbetti, M. (2004). Sourdough Bread Made from Wheat and Nontoxic Flours and Started with Selected Lactobacilli Is Tolerated in Celiac Sprue Patients. [PubMed]. *Applied and Environmental Microbiology*, *70*(2), 1088–1096. doi:10.1128/AEM.70.2.1088-1096.2004

Fernández-Bañares, F., Carrasco, A., García-Puig, R., Rosinach, M., González, C., Alsina, M., Loras, C., Salas, A., Viver, J. M., & Esteve, M. (2014). Intestinal intraepithelial lymphocyte cytometric pattern is more accurate than subepithelial deposits of anti-tissue transglutaminase IgA for the diagnosis of celiac disease in lymphocytic enteritis. [PubMed]. *PLoS One*, *9*(7), e101249. Advance online publication. doi:10.1371/journal.pone.0101249

Freeman, H. J. (2010). Risk factors in familial forms of celiac disease. *World Journal of Gastroenterology*, *16*(15), 1828–1831. doi:10.3748/wjg.v16.i15.1828

Growth Charts for Children with Down Syndrome. (n.d.). Retrieved April 21, 2020, from https://www.cdc.gov/ncbddd/birthdefects/downsyndrome/growth-charts.html

Gujral, N., Freeman, H. J., & Thomson, A. B. R. (2012). Celiac disease: Prevalence, diagnosis, pathogenesis and treatment. [PubMed]. *World Journal of Gastroenterology*, *18*(42), 6036–6059. doi:10.3748/wjg.v18.i42.6036

Leffler, D. A., Dennis, M., Hyett, B., Kelly, E., Schuppan, D., & Kelly, C. P. (2007). {A figure is presented}Etiologies and Predictors of Diagnosis in Nonresponsive Celiac Disease. [PubMed]. *Clinical Gastroenterology and Hepatology*, *5*(4), 445–450. doi:10.1016/j.cgh.2006.12.006

Ludvigsson, J. F., & Fasano, A. (2012). Timing of introduction of gluten and celiac disease risk. [PubMed]. *Annals of Nutrition & Metabolism*, *60*(s2), 22–29. doi:10.1159/000335335

Macdonald, S. (2007). Sarah Macdonald. 90–124.

Manhan, K., & Janice, R. (2017). *Krause's Food & Nutrition Care Process* (14th ed.). ELSEVIER.

Matysiak-Budnik, T., Candalh, C., Cellier, C., Dugave, C., Namane, A., Vidal-Martinez, T., Cerf-Bensussan, N., & Heyman, M. (2005). Limited efficiency of prolyl-endopeptidase in the detoxification of gliadin peptides in celiac disease. [PubMed]. *Gastroenterology*, *129*(3), 786–796. doi:10.1053/j.gastro.2005.06.016

Rostami, K., Malekzadeh, R., Shahbazkhani, B., Akbari, M. R., & Catassi, C. (2004). Coeliac disease in Middle Eastern countries: A challenge for the evolutionary history of this complex disorder? [PubMed]. *Digestive and Liver Disease*, *36*(10), 694–697. doi:10.1016/j.dld.2004.05.010

Saeed, A., Assiri, A., Assiri, H., Ullah, A., & Rashid, M. (2017). Celiac disease in Saudi children: Evaluation of clinical features and diagnosis. [PubMed]. *Saudi Medical Journal*, *38*(9), 895–899. doi:10.15537mj.2017.9.20808

Sams, A., & Hawks, J. (2014). Celiac disease as a model for the evolution of multifactorial disease in humans. [PubMed]. *Human Biology*, *86*(1), 19–36. doi:10.3378/027.086.0102

Shaw, V. (2014). *Clinical Paediatric Dietetics* (4th ed.)., doi:10.1002/9781118915349

Singh, P., Arora, A., Strand, T. A., Leffler, D. A., Catassi, C., Green, P. H., Kelly, C. P., Ahuja, V., & Makharia, G. K. (2018). Global Prevalence of Celiac Disease: Systematic Review and Meta-analysis. [PubMed]. *Clinical Gastroenterology and Hepatology*, *16*(6), 823–836.e2. doi:10.1016/j.cgh.2017.06.037

UCSF. (2008). Food Exchange Lists. Choose Your Foods: Exchange Lists for Diabetes, 1–17. https://dtc.ucsf.edu/pdfs/FoodLists.pdf

United States Department of Agriculture. (n.d.). Retrieved April 24, 2020, from https://fdc.nal.usda.gov/

Vege, S. S., Ziring, B., Jain, R., Moayyedi, P., Adams, M. A., Dorn, S. D., Dudley-Brown, S. L., Flamm, S. L., Gellad, Z. F., Gruss, C. B., Kosinski, L. R., Lim, J. K., Romero, Y., Rubenstein, J. H., Smalley, W. E., Sultan, S., Weinberg, D. S., & Yang, Y.-X. (2015). American gastroenterological association institute guideline on the diagnosis and management of asymptomatic neoplastic pancreatic cysts. [PubMed]. *Gastroenterology*, *148*(4), 819–822. doi:10.1053/j.gastro.2015.01.015

Volta, U., & Villanacci, V. (2011). Celiac disease: Diagnostic criteria in progress. [PubMed]. *Cellular & Molecular Immunology*, *8*(2), 96–102. doi:10.1038/cmi.2010.64

Width, M., & Reinhard, T. (2018). *The Essential Pocket Guid for Clinical Nutrition*. Second.

KEY TERMS AND DEFINITIONS

Autoimmune Disorder: a condition in which the immune system mistakenly attacks the body itself.

Down Syndrome: a genetic disorder that results from the presence of all or part of the third copy of chromosome 21. It is usually connected to delays in growth and physical development, mild to moderate intellectual disability and characteristic facial features.

Gliadin: (a type of prolamin) a class of proteins present in wheat and cereals within the grass genus, Triticum. Gliadins, which are a component of gluten, enable bread to rise during baking. Both gliadins and glutenins are the main elements of the gluten fraction of the wheat seed, whereby gluten is typically found in products such as wheat flour. Gluten is split evenly between gliadins and glutenins, although variations are found in different sources.

Gluten: proteins found in wheat, rye, and barley that help food maintain their shape, acting as an adhesive that holds food together.

Hyperthyroidism: (overactive thyroid) a condition that arises when the thyroid gland produces too much of the hormone "thyroxine."

Insulin-Dependent Diabetes Mellitus: an autoimmune disease that destroys insulin-producing cells in the pancreas.

Lactobacilli: gram-positive, fermentative, facultative anaerobic bacteria that normally live in the digestive, urinary, and genital systems without causing diseases.

Meta-Analysis: a statistical method used to combine research study data to summarize the results of multiple studies.

APPENDIX: ABBREVIATIONS

BPM: Beat per minute
CD: Celiac disease
cm: Centimeter
GF: Gluten-free
GFD: Gluten-free diet
GI: Gastrointestinal
gm: Gram
H: High
Hb: Hemoglobin
HbA1C: Glycated hemoglobin
IDDM: Insulin dependent diabetes mellitus
IgA: Immunoglobulin A
IU: International unit
Kcal: Kilo Calorie
Kg: Kilogram
KSA: Kingdom of Saudi Arabia
L: Liter
L: Low
MCH: Mean corpuscular hemoglobin
mg: Milligram
mmHg: Millimeter mercury
MNT: Medical Nutrition Therapy
RBC: Red blood cells
RDN: Registered dietitian nutritionist
tbs: Tablespoon
TIBC: Total iron binding capacity
TSH: Thyroid stimulating hormone
tsp: Teaspoon
tTG: Tissue transglutaminase
USDA: United States Department of Agriculture
WBC: White blood cells

Chapter 6
Lactose Intolerance

Jomanah Abduljalil H. Bakhsh
King Abdulaziz University, Saudi Arabia

EXECUTIVE SUMMARY

This chapter presents a case scenario of lactose intolerance. Lactose intolerance is the inability to digest and absorb lactose, which is the sugar in milk, due to deficiency of the enzyme lactase. This condition commonly occurs after weaning, and it results in various gastrointestinal symptoms such as diarrhea. In addition, it may result in nutritional deficiencies. Management of lactose intolerance requires diet manipulations. This case study provides the needed information to implement the appropriate intervention such as patient's details and case history. Moreover, the case analysis section discusses in detail the disease pathophysiology and the medical nutrition therapy goals. This comprehensive analysis will allow the dietetic professional to follow the nutrition care process (NCP) framework (assessment, diagnosis, intervention, and monitoring and evaluation) to properly intervene and deal with the case. This case study will show the importance of the medical nutrition therapy for the management of lactose intolerance.

INTRODUCTION

Lactose is a disaccharide consisting of glucose and galactose, and it is the main sugar in milk. In addition, lactose has several uses in the food industry such as for confectionary and baked goods; this is due to its physiological properties. Lactose digestion occurs in the small intestine by the brush border enzymes. Lactase also called lactase-phlorizin hydrolase (LPH) is the enzyme specifically responsible for lactose hydrolysis into its constituent two monosaccharides. The ability to digest lactose is considered essential during the first year of life because it provides almost

DOI: 10.4018/978-1-7998-3802-9.ch006

50% of the required energy for infants. The largest quantities of lactase are found in the jejunum, and since lactase is found on the surface of the intestinal villi, this makes it more vulnerable than other deeper enzymes to be affected by intestinal cell damage (Robayo-Torres & Nichols, 2007; Shaukat et al., 2010; Vesa, Marteau, & Korpela, 2000).

EPIDEMIOLOGY

All newborn mammals are born with sufficient concentrations of lactase in the small intestine, and only around 50% of the enzyme lactase is needed to be active for effective lactose digestion. However, around 75% of people worldwide experience a decrease in lactase synthesis (Mahan & Raymond, 2017; Morelli, Amrani, Goulet, & Lukito, 2019). Lctose intolerance is highly prevalent among Asians, Africans, and South Americans with prevalence above 50% in those populations; moreover, in some Asian countries, the prevalence almost reaches 100% (Vesa et al., 2000). On the other hand, people of European descent have relatively low percentages of lactose intolerance. Studies show that 75-85% of white adults of European origin retain high levels of the enzyme LPH which is a trait called the lactase persistence phenotype. In such case, levels of lactase retained are about half the amount of other saccharidases. Lactose intolerance is not common among children before the age of six (Mahan & Raymond, 2017; Robayo-Torres & Nichols, 2007).

ETIOLOGY AND PATHOPHYSIOLOGY

There are three types of lactose intolerance: primary, secondary, and congenital. Figure 1 is a mind map that shows the etiology, pathophysiology, symptoms and medical nutrition therapy (MNT) of lactose intolerance. Primary lactose intolerance, also called adult hypolactasia, is the most common, and it is the decline of lactase or LPH synthesis after infancy (Deng, Misselwitz, Dai, & Fox, 2015; Mahan & Raymond, 2017; Swagerty, Walling, & Klein, 2002). This type is closely related to ethnicity and increasing age (Mayo Clinic Organization, 2020). In other words, the activity of LPH is known to be low before 24 weeks of gestation, and then it increases during the third trimester to reach levels that are comparable to infants' levels who are at the age of two to eleven months. After this phase, the genetic makeup determines what happens next. In most of the cases, the activity of this enzyme starts to decrease at ages around five years, and this is categorized as lactase non-persistence phenotype. This type of lactose intolerance is characterized by low levels of lactase activity in the jejunum as well as poor proximal digestion of lactose.

A minority of individuals with non-persistent lactase have been reported to have defects in the intracellular processing of the produced lactase protein. On the other hand, the pathophysiology that occurs mostly relies on the LCT gene (also called lactase-glycosylceramidase) regulation; it is the gene that provides information for the synthesis of the enzyme lactase. In fact, adult hypolactasia is inherited in an autosomal recessive pattern which means these subjects must have two of the recessive alleles to show symptoms (Genetics Home Reference, 2020; Pray, 2000; Robayo-Torres & Nichols, 2007).

As mentioned earlier, the location of the lactase enzyme is on the outermost surface of the intestine, and therefore it is vulnerable to damage in case of any insult or injury occurring in the small intestine (Pray, 2000). Secondary lactose intolerance, also known as acquired hypolactasia, occurs as a result of other conditions affecting the intestinal tissue (Mahan & Raymond, 2017; Swagerty et al., 2002). This intestinal damage mainly affects either the amount of lactase or its activity time. In essence, the insult would leave insufficient intestinal surface to produce the required amount of lactase or would accelerate the gastrointestinal movement thus reducing the transit time (Pray, 2000). Conditions that result in secondary lactose intolerance include inflammatory diseases, malnutrition, celiac disease, sprue syndromes, and human immunodeficiency virus (HIV). In children, this type is commonly secondary to viral or bacterial infections. In addition, intestinal resections that would result in short bowel syndrome increase the intestinal passage rate and therefore might cause lactose intolerance. Moreover, chemotherapy, intestinal radiation and some medications such as antimetabolites and neomycin may induce secondary lactose intolerance. Regardless, further investigation for these individuals is required to determine the primary condition, and treating the underlying problem would help to achieve regeneration of the intestinal tissue in many of the secondary lactose intolerance cases, and lactase may return to pre-damage levels and thus improve lactose tolerance (Mahan & Raymond, 2017; Pray, 2000; Swagerty et al., 2002).

Finally, congenital lactose intolerance is a very severe inborn condition that is extremely rare, occurring mostly in Finland (Deng et al., 2015; Robayo-Torres & Nichols, 2007). This condition is caused by mutations in the LCT gene, thus interfering with the function of lactase, and mutations are inherited in an autosomal recessive pattern. Congenital lactose intolerance is characterized by an almost complete absence of lactase enzyme activity in the jejunum. The mucosa in the intestine shows normal structure and activity of the other disaccharidases. As mentioned above, lactase is essential during infancy to be able to digest lactose in breast milk or formula. Therefore, absence of lactase may result in severe dehydration, acidosis, and weight loss that can be fatal if not recognized and treated appropriately after birth. Usually, it is diagnosed at a mean age of 36 days. Following a lactose-restricted diet would alleviate symptoms, and consequently these infants will have the ability to grow and develop normally (Deng et al., 2015; Genetics Home Reference, 2020; Robayo-Torres & Nichols, 2007).

SIGNS AND SYMPTOMS

In the past 60 years, the clinical symptoms of lactose intolerance have been identified; before that, they were only described in a general sense (Morelli et al., 2019). Lactose intolerance is a condition that does not cause any discomfort unless dietary lactose is ingested (Mattar, de Campos Mazo, & Carrilho, 2012), and symptoms usually appear after 30 minutes to two hours from consuming lactose containing food (Mayo Clinic Organization, 2020). They are usually gut symptoms; however, there are studies suggesting that symptoms may not be restricted to only gastrointestinal problems but also systematic symptoms which include headache, muscle and joint pain, vertigo, urinary difficulties, sore throat, and cardiac arrhythmia (Deng et al., 2015; Mattar et al., 2012). In lactose intolerance, undigested lactose acts osmotically and increases the influx of fluids into the bowel lumen; this approximately triples the predicted intestinal tract volume as well as the fecal water content based on the sugar content osmolality (Deng et al., 2015; Swagerty et al., 2002). In addition, due to osmosis, the intestinal lumen dilates and thus accelerates the intestinal motility. Reducing the gastrointestinal transit time induces lactose maldigestion because it results in decreasing the contact time between lactose and the remaining lactase (Vesa et al., 2000).

After that, lactose passes into the colon, and it increases acidity in the colon (Mattar et al., 2012). The colonic microbiota ferment lactose into short chain fatty acids (SCFA's), carbon dioxide (CO2), hydrogen (H2), and methane (CH4). The fermentation process results in the cleavage of the sugar lactose into its constituent monosaccharides. Not only are these hydrolyzed simple sugars not absorbed by the mucosa in the colon, they also attract more fluids to the lumen. Consequently, gastrointestinal (GI) symptoms appear in intolerant individuals; symptoms of lactose intolerance include diarrhea, abdominal pain, flatulence, bloating, nausea, and borborygmi. There is conflicting evidence whether the origin of these symptoms is the small intestine or the colon; regardless, it is generally possible that symptoms originate from both intestinal and colonic conditions (Deng et al., 2015; Mahan & Raymond, 2017; Swagerty et al., 2002; Vesa et al., 2000). Normally, the stool in lactose intolerance would be described as foamy, watery, and voluminous. In some cases, constipation occurs possibly due to the production of methane as this gas may reduce the intestinal motility (Mattar et al., 2012).

The severity of symptoms varies depending on many factors; these include the amount of lactose ingested, the activity of the remaining lactase enzyme, the food ingested along with lactose, the ability to ferment lactose, and the sensitivity to lactose fermentation byproducts (Mahan & Raymond, 2017). Ethnicity and age also affect the severity of symptoms; for instance, older individuals are susceptible to more severe problems (Swagerty et al., 2002). As mentioned above, consuming other foods along with lactose may help reduce the severity of symptoms, and one way to explain that is the effect of food on the gastrointestinal emptying speed. For example, the presence of fat has been shown to slow gastric emptying; consequently, more time will be available for lactose to be in contact with intestinal lactase. Thus, delayed gastric emptying has been proposed to improve the digestion and tolerance of lactose. This correlation was reported in studies comparing full-fat with fat-free milk; however, other studies have shown no significant improvements (Vesa et al., 2000).

DIAGNOSIS

Lactose intolerance is preferred to be objectively diagnosed since half of the cases diagnosed subjectively proves to be false. This is because most of lactose intolerance symptoms can be confused with other gastrointestinal problems such as irritable bowel syndrome (IBS) or other food sensitivities that might induce similar symptoms as a result of ingestion of foods other than lactose. Therefore, lactose intolerance can be diagnosed by various methods, and the most invasive is intestinal biopsy. This test measures the lactase activity and the ratio of sucrase to lactase. This test is not in use anymore because lactase levels are poorly correlated to the appearance of symptoms; moreover, lactose intolerance is not considered a harmful nor severe disease so no need for such an invasive method (Mattar et al., 2012; Morelli et al., 2019). Lactose intolerance is currently most commonly diagnosed by either of two tests: lactose tolerance test or hydrogen breath test (Swagerty et al., 2002).

Lactose tolerance tests involve the ingestion of a specified oral dose of lactose, and blood glucose levels are measured before and after lactose administration at specific time intervals (Mattar et al., 2012). The lactose amount is roughly 1 to 1.5 gram per kilogram of body weight (Swagerty et al., 2002). Oral ethanol is given before the test to inhibit the metabolism of galactose which allows the determination of the test results. Maximum blood glucose rises of less than 20 mg/dL and galactose of less than 10 mg/dL indicate lactose intolerance. This indicates the inability to hydrolyze and absorb lactose in the intestine. Moreover, the measure of galactose along with glucose improves the connection between the test results and the lactase activity more than using the blood glucose level alone (Mattar et al., 2012). However, 20 percent of those tested get false results, whether positive or negative, due to variations in gastric emptying and metabolism (Swagerty et al., 2002).

Currently, the test that is considered the best for population screening of lactose intolerance is the hydrogen breath test (Mattar et al., 2012). The sensitivity and specificity of this test, which has become widely available, is more than the lactose tolerance test, and it is cost effective and non-invasive (Morelli et al., 2019; Swagerty et al., 2002). The hydrogen breath test is based on the principle of the fermentation of lactose by the colonic microbiota which produces gases including hydrogen along with other byproducts. It is believed that these gases get absorbed and excreted by the lungs (Mattar et al., 2012); thus, hydrogen can be detected in the pulmonary excretion after lactose ingestion to identify lactose intolerance. The test result reveals the amount of hydrogen eliminated through the lungs after ingesting a specific amount of lactose, approximately 25 to 50 g, and if the amount of hydrogen in the breath rises by 20 ppm or more over the baseline, it indicates deficiency of the lactase enzyme (Swagerty et al., 2002).

The reliability of the hydrogen breath test depends on various factors. For instance, the activity of the colonic microflora plays a significant role, and this can be affected by a recent use of antibiotics, high colonic acidity, or colonic adaptation to lactose due to continuous exposure. Any of the previous three conditions might cause false negative results (Mattar et al., 2012). There are other factors that are not related to lactose ingestion which may increase the hydrogen excretion such as smoking, sleeping, exercising, and using aspirin (Swagerty et al., 2002). In addition to that, the dosage of 50 g of lactose is equivalent to four or five cups of milk which is considered much more than a usual reasonable amount that might be ingested at once (Mattar et al., 2012). Therefore, a more physiologic and appropriate dose of 20 to 25 g of lactose was recommended to be used in the hydrogen breath test (Morelli et al., 2019).

MEDICAL NUTRITION THERAPY

There is no treatment that helps the body to synthesize more lactase enzyme (Mayo Clinic Organization, 2020). The main goal of the treatment in lactose intolerance should be to improve the gastrointestinal symptoms and not solely to reduce malabsorption (Deng et al., 2015). Managing symptoms of lactose intolerance requires changing in the diet; hence, patient education is a very crucial and useful part of the management protocol (Mahan & Raymond, 2017; Swagerty et al., 2002). At the initial phase, it is recommended to temporarily avoid dairy products that contain lactose; this restricted diet is followed with the aim of achieving remission of symptoms. Most lactose intolerant subjects tolerate up to 12 grams of lactose without experiencing significant gastrointestinal symptoms (Mattar et al., 2012). Table 1 shows lactose content in common foods that individuals can look out for. In addition, many medications contain lactose but rarely over 500 mg, so mostly they are well tolerated and won't need to be avoided (Escott-Stump, 2012).

A systematic review has shown that, in comparison to control subjects, symptoms did not significantly increase when ingesting less than 15 grams of lactose. A significant increase in symptoms was exhibited when participants consumed 20 grams or more. More severe symptoms were reported in tolerance testing involving the ingestion of 50 grams (Shaukat et al., 2010). However, it is difficult to quantify and gauge the contribution of a single food component, such as lactose, towards causing symptoms because there are other components in the food ingested, such as fat, that might cause similar gastrointestinal symptoms (Deng et al., 2015). Individuals with very low lactose tolerance should be informed about hidden sources of lactose; prepared food products, even though labeled as nondairy, sometimes contain ingredients that have lactose such as whipped toppings (Swagerty et al., 2002).

After the initial phase, it is recommended to gradually reintroduce lactose to the diet until achieving the patient's tolerance level. It is the individual threshold in which gastrointestinal symptoms appear (Mattar et al., 2012). Increments of the amount of lactose introduced can be achieved over several weeks; regular consumption of lactose containing food might increase the patient's threshold to diarrhea (Mahan & Raymond, 2017). To facilitate lactose tolerance, various measures can be taken such as distributing lactose consumption over the day instead of having it all at once (Mattar et al., 2012). Ingesting lactose with other foods has been shown to be associated with less symptoms. In addition, fermented dairy products are tolerated well among intolerant individuals; these products such as yogurt, sour cream, and aged cheese contain bacterial galactosidase which is an enzyme produced by the bacterial cultures in fermented food. Galactosidase facilitates the digestion of lactose in the intestine and therefore improves lactose tolerance. However, the processing method of foods affects the presence of galactosidase; due to its sensitivity to freezing, frozen yogurt might not be as tolerated as regular yogurt (Mahan & Raymond, 2017).

MEDICAL MANAGEMENT

There are pharmacological approaches that might aid in alleviating lactose intolerance symptoms. For instance, lactase enzyme supplements are available to help reduce gastrointestinal problems after lactose ingestion especially for patients with mild malabsorption, and these supplements can be in tablets or liquid forms. Milk products can be treated with lactase enzymes such as Lactaid. However, commercial variations in the preparation processes of these enzymes may affect their efficiency (Mahan

& Raymond, 2017; Swagerty et al., 2002). One double-blind placebo-controlled crossover study has reported that exogenous lactase obtained from Kluyveromyces lactis can be used as a valid therapeutic approach for lactose intolerant subjects and without side effects (Montalto et al., 2005). Nevertheless, patients must be aware that lactase supplements are an adjunct approach but not a substitute to the diet restriction as symptoms may not be totally relieved (Swagerty et al., 2002).

Another pharmacological strategy is the use of probiotics, and it is based on the principle of altering the intestinal microbiota. One study showed that consumption of the probiotics, Lactobacillus casei Shirota and Bifidobacterium breve Yakult, reduced lactose intolerance gastrointestinal symptoms. Subjects were consuming these probiotics for four weeks, and the effects stayed for three months or more after suspension. On the other hand, another study involved self-reported lactose intolerant participants who consumed milk that contains Lactobacillus acidophilus, but this study did not show any positive effects regarding alleviating the symptoms in comparison to the control subjects (Deng et al., 2015). A systematic review reported that the relationship between probiotics and lactose intolerance is overall positive with varying degrees of effectiveness (Oak & Jha, 2019). However, other studies conducted on the efficacy of probiotics to alleviate lactose intolerance symptoms have shown conflicting results, and the role is still uncertain (Mattar et al., 2012). Therefore, further studies are required to provide strong evidence in order to support probiotics' pharmacologic effect.

CALCIUM AND VITAMIN D

Calcium is a crucial nutrient for the development of the human skeletal system and also for the protection from osteoporosis which is a disease that involves thinning of the bones. Osteoporosis is considered a major public health problem. The major dietary source of calcium is dairy products, and one serving of milk, cheese, or yogurt provides 300 mg of calcium (Deng et al., 2015; Jackson & Savaiano, 2001). Generally, the dietary calcium recommendation for adolescents and young adults is 1200 to 1500 mg per day, and for adults, the amount depends on two factors which are gender and menopausal status (Mattar et al., 2012). Subjects who self-reported lactose intolerance tend to obsessively restrict other unrelated food elements along with lactose due to their general anxiety about their health. This is considered stressful and negatively affect their quality of life and could result in malnutrition (Deng et al., 2015). One study revealed that participants who perceived themselves to be lactose intolerant experienced self-imposed dairy restrictions that were correlated with lower spinal bone mineral content values; in the long term, this might be associated with higher risk of osteoporosis (Matlik et al., 2007).

It is considered a logical and reasonable approach to recommend individuals who restrict dairy intake to increase their consumption of calcium through other dietary sources or supplements especially if they are at risk of osteoporosis (Deng et al., 2015). So, calcium should be supplemented if required (Mattar et al., 2012). However, recent evidence suggests that lactose intolerant patients can achieve the amount of dairy recommended by the American Dietetic Association without experiencing symptoms (Swagerty et al., 2002). The 2015–2020 Dietary Guidelines for Americans recommend adults to consume 3 servings of dairy per day (HHS & USDA, 2015). Following the measures mentioned in the paragraphs above that enhance lactose tolerance such as the gradual introduction and repeated consumption of lactose might aid in achieving this recommended amount of daily servings. In addition, the Dietary Guidelines for Americans suggests the use of lactose free dairy products as well as fortified soy beverages as substitutes (Hodges, Cao, Cladis, & Weaver, 2019).

In addition, vitamin D is required for healthy bone mineralization and calcium absorption. Its metabolite, 1,25$(OH)_2$-D-3, acts as a hormone in the human body to regulate calcium and phosphate metabolism. Vitamin D has been shown to be crucial for the development of muscles as well. In the United Sates, the Recommended Dietary Allowance (RDA) of vitamin D for both males and females between the age of 9 to 70 years is 600 IU per day (Itkonen, Erkkola, & Lamberg-Allardt, 2018; Schmid & Walther, 2013). While vitamin D is naturally found in limited food choices mainly of animal origin such as oily fish and oils from fish, exposure to sunlight is considered a major source (Holick & Chen, 2008). However, most activities nowadays are carried indoors, thus preventing sufficient exposure to sunlight. Although most non-fortified dairy products contain low amounts of vitamin D, there are countries like the United States, Canada, and Finland that placed a national policy for milk fortification. This approach has been shown to contribute to the 25(OH)D status and vitamin D intake (Itkonen et al., 2018; Schmid & Walther, 2013). Therefore, monitoring of vitamin D intake among lactose intolerant individuals is crucial, and supplementation might be required (Mattar et al., 2012).

LACTOSE INTOLERANCE AND OTHER DISEASES

Cow's milk allergy and lactose intolerance can be confusing for many people; however, these two terms cannot be used interchangeably because they are two distinct conditions. The main difference from lactose intolerance is that cow's milk allergy involves the immune system, and it is an immunological reaction against the protein in milk. There are two types of cow's milk allergy: immunoglobulin E (IgE) and non-IgE mediated milk allergy. The latter is the one that often be mistakenly confused with lactose intolerance; its symptoms are delayed which means that they occur after up to 48 hours of milk exposure. However, the IgE mediated symptoms usually appear immediately. Symptoms of milk allergy involves not only gastrointestinal symptoms as is the case in lactose intolerance but also skin or respiratory symptoms as well. The management of milk allergy requires exclusion of all cow's milk and it its products from the diet (diet free from cow's milk protein) (Walsh, Meyer, Shah, Quekett, & Fox, 2016).

There is conflicting evidence regarding the association between lactose digestion ability and the risk of diseases. For instance, it has been proposed that ingesting milk in individuals with lactase persistence is correlated with increasing the risk of cataract formation. This was shown in humans who have congenital defect in the metabolism of galactose which is a substantial decrease or even absence of the hepatic galactokinase. Diabetes was suggested to act as an accelerating factor in this mechanism. Nevertheless, there are other studies that disproved the existence of this relationship. In addition, ovarian cancer has also been linked to lactose digestion; this correlation is based on the suggestion that galactose is considered a toxin to the oocytes. However, as in the case of cataract formation, opposing studies have shown the lack of this relationship between galactose consumption and ovarian cancer (Vesa et al., 2000).

SETTING THE STAGE

The data of this case study were collected from a gastroenterology clinic in a private hospital in Jeddah, Saudi Arabia. The case was evaluated and medically managed by a specialized gastroenterologist, and the patient was referred to a dietitian for nutrition assessment and intervention. Appropriate diet prescription and recommendations were delivered to the patient to help alleviate lactose intolerance symptoms. The patient did not receive any financial support to report the case in this chapter; therefore, there was no conflict of interest.

CASE DESCRIPTION

Patient's Details

- Age: 22 years old
- Gender: Female

Case History

Case description: The patient is in her last year in college, and she has been suffering from recurrent abdominal cramps and diarrhea after meals that is starting to affect her academic performance. Last week, she went to her friend's party and enjoyed her time. Unfortunately, after one hour of eating dinner, she had to leave due to discomfort and pain. She had eaten steak and mac-and-cheese, and she ended the meal with a large cup of vanilla ice-cream milkshake. She experienced abdominal pain that reached a new peak, and she had watery diarrhea more than three times a day that lasted for three days. Moreover, she started to have headaches frequently. Although her appetite did not change, she lost 3 kg in the last month. The patient couldn't tolerate more, so she visited a gastroenterologist After asking her about her complains, the doctor suspected a digestive problem: irritable bowel syndrome or other food sensitivities. Thus, he performed medical investigations that included the hydrogen breath test and lactose tolerance test. Results indicated her diagnosis with lactose intolerance.

- Medical history: medically free
- Surgical history: Laparoscopic Ovarian Cyst Removal
- Smoking: nonsmoker
- Family history: Mother is diabetic, and father is hypertensive.

Main Medical Diagnosis

Lactose Intolerance

Demographics

- Marital status: single - lives with her mother, father, and two siblings
- Education: graduating from college this year - majoring in computer science
- Occupation: student
- Ethnicity and religion: Asian and Muslim

Anthropometry

- Current weight: 57 kg
- Admission weight: 57.3 kg
- Usual body weight (UBW): 60 kg
- Height: 160 cm

Table 1. Biochemical Data

Parameter	Patients Results	Reference
Albumin	5.5 g/dL	3.5-5.0 g/dL
Total Protein	8.3 g/dL	6.4-8.3 g/dL
Blood Urea Nitrogen (BUN)	22 mg/dL	10-20 mg/dL
Creatinine (Cr)	1 mg/dL	0.5-1.1 mg/dL
Calcium (Ca)	7.5 mg/dL	9.0-10.5 mg/dL
Magnesium (Mg)	0.6 mmol/L	0.65-1.05 mmol/L
Sodium (Na)	135 mmol/L	136-145 mmol/L
Chloride (Cl)	100 mmol/L	98-106 mmol/L
Potassium (K)·	3.3 mmol/L·	3.5-5.0 mmol/L·

Nutritional-Focused Physical Examination

- General appearance: normal weight, 22 years old female, pale looking
- Vital Signs: pulse 85 BPM, temperature 37.1 C^0, blood pressure 117/80 mm Hg, respiratory rate 15 BPM
- Skin, hair, and nails: dry skin, normal hair and nails
- HEENT: normal
- Cardiopulmonary system: regular heart rate, normal sound, and clear chest
- Extremities, muscles, and bones: no edema, normal strength
- Digestive system: bloated abdomen
- Nerves and cognition: oriented and alert

Food/Nutrition-Related History

Patient states that she has a good appetite, and she consumes 3 meals and 1-2 snacks per day. She reports eating a variety of fruits, vegetables, grains, proteins, and dairy sources. She drinks around two liters of water daily, and she walks for 30 minutes three days a week. She is complaining of watery diarrhea, flatulence, and abdominal pain especially after meals. In the past month, she lost 3 kg of her usual body weight.

- Food allergies/intolerances: Diagnosed Lactose Intolerance
- Food purchase/preparations: She frequently uses condensed milk with coffee and tea and in preparing sweets.
- Vitamin and mineral supplementation: not applicable

Table 2. 24-Hour Recall

Time	Food Items and Quantities
8:00 am	1 cup of cornflakes with 1 cup of milk; 1 tbsp honey; ½ cup of strawberries
12:00 pm	1 blueberry muffin; 3 scoops of vanilla ice-cream
3:00 pm	1 beef cheeseburger; ½ cup of fried potato fries
8:00 pm	1 medium turkey and cheese sandwich; 1 orange; 1 cup of tea
11:30 pm·	6 oz fried chicken; 1 cup of bulgur salad; 1 cup of creamy pasta·

Medications (If Any)

Not applicable

Nutritional Management

Disease Pathophysiology and Management Mind Map

Figure 1. Lactose Intolerance etiology, pathophysiology, symptoms and medical nutrition therapy mind map.
Developed by Khalifa, N 2020

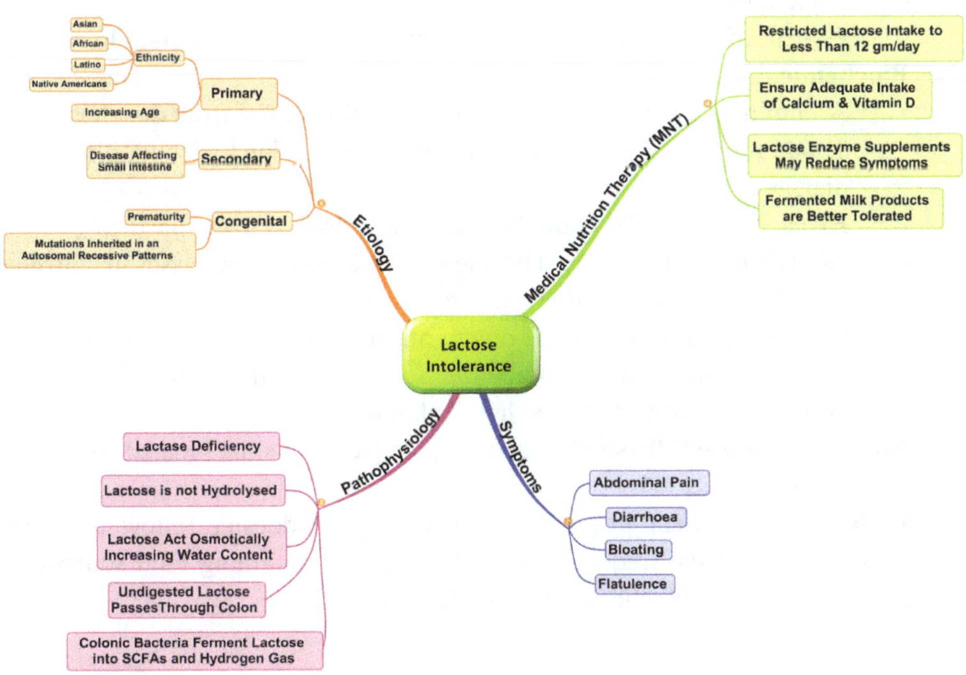

Main Aim of the Nutrition Therapy

Reduce and control intake of lactose containing food to alleviate symptoms. However, as mentioned above, strict avoidance of all dairy products is not necessary as most maldigesters tolerate up to 12g of lactose (the amount equivalent to a cup of milk).

Maintain sufficient intakes of calcium and vitamin D from non-lactose foods and other approaches especially for pregnant women and children and may consider supplement use if required.

ADIME Note

Assessment: The patient is a 22-year-old female patient diagnosed with lactose intolerance, and she has been complaining of recurrent abdominal cramps and diarrhea after meals.

- **Anthropometry:**
    - Weight: 57 kg
    - Height: 160 cm
    - Body Mass Index (BMI): 22.3 kg/m2 (normal weight)
    - Ideal Body Weight (IBW): 52.3 kg
    - Usual Body Weight (UBW): 60 kg
    - Percent of UBW: 95% (not at risk)
    - Percent of Weight change: 5% in 1 month (significant weight loss)
- **Biochemical:**
    - Albumin: 5.5 g/dL (H) could be due to dehydration from diarrhea
    - Total Protein: 8.3 g/dL (borderline H) could be due to dehydration from diarrhea
    - BUN: 22 mg/dL (H) could be due to dehydration from diarrhea
    - Na: 135 mmol/L (L) could be due to increased sodium losses in diarrhea
    - K: 3.3 mmol/L (L) could be due to diarrhea
    - Ca: 7.5 mg/dL (L) could be due to malabsorption in lactose intolerance
    - Mg: 0.6 mmol/L (L) could be due to malabsorption, excessive loss of body fluids in diarrhea, and hypokalemia
- **Nutrition-Focused Physical Findings:** pale face, dry skin, bloated abdomen, and headache
- **Dietary:** The patient has a good appetite. She doesn't follow any diet restrictions, and she frequently includes lactose-containing food sources in her diet such as milk, cheese, and condensed milk.

Diagnosis

Altered GI function (NC[1]-1.4[2]) related to diagnosis of lactose intolerance as evidenced by watery diarrhea, bloated abdomen, and abnormal lactose tolerance test.

Impaired nutrient utilization (NC[1]-2.1[3]) related to intestinal malabsorption due to lactose intolerance diagnosis as evidenced by watery diarrhea and low levels of Ca (7.5 mg/dL), Mg (0.6 mmol/L), Na (135 mmol/L), and K (3.3 mmol/L).

Altered nutrition-related laboratory values (Albumin and BUN) (NC[1]-2.2[4]) related to dehydration due to impaired intestinal absorption as evidenced by recurrent watery diarrhea and high levels of Albumin (5.5 g/dL) and BUN (22 mg/dL).

Unintended weight loss (NC[1]-3.2[5]) related to intestinal malabsorption due to lactose intolerance diagnosis as evidenced by significant weight loss with 5% loss of the usual body weight in the past month.

Intervention

- **Diet Prescription:** Lactose Restricted Diet, 1750 kcal/d, 80 g/d CHON, 250 g/d Carbohydrates, 50 g/d Fat, 2,000 mL/d Fluids
- **Energy:**
  - Using Harris-Benedict (UBW): 1,329 kcal/d with Activity Factor: 1.3 (ambulatory) = 1,727 kcal/d
  - Using Normal Energy Requirements (UBW): 25-30 kcal/kg/d = 1,500 - 1,800 kcal/d
- **Carbohydrates:**
  - 45-65% of total energy intake = 787.5-1,137 kcal/d = 197-284 g/d
- **Protein:**
  - Normal maintenance: 0.8-1 g/kg/d = 48-60 g/d
  - 10-35% of total energy intake: 175-612 kcal/d = 44-153 g/d
- Fat: 20-35% of total energy intake: 350-612 kcal/d = 39-68 g/d
- Fluid: Average adult Requirement: 30-35 mL/kg/d = 1,800-2100 mL/d

Recommendations

- Initially restrict lactose consumption from food such as milk to less than 12 g/d (depending on tolerance), and then after remission, gradually reintroduce as tolerated until achieving the patient's threshold.
- To improve tolerance, let the patient try lactose with other foods and try to distribute its consumption over the day.
- Educate the patient about reading food labels to distinguish lactose in food products and the hidden sources as well.

- Encourage the patient to use lactose-free food products as alternatives.
- Encourage the patient to consume calcium and vitamin D from non-lactose containing foods and fortified products, and to ensure adequate sunlight exposure for vitamin D.
- Consider calcium and vitamin D supplements if needed.
- Let the patient try fermented milk products (such as yogurt, kefir, laban, labneh, sour cream, cottage cheese and aged cheese) as they are better tolerated due to their low amounts of lactose.
- Educate the patient to replace fluid losses by using Oral Rehydration Solution (ORS) for a few days and by drinking sufficient amounts of fluids every day.

Monitoring/Evaluation

- Monitor GI symptoms (such as diarrhea and abdominal pain)
- Control weight change (to ensure no further weight loss)
- Monitor lab results (such as Albumin, Total Protein, Blood Urea Nitrogen, Na, K, Ca, Mg)
- Monitor dietary intake (adherence to the prescribed plan)

REFERENCES

American Dietetic Association. (2011). *International Dietetics and Nutrition Terminology (IDNT) Reference Manual: Standardized Language for the Nutrition Care Process*. American Dietetic Association.

Deng, Y., Misselwitz, B., Dai, N., & Fox, M. (2015). Lactose Intolerance in Adults: Biological Mechanism and Dietary Management. *Nutrients*, *7*(9), 8020–8035. doi:10.3390/nu7095380 PMID:26393648

Escott-Stump, S. (2012). Nutrition and Diagnosis-Related Care (7th ed.). Wolters Kluwer: Lippincott Williams & Wilkins.

Genetics Home Reference. (2020). *Lactose Intolerance*. Retrieved from https://ghr.nlm.nih.gov/condition/lactose-intolerance

HHS & USDA. (2015). *Dietary guidelines for Americans 2015-2020* (8th ed.). Government Printing Office.

Hodges, J. K., Cao, S., Cladis, D. P., & Weaver, C. M. (2019). Lactose Intolerance and Bone Health: The Challenge of Ensuring Adequate Calcium Intake. *Nutrients, 11*(4), 718. Advance online publication. doi:10.3390/nu11040718 PMID:30925689

Holick, M. F., & Chen, T. C. (2008). Vitamin D deficiency: A worldwide problem with health consequences. *The American Journal of Clinical Nutrition, 87*(4), 1080s–1086s. doi:10.1093/ajcn/87.4.1080S PMID:18400738

Itkonen, S. T., Erkkola, M., & Lamberg-Allardt, C. J. E. (2018). Vitamin D Fortification of Fluid Milk Products and Their Contribution to Vitamin D Intake and Vitamin D Status in Observational Studies-A Review. *Nutrients, 10*(8), 1054. Advance online publication. doi:10.3390/nu10081054 PMID:30096919

Jackson, K. A., & Savaiano, D. A. (2001). Lactose maldigestion, calcium intake and osteoporosis in African-, Asian-, and Hispanic-Americans. *Journal of the American College of Nutrition, 20*(2, Suppl), 198s–207s. doi:10.1080/07315724.2001.10719032 PMID:11349943

Mahan, L. K., & Raymond, J. L. (2017). *Krause's Food and the Nutrition Care Process* (14th ed.). Elsevier.

Matlik, L., Savaiano, D., McCabe, G., VanLoan, M., Blue, C. L., & Boushey, C. J. (2007). Perceived milk intolerance is related to bone mineral content in 10- to 13-year-old female adolescents. *Pediatrics, 120*(3), e669–e677. doi:10.1542/peds.2006-1240 PMID:17766507

Mattar, R., de Campos Mazo, D. F., & Carrilho, F. J. (2012). Lactose intolerance: Diagnosis, genetic, and clinical factors. *Clinical and Experimental Gastroenterology, 5*, 113–121. doi:10.2147/CEG.S32368 PMID:22826639

Mayo Clinic Organization. (2020). *Lactose Intolerance*. Retrieved May 26, 2020, from https://www.mayoclinic.org/diseases-conditions/lactose-intolerance/symptoms-causes/syc-20374232

Montalto, M., Nucera, G., Santoro, L., Curigliano, V., Vastola, M., Covino, M., Cuoco, L., Manna, R., Gasbarrini, A., & Gasbarrini, G. (2005). Effect of exogenous β-galactosidase in patients with lactose malabsorption and intolerance: A crossover double-blind placebo-controlled study. *European Journal of Clinical Nutrition, 59*(4), 489–493. doi:10.1038j.ejcn.1602098 PMID:15674309

Morelli, L., Amrani, N., Goulet, O., & Lukito, W. (2019). Lactose Intolerance: Clinical Symptoms, Diagnosis and Treatment. *Global Dabetes Open Access Journal, 1*(1), 1–10.

Oak, S. J., & Jha, R. (2019). The effects of probiotics in lactose intolerance: A systematic review. *Critical Reviews in Food Science and Nutrition*, *59*(11), 1675–1683. doi:10.1080/10408398.2018.1425977 PMID:29425071

Pray, W. (2000). Lactose Intolerance: The Norm Among the World's Peoples. *American Journal of Pharmaceutical Education*, *64*, 205–207.

Robayo-Torres, C. C., & Nichols, B. L. (2007). Molecular Differentiation of Congenital Lactase Deficiency from Adult-Type Hypolactasia. *Nutrition Reviews*, *65*(2), 95–98. doi:10.1111/j.1753-4887.2007.tb00286.x PMID:17345962

Schmid, A., & Walther, B. (2013). Natural Vitamin D Content in Animal Products. *Advances in Nutrition*, *4*(4), 453–462. doi:10.3945/an.113.003780 PMID:23858093

Shaukat, A., Levitt, M., Taylor, B., MacDonald, R., Shamliyan, T., Kane, R., & Wilt, T. (2010). Systematic Review: Effective Management Strategies for Lactose Intolerance. *Annals of Internal Medicine*, *152*(12), 797–803. doi:10.7326/0003-4819-152-12-201006150-00241 PMID:20404262

Swagerty, D., Walling, A., & Klein, R. (2002). Lactose Intolerance. *American Family Physician*, *65*(9), 1845–1851. PMID:12018807

Vesa, T. H., Marteau, P., & Korpela, R. (2000). Lactose Intolerance. *Journal of the American College of Nutrition, 19*(sup2), 165S-175S. doi:10.1080/07315724.2000.10718086

Walsh, J., Meyer, R., Shah, N., Quekett, J., & Fox, A. T. (2016). Differentiating Milk Allergy (IgE and Non-IgE Mediated) from Lactose Intolerance: Understanding the Underlying Mechanisms and Presentations. *The British Journal of General Practice*, *66*(649), e609–e611. doi:10.3399/bjgp16X686521 PMID:27481986

KEY TERMS AND DEFINITIONS

Diarrhea: It is defined by the World Health Organization as the passage of loose or liquid stool for three or more times per day (or more frequent than what is normal for the individual).

Gene Mutation: It is an alteration in the sequence of the deoxyribonucleic acid (DNA) that makes up a gene.

Hydrogen Breath Test: It is a diagnostic test that is specific and sensitive to diagnose carbohydrate malabsorption or small intestine bacterial overgrowth.

Lactase: It is the enzyme responsible to digest and hydrolyze lactose, the sugar in milk, into glucose and galactose.

Lactose Tolerance Test: It is a diagnostic test that reveals the body's ability to break down lactose; that if lactose is digested and absorbed, this will result in rise of blood sugar.

Oral Rehydration Solution (ORS): It is a fluid that contains glucose and salts used to replace fluid losses and correct dehydration as in the case of diarrhea.

Preterm Infant: It is an infant born before the completion of 37 weeks of gestation.

Short Chain Fatty Acids (SCFA's): They are produced by the intestinal microbiota in the fermentation process (e.g., acetic, butyric, and propionic acids).

ENDNOTES

1 NC refers to the Clinical domain in the Nutrition Diagnostic Terminology, and it is defined as "nutritional findings/problems identified that relate to medical or physical conditions." (American Dietetic Association, 2011)

2 This number is the code of the problem inside the Clinical domain in which number 1 refers to Functional defined as "change in physical of mechanical functioning that refers with or prevents desired nutritional consequences." Number 4 refers to the problem (altered GI function). (American Dietetic Association, 2011)

3 This number is the code of the problem inside the Clinical domain in which number 2 refers to Biochemical defined as "change in capacity to metabolize nutrients as a result of medications, surgery, or as indicated by altered lab values." Number 1 refers to the problem (impaired nutrient utilization). (American Dietetic Association, 2011)

4 This number is the code of the problem inside the Clinical domain in which number 2 refers to Biochemical defined as "change in capacity to metabolize nutrients as a result of medications, surgery, or as indicated by altered lab values." Number 2 refers to the problem (altered nutrition0related laboratory values). (American Dietetic Association, 2011)

5 This number is the code of the problem inside the Clinical domain in which number 3 refers to Weight defined as "chronic weight or changed weight status when compared with usual or desired body weight." Number 2 refers to the problem (unintended weight loss). (American Dietetic Association, 2011)

APPENDIX 1

Table 3. Lactose content in common foods

Food Product	Serving Size	Estimated Lactose Content
Milk	1 cup	10-12 g
Cheese	1 once	0-2 g
Heavy Cream	½ cup	3-4 g
Evaporated Milk	1 cup	24 g
Ice cream	½ cup	6 g
Nonfat dry milk powder	1 cup	62 g
Sweetened condensed milk	1 cup	40 g
Yogurt	1 cup	5-10 g

(Data Source: Mahan & Raymond, 2017)

APPENDIX 2: ABBREVIATIONS

BMI: Body Mass Index
BUN: Blood Urea Nitrogen
Ca: Calcium
Cl: Chloride
Cr: Creatinine
GI: gastrointestinal
HIV: human immunodeficiency virus
IBS: irritable bowel syndrome
IBW: Ideal Body Weight
IgE: immunoglobulin E
K: Potassium
Kg: Kilogram
LPH: lactase-phlorizin hydrolase
Mg: Magnesium
MNT: medical nutrition therapy
Na: Sodium
ORS: Oral Rehydration Solution
Oz: Ounce
RDA: Recommended Dietary Allowance
SCFA's: short chain fatty acids
Tbsp: tablespoon
UBW: Usual Body Weight

Chapter 7
Inflammatory Bowel Diseases (Crohn's Disease)

Sarah Ajabnoor
King Abdulaziz University, Saudi Arabia

Hebah Khayat
King Abdulaziz University Hospital, Saudi Arabia

EXECUTIVE SUMMARY

The case study presented in this chapter is related to Crohn's disease (CD). CD is a type of inflammatory bowel diseases (IBD) affecting both small and large bowels. Several factors are involved in the aetiopathogenesis of CD. Individuals diagnosed with CD will typically experience periods of relapse and remission. Therefore, the main aim of medical therapy in CD is to induce and maintain remission. The case presented in this chapter will demonstrate the role of medical nutrition therapy in a recently diagnosed patient with CD who was admitted with abdominal pain for 6 weeks and acute flare for the disease, which is complicated by weight loss. Overall, the case study will assist the practice of clinical dietitians who are dealing with IBD patients. Mainly, it will allow them to assess the symptoms and associated nutritional complications of CD, and develop a nutrition support intervention plan. Also, it will support the process of patient's education for dietary modification to help alleviate the symptoms in CD.

DOI: 10.4018/978-1-7998-3802-9.ch007

INTRODUCTION

Inflammatory bowel disease (IBD), including Crohn's Disease (CD) and ulcerative colitis (UC), are chronic inflammatory conditions primarily mediated by the immune response. Compared to UC, CD can affect any part of the gastrointestinal tract and is characterized by a discontinuous and transmural (all layers of the intestinal mucosa are affected) pattern of inflammation. The inflammation in CD can be stricturing and penetrating, and can also be associated with fistula and abscess formation. Patients with a confirmed diagnosis of CD will usually experience periods of relapse and remission. The treatment of CD depends on the disease activity and location. The main goal of medical therapy in CD is to induce and maintain the state of remission, restore the damaged mucosa, and improve the patient's overall quality of life. However, in cases where the disease is complicated and advanced, surgical intervention is required. The disease imposes a considerable burden on the quality of life of patients (i.e. frequent hospitalizations, surgery, and work productivity). The incidence and prevalence of CD varies around the globe. The incidence rate of CD is considered to be the highest in western countries (Ashwin N Ananthakrishnan, 2015). However, over the last few decades, the epidemiological trends in CD have altered substantially. The incidence rate for CD is increasing in Western populations as well as in non-Western populations living in Asia. Countries like Japan, Hong Kong, Korea, and Saudi Arabia have all reported a rising incidence rate of the disease (Al-Mofarreh & Al-Mofleh, 2013; Ashwin N Ananthakrishnan, 2015).

The cause of CD is complicated and thought to be multifactorial. The interaction between environmental triggers, genetic predisposition, gut microbiome, and host immune response may contribute to the aetiology and pathophysiology of CD. The risk of CD has been linked with several environmental factors which include: smoking, vitamin D deficiency, infections, the use of certain drugs (e.g. antibiotics, nonsteroidal anti-inflammatory drugs (NSAIDs), and oral contraceptives), exposure to early life factors (i.e. breastfeeding), and diet. The role of diet in the disease's pathogenesis is still evolving. Alterations in the composition of intestinal microbiome and gut barrier functions, the presence of antigens, enhancing immune response, over nutrition, and the modification of prostaglandin are all possible mechanisms of action that could support the role of diet in CD incidence (Hou, Abraham, & El-Serag, 2011). A Western diet, reduced fruit and vegetable intake, and the intake of certain food additives are all suggested dietary risk factors for CD. A high intake of sugar and dietary fat is generally correlated with a high risk of CD, while a high intake of fruit, vegetables and fibre is associated with a protective effect against CD (Hou et al., 2011). Regarding the role of dietary fat, studies have shown that a high intake of omega-3 polyunsaturated fatty acids is correlated with a low risk of ulcerative colitis but not CD, while the consumption of trans fats could increase the disease risk (Ananthakrishnan et al., 2014). However, the dietary intake of fibre (24 g per day) was found to be correlated with up to a 40% reduction in the incidence rate of CD (Ananthakrishnan et al., 2013).

Generally, the location and extent of CD will influence the severity of the symptoms. Commonly reported CD symptoms include: diarrhoea resulting from malabsorption, abdominal pain, rectal bleeding, fever, fatigue, reduced oral intake, and weight loss (Veauthier & Hornecker, 2018). In chronic and severe cases, the disease can be complicated by fistula (abnormal opening between the skin and internal organs), intestinal obstruction (resulting from the thickened intestinal wall due to swelling and development of scar tissues), and abscess formation. The inflammatory burden of CD can affect other organs (not including the gastrointestinal tract), leading to extraintestinal manifestations. Some CD patients present with conditions like anaemia, joint arthritis, eye conditions (i.e. uveitis, iritis, episcleritis), and skin conditions (i.e. erythema nodosum, and pyoderma gangrenosum) (Veauthier & Hornecker, 2018). In paediatric patients, CD can result in growth failure.

CD diagnosis is usually based on several key findings. A combination of clinical, laboratory, radiological, endoscopic, and pathological findings can confirm the final diagnosis of the condition. Radiological imaging and endoscopic studies will help to identify the severity and extent of the disease. Overall, the findings from these investigations will guide gastroenterologists with regard to the management of CD. Clinical diagnostic tools are used to assess the activity of the disease (e.g. Crohn's Disease Activity Index (CDAI) is one of the widely used clinical assessment tool) (Walsh, Bryant, & Travis, 2016). Generally, CD diagnostic scoring tools are usually based on subjective and objective data, which include the patient's symptoms, quality of life, presence of fatigue, levels of biomarkers (i.e. C-reactive protein (CRP) and faecal calprotectin), and disease severity level (e.g. history of intestinal resection, relapse rate, and occurrence of extraintestinal manifestations) (Peyrin-Biroulet et al., 2016; Walsh et al., 2016).

The medical management of CD is considered challenging. The main goal of treatment in CD is to induce and maintain remission, achieve mucosal healing, and improve quality of life by reducing the negative outcomes of the disease. Typically, the decision regarding therapy will depend on the patient's condition and the severity of the disease. Over the past several years, many types of medications have been used to treat CD patients, which include steroids, immunomodulators, biologics, and 5-aminosalicylic containing agents (Veauthier & Hornecker, 2018). To manage the symptoms, corticosteroids are commonly used, but these are associated with many side effects, which make them less effective for maintaining remission. However, immunomodulators and biologics are considered effective in inducing remission (Veauthier & Hornecker, 2018). Surgical intervention is indicated for patients with advanced CD and who are resistant to medical therapy. About half of CD patients will need surgical intervention within the first 10 years of their diagnosis (Frolkis et al., 2013).

There are several factors related to disease symptoms, complications, medical therapy, and management plan that can affect the nutritional status of CD patients. Malnutrition in CD is mainly caused by the presence of weight loss, anorexia, nutrient malabsorption, nutrient loss from the intestines, medication interactions, and intestinal resections (Jansen, Prager, Valentini, & Büning, 2016). Malnutrition is commonly reported in CD patients. In active CD, malnutrition is associated with a high rate of morbidity and mortality (Norman, Pichard, Lochs, & Pirlich, 2008). Thus, the role of medical nutrition therapy (MNT) in CD management is considered very important. Generally, the aims of MNT in CD are to restore and maintain nutritional status, help in inducing and maintaining remission, manage symptoms, and probably decrease the inflammatory response.

Restoring and maintaining the nutritional status in malnourished CD individuals can be achieved via appropriate nutrition support practice, which involves the provision of oral nutritional supplements (ONS), enteral nutrition (EN), or parenteral nutrition (PN). The decision regarding the most appropriate route of nutrition support in CD patients can be complex and challenging. Nutrition support dietitians should be able to determine the patient's ability to tolerate oral intake, determine the intestinal absorptive capacity, assess the patient's nutritional status, and establish treatment goals. ONS is usually the first choice for delivering nutrition support. It is recommended that up to 600 kcal/day can be provided by ONS in addition to the normal oral intake (Bischoff et al., 2020). For patients unable to tolerate oral intake and with a functioning gut, EN via tube feeding is considered. EN can be provided partially (supplementary to normal food intake) or exclusively (food intake is completely excluded). Enteral nutritional supplements used by CD patients can be either polymeric (whole protein-based), elemental (amino acid-based), or semi-elemental (peptide-based). Due to their palatability, polymeric formulae have been more favoured by patients, resulting in high compliance with EN. However, there remains no valid recommendation regarding the selection of the appropriate EN feed composition in CD (Di Caro et al., 2019). Recent studies have shown no differences in the incidence rates of remission and adverse effects between the three types of enteral feeds (Narula et al., 2018). In paediatric patients with CD, EN has been recommended as the primary therapy for inducing remission (Di Caro et al., 2019). However, in adult patients, the use of EN to induce remission is less effective than corticosteroids. It is suggested that EN should be indicated for: paediatric patients, adults who find the feeds palatable and are able to take them orally with good compliance, adults who can tolerate an enteral tube, or when corticosteroid therapy is not well tolerated by the patient (Narula et al., 2018). The mechanism of action of EN in CD has not yet been fully explained. Modulating the gut inflammatory response and microbiome are suggested mechanisms of action that have been investigated by several studies (Di Caro et al., 2019). In cases where the gastrointestinal tract is poorly functioning (e.g. intestinal obstruction where an enteral tube cannot be inserted, short bowel syndrome leading to a high degree of malabsorption, and the presence of high output intestinal fistula), total or supplementary PN is indicated. PN is administered via central or peripheral line, depending on the duration of the treatment. Generally, PN is not recommended as a first line of therapy in CD patients (Van Gossum et al., 2009). The management of PN can be complex and challenging. PN monitoring should be appropriately managed and closely evaluated in malnourished CD patients who are at a high risk of developing metabolic and electrolytes imbalances (refeeding syndrome) (Alastair, Emma, & Emma, 2011). When applied, PN can improve the quality of life of CD malnourished patients by restoring their nutritional status and preventing the complications associated with malnutrition.

Assessing the energy and macronutrient requirements in CD patients is considered one of the goals of medical nutrition therapy for restoring and maintaining nutritional status. In CD, the total energy requirements are generally considered similar to those of healthy individuals (Bischoff et al., 2020). However, patients with significant weight loss who are severely malnourished should be carefully monitored before any nutritional plan is initiated to avoid the risk of refeeding syndrome. For such patients, the feeding protocol should be adjusted, aiming to start with a lower rate of caloric intake (25-50% of the estimated energy requirements) and closely monitored before reaching the higher goal of the estimated energy requirements (Boullata et al., 2009; Eiden, 2003). For protein requirements, 1-1.5 g/kg/day is generally recommended, depending on the activity of the disease (Bischoff et al., 2020). In active CD, it is recommended that the protein requirements should be 1.2-1.5 g/kg/day while, for patients in remission, protein requirements of 1 g/kg/day can be adequate (Bischoff et al., 2020).

Managing micronutrient deficiencies is another key factor for restoring and maintaining the nutritional status in malnourished CD individuals. The most common nutrient deficiency is that associated with anaemia and osteoporosis. However, magnesium and zinc deficiencies have also been reported in CD patients (Geerling, Badart-Smook, Stockbrügger, & Brummer, 1998; O'Sullivan & O'Morain, 2006). Frequent diarrhoea, intestinal malabsorption, the presence of high out-put stoma/fistula, and intestinal resections are possibly related to the development of magnesium and zinc deficiencies (Lomer, 2011). Anaemia is considered a common extraintestinal feature present in CD patients, which is mostly related to iron deficiency. In CD, the incidence of anaemia is linked to multiple factors, which include intestinal blood loss, inflammatory burden, and an inadequate intake of dietary iron (Lomer, 2011). To help to restore serum iron and haemoglobin, supplementation with iron is recommended for all CD patients with iron deficiency (Bischoff et al., 2020). Iron supplementation can be provided orally or intravenously, depending on the patient's condition and the severity of the disease. Vitamin B_{12} and folic acid deficiencies are other possible causes for developing anaemia in CD, which result from poor diet, malabsorption, the use of anti-inflammatory drugs (e.g. sulphasalazine), and the intestinal resection of terminal ileum (Lomer, 2011). Adequate supplementation of these micronutrients should be provided as well. Moreover, osteoporosis is highly reported, with CD resulting in an increased risk of fractures among diagnosed patients (Lo et al., 2020). The aetiology of osteoporosis in CD can be related to many factors, including weight loss >10% of body weight, BMI less than 20, malabsorption, vitamin D and calcium deficiency, steroid therapy, inflammatory response, and ageing (Lomer, 2011). Therefore, patients with active CD who are treated with corticosteroids should be regularly assessed and evaluated regarding their vitamin D and serum calcium status. If necessary, the supplementation of vitamin D should be provided to avoid low bone mineral density.

Several dietary approaches for managing the symptoms of CD have been suggested, yet there is no single specific diet that can be prescribed for CD patients (Bischoff et al., 2020). Therefore, the dietitians' advice for managing the symptoms of active CD should be individualized. Modifying food intake according to the patient's perceptions of food intolerances is one way to help manage his exacerbating symptoms. For example, some patients could benefit from restricting their dietary fat, dairy products, and gluten-containing foods. Also, dietary fibre could be restricted in CD, particularly in patients with bowel obstruction. Furthermore, the use of a diet that is low in fermentable oligo-, di, mono-saccharides, and polyols (FODMAP) to reduce functional symptoms is a newly investigated dietary approach in CD. FODMAPs are poorly absorbed short-chain carbohydrates that can lead to intestinal fluid retention and bacterial fermentation, leading to increased gas formation. Recent findings support the positive effect of low FODMAP for safely managing abdominal symptoms in CD patients (Cox et al., 2020). However, because of the restrictive nature of the diet, a close assessment and monitoring of patient's intake and nutritional status are warranted.

The possible role of diet in reducing inflammation in CD is limited by the current evidence. The proposed anti-inflammatory effect of omega-3 polyunsaturated fatty acids both in health and in disease was investigated in the context of CD. However, several studies have found no significant effect of supplementation with omega-3 polyunsaturated fatty acids in terms of inducing remission and disease activity (Chiara, Franco, Marco, Antonio, & Donato, 2020). Future investigation is still needed to address the therapeutic potential of omega-3 polyunsaturated fatty acids and other promising anti-inflammatory nutrients in CD.

In summary, the aetiopathogenesis of CD is complex. Managing patients with CD could be challenging. The plan for medical nutrition therapy should be initiated early and individualized according to the patient's condition.

CASE STUDY

Setting the Stage

The following case study mimics some of the real case scenarios in gastroenterology that are usually referred to clinical dietitian in hospital ward for nutritional support and management. Patients with IBD usually undergo several stages of medical evaluation. A combination of clinical, laboratory, radiological, endoscopic, and pathological findings are required to confirm the final diagnosis of IBD. Nutritional evaluation is an integral part of the management plan for IBD patients. This case study mainly presents the challenges associated with nutrition support in patients with Crohn' disease. Both of the authors don't have any conflict of interest to be declared.

Patient's Details

- Age: 19
- Gender: Male

Case History

Medical history: Recently diagnosed with CD (4 months ago). Admitted with severe abdominal pain for the last six weeks and active CD with history of diarrhoea 2-3 times/day for the last week. Last report from colonoscopy indicated patches of ulceration with exudation in the rectum, sigmoid and descending colon; severely inflamed and strictured coecum and terminal ileum.

- Surgical history: No previous surgery
- Smoking: Non-smoker
- Family history: No family history of CD

Main Medical Diagnosis

Recently diagnosed CD

Demographics

- Marital status: Single, living with his parents
- Years of education: 12 years
- Occupation: Student
- Ethnicity: Arab
- Religion: Muslim

Anthropometry

- Current weight: 32 kg (Weight on admission)
- Usual weight: 47 kg (4 months ago). Lost weight due to significant reduction in oral intake resulting from abdominal pain
- Height: 157 cm

Table 1. Biochemical Data

Parameter	Patients Results	Reference
Chemistry		
Sodium	138	136- 145 mmol/L
Potassium	2.91 ↓	3.5- 5.1 mmol/L
Chloride	104	98- 107 mmol/L
BUN	1.8 ↓	2.5- 6.4 mmol/L
Creatinine serum	36 ↓	53- 115 umol/L
Glucose	5.4	3.9- 6.7 mmol/L
HIL index	111	-
Calcium	2.17	2.12 – 2.52 mmol/L
Phosphate	1.11	0.81 – 1.58 mmol/L
Total Protein	67	64 – 82 g/L
Albumin	19.5 ↓	40.2 – 47.6 g/L
Alkaline Phosphatase (ALPI)	58	40 – 150 U/L
Aspartate Amino Transferase (AST)	18	15 – 37 U/L
Alanine Amino Transferase (ALTI)	13	12 – 78 U/L
Gamma-glutamyl Transferase (GGT)	6	5 – 85 U/L
Bilirubin - Total	4	0 – 17 umol/L
C-Reactive Protein (CRP)	187 ↑	0 – 3 mg/L
Lactic Acid	0.8	0.4 - 2

continues on following page

Table 1. Continued

Parameter	Patients Results	Reference
Cholesterol	3.54	0- 5.20 mmol/L
Triglycerides	0.76	0.30- 2.30 mmol/L
Haematology		
White Blood Cell Count (WBC)	7.70	4.5 – 11.5 K/uL
Red Blood cell count (RBC)	3.08 ↓	4.00 – 5.40 M/uL
Haemoglobin (Hb)	8.7 ↓	12.0 – 15.0 g/dL
Hematocrit (HCT)	26.5 ↓	35 – 49%
Mean Cell Volume (MCV)	89	80 – 94 fL
MCH (Mean Cell Haemoglobin)	29 ↓	32 – 36 pg
MCHC	32.0	32 – 36%
RDW-CV	14.2	-
Platelets	325	150 – 450 K/uL
Automated Basophils	0.4	0 – 2%
Automated Neutrophils	4.30	2 – 7.5 K/uL
Automated Lymphocytes	2.0	1.5 – 4 K/uL
Automated Monocytes	0.99	0.4 – 1.0 K/uL
Automated Eosinophils	0.18	0.04 – 0.4 K/uL
Automated Basophils	0.01	0.01 – 0.08 K/uL
MPV	10	0.0 – 100 fL
PDW	8.8	-
P-LCR	18.4	-
Plateletcrit	0.3	- %
Automated Neutrophils	56.1	50 – 70%
Neuleated RBC	0.0	- %
Automated Immature Granulocytes	1.0	0.0 – 1.1
Automated Lymphocytes	28.0	20 – 45%
Automated Monocytes	11.0	2 – 11%
Automated Eosinophils	2.6	1 – 3%
Automated Immature Granulocytes	0.06	0.0 – 0.07
Neucleated RBC	0.0	- K/uL
Vitamin D total (25-OH-Vitamin D3)	57 ↓	75 – 250 nmol/L

Nutritional-Focused Physical Examination

- General appearance: Patient looking pale and in pain with muscle wasting (cachectic appearance); alert and oriented x3.
- Heart: Normal rate and rhythm
- HEENT: All clear
- Genitalia: Normal
- Neurologic: Alert, aware, and oriented
- Extremities: Normal
- Skin: Looks pale
- Chest/lungs: Clear with normal respirations
- Peripheral vascular: Normal with no peripheral oedema
- Abdomen: Active bowel sounds; positive history of diarrhoea 2-3 times/day for the last week

Vital Signs

- Pulse: 80 BPM
- Temp: 36.7 °C
- Blood pressure: 94/65 mmHg
- Respiratory rate: 19 BPM

Malnutrition Screening

According to the Nutritional Risk Screening score (NRS (2002)) (Hersberger et al., 2019; Kondrup, Rasmussen, Hamberg, STANGA, & Group, 2003), the patient is considered at risk for malnutrition (score= 4).

Food/Nutrition-Related History

Patient is complaining of a poor appetite. No chewing or swallowing difficulties were reported. He said that he is not eating well and has lost weight, mainly due to his abdominal pain. According to his three day food record, he eats about 500 kcal/day (Table 2).

- Food allergies/intolerances: None
- Food purchase/preparations: Family
- Vitamin and mineral supplementation: None

Table 2. Recent Dietary Intake (3 Days Food Record)

	Meal	Food Items and Quantities
Day 1	*Meal 1*	1 boiled egg and two slices of toast bread
	Meal 2	1 Doughnut and half cup of juice
	Meal 3	3 pieces of small pizza (bite-size) and grilled potato
	Meal 4	
	Meal 5	
	Meal 6	
Day 2	*Meal 1*	1 boiled egg
	Meal 2	
	Meal 3	
	Meal 4	
	Meal 5	
	Meal 6	
Day 3	*Meal 1*	
	Meal 2	Half sandwich (cheese)
	Meal 3	Bechamel pasta (half plate)
	Meal 4	
	Meal 5	2 pieces of small pizza (bite-size)
	Meal 6	

Medications

- Heparin (40 mg)
- Tramadol (100 mg)
- Prednisolone (40 mg)

Medical Plan

- MRI for abdomen
- Initiate TPN via PICC line (patient cannot tolerate adequate enteral feeding)
- Surgical consultation
- Nutrition support team consultation

Nutritional Management

Disease Pathophysiology and Management Mind Map (Figure 1)

Figure 1. Crohn's Disease aetiology, pathophysiology, clinical manifestation, and medical nutrition therapy map
(Developed by: Khalifa, N 2020).

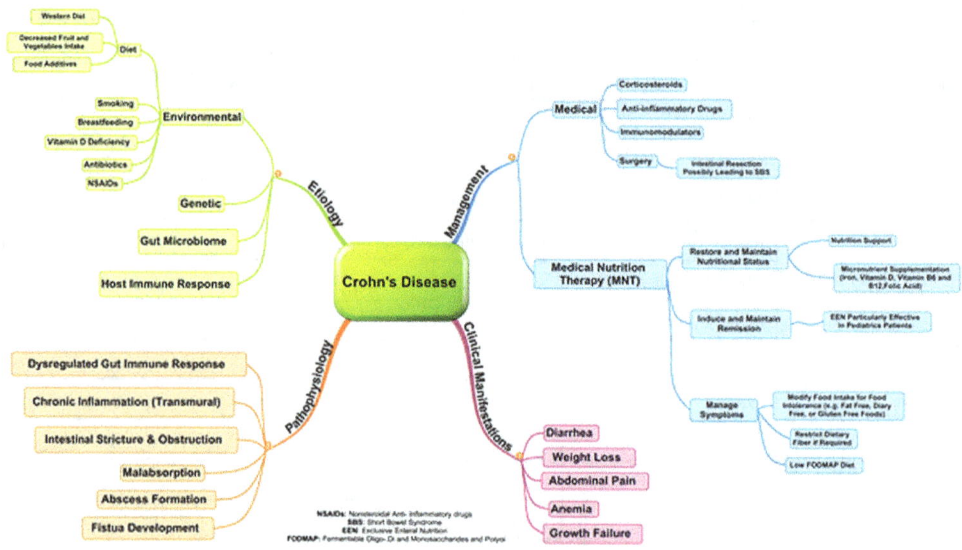

Main Aim of the Nutrition Therapy

- Provide nutrition support due to inadequate oral intake
- Provide adequate energy and protein via nutrition support to help gain weight
- Manage micronutrient deficiency resulting from malabsorption
- Modify the food intake according to the patient's tolerance to help to alleviate the symptoms

ADIME Note

Assessment

- **Anthropometry:**
    - Current BMI = 13 (underweight)
    - Percentage weight loss = 32% (severe weight loss in last 4 months)
    - Ideal body weight = 53.1 kg
    - Biochemical Data: Here we identified the most important and abnormal measurements from the patient's laboratory results with an explanation of the relevant mechanisms for the abnormal values (see Table 3).

Table 3.

Parameter	Patients Results	Reference	Possible Mechanisms for Abnormal Values
Potassium	2.91 ↓	3.5- 5.1 mmol/L	Reduced levels is possibly related to the diarrhoea.
BUN	1.8 ↓	2.5- 6.4 mmol/L	Reduced level is possibly due to the negative nitrogen balance
Creatinine serum	36 ↓	53- 115 umol/L	Reduced level is possibly due to malnutrition
Albumin	19.5 ↓	40.2 – 47.6 g/L	Depletion in visceral protein could be related to the ongoing inflammation
C-Reactive Protein (CRP)	187 ↑	0 – 3 mg/L	Inflammation is associated with a higher synthesis level of acute-phase proteins like CRP.
Red Blood cell count (RBC)	3.08 ↓	4.00 – 5.40 M/uL	Reduced level is possibly associated with the iron-deficiency anaemia
Haemoglobin (Hb)	8.7 ↓	12.0 – 15.0 g/dL	Reduced levels is possibly associated with the iron malabsorption and the consequences related to the underlying intestinal ulceration.
Hematocrit (HCT)	26.5 ↓	35 – 49%	Reduced levels is possibly associated with the iron malabsorption and the consequences related to the underlying intestinal ulceration.
MCH (Mean Cell Hemoglobin)	29 ↓	32 – 36 pg	Reduced level is possibly associated with the iron-deficiency anaemia
Vitamin D total (25-OH-Vitamin D3)	57 ↓	75 – 250 nmol/L	Reduced levels is possibly related to the malabsorption syndrome associated with Crohn's disease

  - Clinical: Abdominal pain and complaining of diarrhoea 2-3 times/day for the last week.
  - Dietary: Reduced oral intake; poor appetite; patient is following a low-fat diet.
- **Diagnosis:** Inadequate oral intake related to poor appetite and abdominal pain as evidenced by:
  - History of severe weight loss in the last four months.
  - Daily caloric intake less than the estimated energy requirements by approximately 60% (according to the three days food record, the patient's food intake is about 500 kcal/day).

Intervention

- **Diet prescription:**
    - Energy: According to the suggested energy requirements based on the patient's BMI (Eiden, 2003; Mueller, 2017), the caloric requirements for the patient is: 36-45 kcal/kg/day = 1152-1440 kcal/day
    - Protein: 1-1.5 gm/kg/day = 32-48 gm/day (Eiden, 2003; Mueller, 2017)
    - Fluid: 30-35 ml/kg/day = 960-1120 ml/day
- **Prescription for parenteral nutrition:** The patient was placed on PN via PICC line and was initiated at a rate of (15-30 kcal/kg/day) (Ayers, Guenter, Holcombe, & Plogsted, 2014). The total calories and macronutrients prescribed for the PN is shown in Table 4.

Table 4.

Day 1	
Energy	15 kcal/kg/day = 480 kcal/day As patient was at risk of refeeding syndrome PN will be initiated slowly at a low rate.
Rate of PN	30 ml/hr
Total volume	22.5 ml/kg/day = 720 ml/day
Dextrose	2.7 gm/kg/day = 88.4 gm/day (62.6% total kcal) GIR: 1.9 mg/kg/min
Amino acids	1.4 gm/kg/day = 44.8 gm/day (37.3% total kcal)
Lipids	No lipids provided at that time
Day 2	
Energy	25 kcal/kg/day = 800 kcal/day
Rate of PN	30 ml/hr
Total volume	27.5 ml/kg/day = 880 ml/day
Dextrose	2.7 gm/kg/day = 88.4 gm/day (37.5% total kcal) GIR: 1.9 mg/kg/min
Amino acids	1.4 gm/kg/day = 44.8 gm/day (22.4% total kcal)
Lipids	1 gm/kg/day = 32 gm/day (40% total kcal) Lipids were infused over 12 hours at a rate of 13.3 ml/hr
Day 3	
Energy	36 kcal/kg/day = 1152 kcal/day Since patient's labs were stable the dextrose was increased to reach his required calories based on his BMI.
Rate of PN	37 ml/hr
Total volume	32.7 ml/kg/day = 1048 ml/day

continues on following page

Table 4. Continued

Dextrose	6 gm/kg/day = 192 gm/day (56.6% total kcal) GIR: 4 mg/kg/min
Amino acids	1.4 gm/kg/day = 44.8 gm/day (15.5% total kcal)
Lipids	1 gm/kg/day = 32 gm/day (27.7% total kcal) Lipids were infused over 12 hours at a rate of 13.3 ml/hr.

Recommendations

Provide adequate energy and protein via parenteral nutrition without causing refeeding syndrome.

Rationale: The provision of adequate energy and protein via nutrition support is important for the patient. However, the patient is considered at risk of refeeding syndrome due to the malnutrition and metabolic stress resulting from CD. Therefore, PN will be initiated slowly at a low rate (15-30 kcal/kg/day), and the total calories will be increased gradually with a close assessment of serum electrolytes. Moreover, according to the physician's medical plan, this patient might be considered a candidate for surgical intervention in the future. Thus, restoring his nutritional status and body weight via nutrition support is paramount for enhancing his postoperative recovery in the future. Inadequate nutritional intake prior to abdominal resection is associated with postoperative complications and mortality. According to the latest guidelines by the European Society for Clinical Nutrition (ESPEN), surgical intervention should be postponed for up to 14 days in malnourished IBD patients, to allow sufficient time to provide intensive nutritional support (Bischoff et al., 2020).

Encourage enteral nutrition or the oral intake of food and beverages as tolerated.

Rationale: Oral supplementation with enteral feeds should always be encouraged. In this case, due to the abdominal pain, the patient was unable to tolerate oral intake once TPN was started. Therefore, once the abdominal pain is resolved, oral nutritional supplement should be prescribed. Patient compliance with oral feeds should be regularly monitored to check for any intolerances. Also, it is important to encourage regular food intake. Once the patient starts tolerating food and oral nutritional supplements with no gastrointestinal complains, plan to start tapering the parenteral nutrition. Aim to provide only half of the requirements via PN while oral nutritional supplements would provide the patient with the rest of his daily requirements. Normal food intake should be regularly encouraged as well. Compared to PN, EN is always considered the preferred route of feeding. However, in situations where patients are unable to meet >60% of their caloric needs via the enteral nutrition route, then supplementary parenteral nutrition is indicated (Bischoff et al., 2020).

Provide low fat, low fibre, and high potassium diet.

Rationale: Once the patient starts tolerating food intake, it is important to discuss the possible effects of diet on gastrointestinal symptoms. There is no single IBD diet that can be prescribed to induce remission in patients with active CD (Bischoff et al., 2020). However, it is suggested that certain components of the diet could worsen the symptoms in patients with active disease. Therefore, individualized dietetic advice and dietary plans should be provided for such patients. Regarding the current case, a low-fat diet is recommended because of the presence of malabsorption and diarrhoea. Reducing the amount of dietary fibre intake is also recommended for this patient. In CD, the intake of dietary fibre is often contradicted due to intestinal strictures and obstruction. Therefore, a modified diet that is low in insoluble fibre is typically recommended for patients experiencing intestinal strictures. Moreover, a high potassium diet is recommended for this patient to help to correct his low serum potassium levels. An electrolytes imbalance is common in IBD patients, which usually results from the reduced intestinal absorption and secretion of electrolytes (Barkas, Liberopoulos, Kei, & Elisaf, 2013). In this case, the reduced serum levels of potassium are possibly related to the diarrhoea, which is associated with dehydration. Therefore, the electrolyte losses should be medically managed by fluid replacement in addition to nutritional management, which may include increasing the intake of food items with high potassium.

Adjust for micronutrients deficiency.

Rationale: Generally, patients with CD are at high risk of micronutrients deficiency as a result of malabsorption from diarrhoea and reduced dietary intake resulting from the active disease. Therefore, the regular monitoring of micronutrients deficiency is recommended, and specific micronutrients supplementation will need to be considered (Bischoff et al., 2020). In the current case, the patient seems to be experiencing anaemia (haemoglobin level is 8.7 g/dL), which is a common extraintestinal manifestation of the disease. In CD, anaemia could mainly result from iron malabsorption, losses in diarrhoea, and long-term severe intestinal inflammation. Serum ferritin should also be checked for the appropriate diagnosis of iron deficiency anaemia. Another common micronutrient deficiency in CD is vitamin D. Several risk factors are associated with vitamin D deficiency in CD, which include: gut losses, malabsorption, reduced food intake associated with anorexia in active disease, and corticosteroids treatment. All of these factors might contribute to increased calcium excretion, leading to osteoporosis. Here, low levels of vitamin D were reported for the patient. It is recommended that serum calcium and vitamin D should be routinely monitored. Regular supplementation is recommended, if necessary, to avoid low bone mineral density and reduce the risk of fracture.

Monitoring/Evaluation

Continuous monitoring is essential for the presented case. There are several elements in the monitoring plan that should be implemented to ensure the best quality and safety of the nutrition care plan. These include the regular monitoring of oral intake, weight changes, biochemical data, and bowel movements.

In conclusion, this case study illustrated the strategy for applying medical nutritional therapy in the context of a CD-based patient scenario. A critical evaluation and application of the current evidence and IBD nutritional guidelines was conducted to provide an individualized nutritional plan according to the patient's requirements.

REFERENCES

Al-Mofarreh, M. A., & Al-Mofleh, I. A. (2013). Emerging inflammatory bowel disease in Saudi outpatients: a report of 693 cases. *Saudi Journal of Gastroenterology: Official Journal of the Saudi Gastroenterology Association, 19*(1), 16.

Alastair, F., Emma, G., & Emma, P. (2011). Nutrition in inflammatory bowel disease. *Journal of Parenteral and Enteral Nutrition, 35*(5), 571–580. doi:10.1177/0148607111413599 PMID:21825089

Ananthakrishnan, A. N. (2015). Epidemiology and risk factors for IBD. *Nature Reviews. Gastroenterology & Hepatology, 12*(4), 205–217. doi:10.1038/nrgastro.2015.34 PMID:25732745

Ananthakrishnan, A. N., Khalili, H., Konijeti, G. G., Higuchi, L. M., de Silva, P., Fuchs, C. S., Willett, W. C., Richter, J. M., & Chan, A. T. (2014). Long-term intake of dietary fat and risk of ulcerative colitis and Crohn's disease. *Gut, 63*(5), 776–784. doi:10.1136/gutjnl-2013-305304 PMID:23828881

Ananthakrishnan, A. N., Khalili, H., Konijeti, G. G., Higuchi, L. M., de Silva, P., Korzenik, J. R., Fuchs, C. S., Willett, W. C., Richter, J. M., & Chan, A. T. (2013). A prospective study of long-term intake of dietary fiber and risk of Crohn's disease and ulcerative colitis. *Gastroenterology, 145*(5), 970–977. doi:10.1053/j.gastro.2013.07.050 PMID:23912083

Ayers, P., Guenter, P., Holcombe, B., & Plogsted, S. (2014). *ASPEN parenteral nutrition handbook*. American Society for Parenteral and Enteral Nutrition.

Barkas, F., Liberopoulos, E., Kei, A., & Elisaf, M. (2013). Electrolyte and acid-base disorders in inflammatory bowel disease. *Annals of Gastroenterology, 26*(1), 23. PMID:24714322

Bischoff, S. C., Escher, J., Hébuterne, X., Kłęk, S., Krznaric, Z., Schneider, S., ... Wiskin, A. E. (2020). ESPEN practical guideline: Clinical Nutrition in inflammatory bowel disease. *Clinical Nutrition (Edinburgh, Lothian)*, *39*(3), 632–653. doi:10.1016/j.clnu.2019.11.002 PMID:32029281

Boullata, J., Brantley, S., Corkins, M., Guenter, P., Krenitsky, J., Lyman, B., . . . Wessel, J. (2009). Enteral Nutrition Practice Recommendations. *Parenteral and Enteral Nutrition, 33*(2).

Chiara, M. M., Franco, S., Marco, P., Antonio, G., & Donato, M. G. A. (2020). Nutrition, IBD and Gut Microbiota: A Review. *Nutrients*, *12*(4), 944. doi:10.3390/nu12040944 PMID:32235316

Cox, S. R., Lindsay, J. O., Fromentin, S., Stagg, A. J., McCarthy, N. E., Galleron, N., . . . Pons, N. (2020). Effects of Low FODMAP Diet on Symptoms, Fecal Microbiome, and Markers of Inflammation in Patients With Quiescent Inflammatory Bowel Disease in a Randomized Trial. *Gastroenterology, 158*(1), 176-188.

Di Caro, S., Fragkos, K. C., Keetarut, K., Koo, H. F., Sebepos-Rogers, G., Saravanapavan, H., Barragry, Rogers, Mehta, & Rahman, F. (2019). Enteral Nutrition in Adult Crohn's Disease: Toward a Paradigm Shift. *Nutrients*, *11*(9), 2222. doi:10.3390/nu11092222 PMID:31540038

Eiden, K. A. (2003). Nutritional considerations in inflammatory bowel disease. *Practical Gastroenterology*, *27*(5), 33–54.

Frolkis, A. D., Dykeman, J., Negrón, M. E., deBruyn, J., Jette, N., Fiest, K. M., ... Panaccione, R. (2013). Risk of surgery for inflammatory bowel diseases has decreased over time: A systematic review and meta-analysis of population-based studies. *Gastroenterology*, *145*(5), 996–1006. doi:10.1053/j.gastro.2013.07.041 PMID:23896172

Geerling, B. J., Badart-Smook, A., Stockbrügger, R. W., & Brummer, R. (1998). Comprehensive nutritional status in patients with long-standing Crohn disease currently in remission. *The American Journal of Clinical Nutrition*, *67*(5), 919–926. doi:10.1093/ajcn/67.5.919 PMID:9583850

Hersberger, L., Bargetzi, L., Bargetzi, A., Tribolet, P., Fehr, R., Baechli, V., . . . Kutz, A. (2019). Nutritional risk screening (NRS 2002) is a strong and modifiable predictor risk score for short-term and long-term clinical outcomes: secondary analysis of a prospective randomized trial. *Clinical Nutrition*.

Hou, J. K., Abraham, B., & El-Serag, H. (2011). Dietary Intake and Risk of Developing Inflammatory Bowel Disease: A Systematic Review of the Literature. *The American Journal of Gastroenterology, 106*(4), 563–573. doi:10.1038/ajg.2011.44 PMID:21468064

Jansen, I., Prager, M., Valentini, L., & Büning, C. (2016). Inflammation-driven malnutrition: A new screening tool predicts outcome in Crohn's disease. *British Journal of Nutrition, 116*(6), 1061–1067. doi:10.1017/S0007114516003044 PMID:27546478

Kondrup, J., Rasmussen, H. H., & Hamberg, O. (2003). Nutritional risk screening (NRS 2002): A new method based on an analysis of controlled clinical trials. *Clinical Nutrition (Edinburgh, Lothian), 22*(3), 321–336. doi:10.1016/S0261-5614(02)00214-5 PMID:12765673

Lo, B., Holm, J. P., Vester-Andersen, M. K., Bendtsen, F., Vind, I., & Burisch, J. (2020). Incidence, Risk Factors and Evaluation of Osteoporosis in Patients With Inflammatory Bowel Disease: A Danish Population-Based Inception Cohort With 10 Years of Follow-Up. *Journal of Crohn's and Colitis.*

Lomer, M. C. (2011). Dietary and nutritional considerations for inflammatory bowel disease. *The Proceedings of the Nutrition Society, 70*(3), 329–335. doi:10.1017/S0029665111000097 PMID:21450124

Mueller, C. M. (2017). *The ASPEN Adult Nutrition Support Core Curriculum* (3rd ed.). American Society for Parenteral and Enteral Nutrition.

Narula, N., Dhillon, A., Zhang, D., Sherlock, M. E., Tondeur, M., & Zachos, M. (2018). Enteral nutritional therapy for induction of remission in Crohn's disease. *Cochrane Database of Systematic Reviews*, 4. doi:10.1002/14651858.CD000542.pub3 PMID:29607496

Norman, K., Pichard, C., Lochs, H., & Pirlich, M. (2008). Prognostic impact of disease-related malnutrition. *Clinical Nutrition (Edinburgh, Lothian), 27*(1), 5–15. doi:10.1016/j.clnu.2007.10.007 PMID:18061312

O'Sullivan, M., & O'Morain, C. (2006). Nutrition in inflammatory bowel disease. *Best Practice & Research. Clinical Gastroenterology, 20*(3), 561–573. doi:10.1016/j.bpg.2006.03.001 PMID:16782529

Peyrin-Biroulet, L., Panés, J., Sandborn, W. J., Vermeire, S., Danese, S., Feagan, B. G., . . . Rycroft, B. (2016). Defining disease severity in inflammatory bowel diseases: current and future directions. *Clinical Gastroenterology and Hepatology, 14*(3), 348-354.

Van Gossum, A., Cabre, E., Hebuterne, X., Jeppesen, P., Krznaric, Z., Messing, B., Powell-Tuck, J., Staun, M., & Nightingale, J. (2009). ESPEN guidelines on parenteral nutrition: Gastroenterology. *Clinical Nutrition (Edinburgh, Lothian), 28*(4), 415–427. doi:10.1016/j.clnu.2009.04.022 PMID:19515465

Veauthier, B., & Hornecker, J. R. (2018). Crohn's Disease: Diagnosis and Management. *American Family Physician, 98*(11), 661–669. PMID:30485038

Walsh, A. J., Bryant, R. V., & Travis, S. P. (2016). Current best practice for disease activity assessment in IBD. *Nature Reviews. Gastroenterology & Hepatology, 13*(10), 567–579. doi:10.1038/nrgastro.2016.128 PMID:27580684

KEY TERMS AND DEFINITIONS

Elemental Feed: A specialized liquid enteral nutritional supplement with amino acids and low-fat content. This type of feed is completely antigen-free.

Exclusive Enteral Nutrition: When enteral nutrition (using a liquid nutritional supplement provided via oral route or feeding tube) completely provide all the nutrient needs with any food intake.

Extraintestinal Manifestations: Clinical features or complications of the disease that is not related to the gastrointestinal tract. It involves other organs, not including the gastrointestinal tract (e.g., joints, eye, and skin).

Fistula: Abnormal connection between two organs, which could result from injury, inflammation, or surgery.

Polymeric Feed: A specialized liquid enteral nutritional supplement with whole protein (from milk, egg, meat, etc.) and high-fat content.

Refeeding Syndrome: Metabolic alterations in electrolytes status which result from rapid provision of calories after a period of caloric deficit.

Relapse: Periods where symptoms are exacerbated (active disease).

Remission: Periods where symptoms are improved or disappear (inactive disease).

Semi-Elemental Feed: A specialized liquid enteral nutritional supplement with oligopeptide (hydrolyzed protein) content.

Stricture: Intestinal stricture is narrowing of the intestinal lumen, which can lead to complete intestinal obstruction.

Transmural Inflammation: All layers of intestinal mucosa are affected and inflamed.

APPENDIX: ABBREVIATIONS

ASPEN: American Society for Parenteral and Enteral Nutrition
CD: Crohn's disease
IBD: Inflammatory bowel disease
NSAIDs: Nonsteroidal anti-inflammatory drugs
PICC: Peripherally inserted central catheter
TPN: Total parenteral nutrition
UC: Ulcerative colitis
ONS: Oral nutritional supplements
EEN: Exclusive enteral nutrition
FODMAP: Fermentable oligo-, di, mono-saccharides, and polyols

Chapter 8
Pediatric Ulcerative Colitis With Extra Intestinal Manifestations:
MNT for Pediatric Ulcerative Colitis

Elham Abbas Aljaaly
King Abdulaziz University, Saudi Arabia

Naglaa Mostafa Elsayed
King Abdulaziz University, Saudi Arabia

EXECUTIVE SUMMARY

Pediatric gastroenterology practitioners adopted different guidelines that focus on high-quality nutrition care for rare disorders such as inflammatory bowel disease in its two main forms: Crohn's disease and ulcerative colitis. This chapter presents a case report of ulcerative colitis with extra intestinal manifestations in the form of right knee arthritis and hypo-chromic microcytic anemia in a 13 years old Egyptian boy who presented to the outpatient services with complains of frequent attacks of right knee pain and swelling, nausea, decreased appetite and food intake, along with significant weight loss. Attacks of diarrhea associated with abdominal cramping and progressive fatigue was reported at the first visit. The authors of this case chapter aimed to share their experience in diagnosing, managing and systematically follow up a pediatric ulcerative colitis patient. The chapter refers to a comprehensive management of the patient's disease who was effectively managed by an integrated multidisciplinary approach.

DOI: 10.4018/978-1-7998-3802-9.ch008

AUTHORS' OVERVIEW OF THE CASE

Inflammatory bowel diseases (IBD) are idiopathic disorders that lead to chronic inflammation of the gastrointestinal tract mucosa. It includes Crohn's disease (CD), ulcerative colitis (UC), and indeterminate colitis (IC) (Hyams, 2005). IBD affects a large parentage of the population in the United States (Kugathasan, et al., 2003). Although earlier studies reported frequent prevalence in Europe and North America, the incidence was either more or the same in countries those are developed or less developed (Soda, et al., 2003).

No exact pathogenesis of UC is known till now. However, genetic, immunologic, and environmental factors may be considered as risk factors (Bradley & Oliva-Hemker, 2012). Up to 25% of UC cases affect children and young adults, and 80% of them have pancolitis (Sawczenko & Sandhu, 2003).

Children with UC usually presented with diarrhea, bleeding per rectum, abdominal pain, and loss of weight (Levine & Burakoff, 2011). This is in addition to psychological and nutritional problems (Bradley & Oliva-Hemker, 2012).

Extra intestinal manifestations (EIMs) affect 25-40% of patients with IBD. EIMs can encompass nearly every body system such as the musculoskeletal, hepato-biliary, ocular, urinary, pulmonary systems as well as the skin. Twenty-five percent of IBD patients have more than one EIM. These manifestations may be primary in the form of inflammation or other effects of disease activity, nearly 100% of IBD patients have an abnormality outside of the gastrointestinal tract. EIMs may precede the onset of colonic symptoms in some patients (Bernstein, Blanchard, Rawsthorne, and Yu,2001).The involvement of joint is the most corporate EIM in children with IBD and may involve 16 -33% of patients at the time of presentation or throughout the follow-up process (Cardile & Romano, 2014).

Arthritis found similarly in males and females and is in general more prevalent in patients with UC than those with CD. Peripheral arthritis classically involves large joints in an asymmetric patterns (Schorr-Lesnick & Brandt, 1988). The knee is the most common affected joint. Treatment of peripheral arthritis depends on the treatment of the underlying UC. Nonsteroidal anti-inflammatory drugs (NSAID) and selective cyclooxygenase-2 (COX-2) inhibitors are used to relieve symptoms (Levine & Burakoff, 2011).

The combination of a complete clinical history, detailed physical examination, radiographic features, endoscopic assessment, and histology of tissue is the best diagnostic approach of UC requires (Bradley & Oliva-Hemker, 2012).

It is crucial to differentiate CD from UC to plan proper treatment for those patients (Evon & Ravikumara M, 2010). There are some points in distinguishing UC and CD. UC starts in the rectum in the form of confluent inflammation and progresses proximally throughout the colon in a continuous and circumferential pattern, while rectal sparing is characteristic of CD (D'Haens, Geboes, Peeters, Baert, Ectors, Rutgeerts, 1997).

Although terminal ileal involvement is in favor with CD, it could also found in some UC patients (Evon & Ravikumara, 2010).

UC affects strictly the large bowel. Therefore, barium study of the upper GIT had a great part in diagnosing small-bowel involvement in IBD and in the differentiation of UC from CD. (Stringer, 1987).

The first line of investigations for children with suspected IBD include both upper and lower gastrointestinal endoscopy using flexible endoscopy, which is harmless and is found to be well tolerated, and valid. This is crucial to differentiate UC from CD (de Bie et al., 2005). Biopsy findings are proved to be a highly sensitive in measuring the disease extent than endoscopy (Williams & Nicholls, 1994). Endoscopy should include the terminal ileum and multiple biopsies should be taken from all segments of the colon whether the mucosa is normal or not (Evon & Ravikumara, 2010). It is important to mention that architectural distortion denoting chronicity in IBD are frequently missing in initial colonic biopsies in children because they are probably to present with a relatively acute onset of symptoms (Glickman, Bousvaros A, Farraye FA, Zholudev A, Friedman S et al., 2004).

In UC, inflammatory changes are characteristically confine to the mucosa, but segmental and deep inflammation is distinctive of CD where the inflammation is transmural, with lymphoid aggregates extending to the subserosa (Evon & Ravikumara, 2010).

Regarding the treatment of UC, no medical cure is present. However, objectives of therapy for pediatric UC should comprise; for acute cases, induction of remission of symptoms, then maintaining long-term remission and preventing recurrence. On the long run, medications are important to prevent cancer development, improve quality of life, growth, and development (Van Limbergen, Russell, Drummond, Aldhous, Round, et al., 2008). The power of treatment differs based on the severity of presented symptoms. Medical therapy for UC includes: 5-aminosalicylates (5-ASAs), corticosteroids, thiopurine immunomodulators, calcineurin inhibitors, antibiotics, probiotics, and anti-tumor necrosis factor (TNF) - agents.-a Biologic therapies, including anti-TNF Agents (Bradley& Oliva-Hemker, 2012). In mild to moderate UC, aminosalicylate is usually used with the dose not exceeding 2-4 g/day (Laharie, 2017).

In case of side effects, better-tolerated 5-ASA preparations (mesalamine, 50-100 g/kg/day; balsalazide 2.25-6.75 g/day) may be used. Sulfasalazine and the 5-ASA preparations efficiently treat active UC and decrease the chances of recurrence. Medications should be continued even during remission. These medications might also reduce the risk of colon cancer development.

Cases of moderate to severe UC or colitis that is unresponsive to 5-ASA therapy should be treated with corticosteroids, with a starting dose of 1-2 mg/kg/day (40-60 mg maximum dose). This medication could be used once daily. In severe colitis, the dose can be divided twice daily and can be given intravenously. Steroids are well thought-out as an effective medication in cases of acute exacerbations. However, they cannot be used as maintenance therapy in children because of their side effects which include growth retardation, osteopenia, glucose intolerance, mood changes, and other complications (Laharie, 2017).

When using medical management, most children with mild manifestations reach remission within three months and may stay in remission on a prophylactic 5-ASA preparation for a long time. However, in 5–10%, remission takes more than 6 months.

Infliximab is active for induction and maintenance therapy in children and adults with moderate to severe disease (Levesque & Sandborn, 2012).

Total colectomy is the treatment of choice in cases with the intractable disease, severe side effects of medications, in addition to fulminant disease that is indifferent to medical treatment. Special procedures are taken during the operation to maintain continence, and a terminal ileostomy is done temporarily for those patients (Mamula, Markowitz, and Baldassano, 2013).

It is important to mention that psychosocial care is an important part of therapy for children with UC as well as their families (Mamula, Markowitz and Baldassano, 2013).

After about 10 years from the onset of symptoms, the risk of development of colon cancer increases dramatically. So, screening colonoscopies beginning after 8-10 years of disease is important. Colectomy should be done in any case with significant dysplasia on biopsy (Beaugerie & Itzkowitz, 2015).

Chronic inflammatory diseases may cause anemia which leads to reduction in hematocrit or red blood cell volume. Besides a reduction in the concentration of blood hemoglobin is caused by anemia. Chronic loss of blood and the use of some medication are respectable causes of anemia. Blood loss from the gastrointestinal tract of small amounts might not be noticed by some patients, particularly children. (Trost et al; 2006).

The size of the average red blood cell is known as the mean corpuscular volume (MCV). Abnormality in the size of cells is called microcytic if the cells are small and for large cells, they termed macrocytic. The mean corpuscular hemoglobin concentration (MCHC) discusses the amount of hemoglobin in the average cell and hypochromic cells are those low in hemoglobin. Microcytic, hypochromic anemia can be caused by a number of diseases including chronic disease (Bain et al; 2006). Iron deficiency is the most common cause of microcytic, hypochromic anemia and inexplicable iron deficiency would have a comprehensive gastrointestinal assessment (Johnson-Wimbley & Graham 2011)

The Medical Nutrition Therapy of diseases recognizes UC as a chronic inflammatory disease of the intestine that is restricted to the colonic and rectal mucosa. The disease course is worse in children, compared with that in adults. Studies found that one third of children population with UC undergo colectomy at 10 years. (Mahan & Raymond, 2016). Malnutrition is common among patients with IBD. However, nutritional problems found in patients with UC are not as severe as in the other IBD such as the CD. This could be due to the lack of involvement of the small intestine.

Pediatric UC in addition to other IBD has a number of concerns to consider when compared to adult IBD. This includes growth, bone health, and psychological influence on the child and his family (Conrad & Rosh, 2017). For example, the height velocity for children with UC is generally average unless they are treated with excessive steroid (Lee et al. 2010). Promotion of optimal growth and development is very important for children and nutritional support for high-energy diet and/or oral nutritional supplements is required if patients with IBD, including UC experienced growth failure or have a significant weight loss (Forbes et al., 2017).

High intake of fats, particularly total fat, Polyunsaturated fatty acids (PUFAs), omega-6 fatty acids in addition to high intake of meats, were reported to be associated with the increase risk of developing UC (Forbes et al., 2017).

Patients with IBD are at risk of vitamin D deficiency and they need a routine measure and supplements' intake as per need (Pappa et al., 2006). As with any pediatric patients with chronic conditions, pediatric UC patients' transition from pediatric to adult care should be an integral part of the UC service. This requires precise attention and cautious planning during the transition process, which is preferable to be with joint clinics that are held between adult and pediatric gastroenterology teams. This will allow pediatric patients to attend these types of clinics for long periods (Abraham & Kahn, 2014). It also allows for better education and development for skills to self-manage the disease during the transition from pediatric to adult care.

Iron-deficiency anemia was reported as the most common cause of anemia in IBD patients. For patients with UC, low iron levels were due to the bleeding during flashes of ulcerative colitis. Other causes include iron absorption problems through the intestines in line for inflammation and diarrhea, and reduced intake of foods that are rich in iron (Laffolie et al., 2017).

Many health organizations developed standards and guidelines that are applied to pediatric patients who receive gastroenterology and nutrition care related services. Guidelines are developed individually or in collaboration with other organizations. Examples include the European Society for Clinical Nutrition and Metabolism (ESPEN) and American Society for Parenteral and Enteral Nutrition (ASPEN), which allowed health professionals in the scope of pediatric gastroenterology combine their resources and proficiency in providing a stronger evidenced-based practice and standardized medical nutrition care. Consequently, this will enhance the quality of services provided to children with nutrition-related medical problems. For example, ESPEN's guidelines in 2018, defined the best effective and safe treatment options of pediatric IBD-associated iron deficiency anemia (IDA). ESPEN released their statement concerning IDA, which recommends iron supplementation for all pediatric IBD patients when IDA is existing. Iron supplementation was recommended to control hemoglobin level and ensure good iron stores for these patients. The ESPEN also considered oral iron supplementation as an effective in IDA IBD pediatric patients who are diagnosed with mild anemia of hemoglobin levels more than 10 g/dL and those with negative inflammatory markers. On the other hand, Intravenous (IV) iron supplementation was recommended for pediatric patients with clinically active IBD. The guidelines also indicated the importance of monitoring the reappearance of iron deficiency (ID) in children with IBD, which could indicate determined intestinal disease activity (Miele et al., 2018).

This chapter presents a report for a case of pediatric UC. The chapter refers to a comprehensive management of a patient with ulcerative colitis who was effectively managed by an integrated multidisciplinary approach. The multidisciplinary team included health professionals who provided medical, nutritional, physiotherapy, psychotherapy and social services. The multidisciplinary team's approach was used for its critical role in conveying benefits to both the patient and the members of the medical team who were handling the case. The approach was used to improve the critical management of the patient's case, enhance health outcomes and patient's satisfaction about the provided health services. On the other hand, to facilitate the team members to efficiently use available resources and to enhance their job satisfaction.

The chapter reviews the case details and includes the patient's information concerning his demographics data and histories for instance medical, surgical, nutritional, and family. The main medical and nutritional diagnoses are also presented in the chapter. Additionally, the present case-based chapter evaluates the patient's growth and nutritional status using anthropometry, hematological and biochemical data. The chapter includes reports on the conducted nutritional-focused physical examination, food/nutrition-related history and food patterns. Solutions and recommendations in managing patient's UC are also untaken to ensure that the patient is better served, his wellness is enhanced to minimize the care needed and to improve his health outcomes. Patient's case management included medications, nutrition therapy, and other related managements. The chapter also presents a report of the case using the ADIME note. ADIME is an abbreviation of Assessment, Diagnosis, Intervention, and Monitoring/Evaluation of the case. The ADIME process is a process used by registered dietitians (RD) to ensure high quality nutrition care to patients and from nutrition professionals. Finally, the chapter will conclude to readers the case study by using a Mindmap to illustrate the whole case based on the

MNT of the disease. The Mindmap concludes the presented case study relating to the etiology of the disease, the pathophysiology, the presented signs and symptoms, and disease management including the medical, physiotherapy, psychological, nutrition support and medical nutrition therapy. *The main aim of this chapter is to describe the comprehensive management of a pediatric patient with ulcerative colitis who was fruitfully managed by an integrated multidisciplinary approach. This is in a hope to guide readers and health professionals in the scope of pediatric gastroenterology in managing similar cases.*

The aim was further explained by the following objectives:

1. To emphasize the importance of managing pediatric UC using a multidisciplinary approach, particularly unlike an adult, medical providers when deal with a child interacts broadly with both the patient and the patient's care provider.
2. To direct the reader in managing similar cases based on the disease location, behavior and the severity of the disease at presentation.
3. To ensure the importance of eliminating the symptoms of the disease, improve the quality of life, and to further avoid hospitalization and surgery when managing similar cases.
4. To confirm the significance of increasing the chance of lasting remission and decreasing the potential for adverse effects of long-standing inflammation, even with the clinical improvement throughout the management period.
5. To give emphasis to the impact on pediatric UC patients' education, school achievement, personal relationships, and social and family life, particularly the disease follows an every so often unpredictable relapsing-remitting course.

SETTING THE STAGE

Data was collected from the patients' archiving system in a pediatric public hospital in Cairo, Egypt. Medical team members involved were a pediatric gastroenterologist, a pathologist, a radiologist, a physiotherapist and the clinical dietitian. Although the multidisciplinary approach was not followed in the hospital, this medical team was formed from health care practitioners who have variable levels of educational, professional and evidence-based training. The team formed had a strong belief that their collaboration and effective communication in managing the patient' disease was essential, particularly to safeguard the patient safety and eliminate the risk for lacking critical information, misunderstanding of information and prescribed medication and other treatment. A consent form was obtained from parents and the child and was signed by the parents to conduct and manage this case. No financial support for reporting this case. Therefore, there is no conflict of interest.

CASE DESCRIPTION

Patient's Details

FA is a 13 years old Egyptian male patient who attended the outpatient pediatric clinic in February 2018 complaining of frequent attacks of right knee pain and swelling that started six months ago. Patient reported nausea, decreased appetite and food intake. The patient and his parents stated that he had recurrent attacks of diarrhea associated with abdominal cramping starting a few months ago. The family also reported unintentional weight loss in 6 months, and progressive fatigue, which later affected his school performance.

On physical examination, FA looked pale and there was swelling, tenderness and limited range of movements involving the right knee joint. No other joint abnormalities. Diagnostic assessment using the X- ray for the right knee showed a mild narrowing of the tibiofemoral joint space with periarticular soft tissue swelling denoting joint effusion, which was also proved by Ultrasonography. Colonoscopy proved pancolitis with inflamed, hyperemic mucosa of the colon and rectum. Changes were in a diffuse, continuous, and superficial pattern. The multiple biopsies revealed superficial mucosal inflammatory changes with no architecture distortion.

Laboratory investigations in the form of complete blood picture, hemoglobin level, ESR (Erythrocytic Sedimentation Rate), CRP (C - reactive protein), autoantibodies including antinuclear antibody, anti-smooth muscle antibody and rheumatoid factor were used to rule out different causes of pediatric arthritis. Stool analysis was normal, but occult blood in stool has to be excluded due to the presence of anemia. Urine analysis showed proteinuria.

At the time of diagnosis, ulcerative colitis was suspected, and a plan was arranged to conduct further investigations by a multidisciplinary team, including detailed related histories and examinations such as physical, nutritional, laboratory, radiographic studies, and colonoscopy as well as the tissue pathology.

Vital Signs

- Pulse: 80 / min.
- Temperature: 37.3 °C
- Blood pressure: 104/60 mm Hg
- Resp. rate: 16/ min.

Case Histories

- **Medical History:** Swollen, painful joints of the right knee. Abdominal pain, along with diarrhea.
- **Surgical History:** None
- **Family History:** No relevant family history was mentioned
- **Diet History:** Dietary patterns reported by the patient and his parents as follows:
  - Three main meals with frequent snacks.
  - High consumption of sweets and fats.
  - Adding sugar to hot and cold drinks.
  - Daily consumption of 2 to 3 cups of milk.
  - Preferences for cheese and eggs.
  - Consumption of processed meats such as sausage, hot dogs and pepperoni.
  - Consumption of fast food (3-4 times/week), which was reduced in the last period because it was accompanied with abdominal colic and diarrhea, particularly when the consumed meals are spicy and/or fatty.
  - Poor appetite, which is combined with diarrhea and abdominal pain.
  - Reduced dietary intake in the last six months, which affected his weight. Parents mentioned a weight loss of 5 Kg in a period of 6 months.
  - Generally have normal bowel habits as 2 times/day. However, when he has diarrhea attacks, his bowel motion could increase to two-three times/day and it is usually associated with abdominal pain.
  - Urine output is normal.
  - No reports for steatorrhea or bloody stool.
  - No food allergy, swallowing or chewing difficulty.

Main Medical Diagnosis

Ulcerative Colitis with extra intestinal manifestations in the form of right knee arthritis. Hypo-chromic microcytic anemia.

Nutrition-Related Assessment, Diagnosis and Consequences

The nutritional status was evaluated by anthropometry, body composition and puberty to assess the malnutrition and growth status, impaired linear growth, as indicators of disease activity. Evaluation of nutritional status also included assessing diet history and dietary intake, biochemical indexes of nutrition.

Growth Status and Weight Change

Tables 1 and 2 represented comparisons of FA's assessed BMI status with the WHO L, M, S parameters and percentiles[1] (Cole, 1990) for body mass index for his age and gender. FA's BMI-for-age measurements when compared to 2007 WHO tables for percentiles, his growth pattern fell between the 25th & 50th percentile curves for the 13 years of age boys. Therefore, the patient' growth status in comparison to WHO reference data (Onis, Mercedes de, et al. 2007) indicated no urgent action is required with regards to his growth status.

Height-for-Age when compared to the WHO tables for percentiles reference, FA's height fell between the 5th & 15th percentile curves for the 13 years of age boys. Therefore, FA was significantly shorter than his healthy peers. This was comparable with the national reference data for the patient as his height falls slightly above the 10th percentile when plotted on the growth charts for Stature-for-Age for Egyptian boys 2 to 21 years **(Figure 1).** Additionally, the patient's weight for age was compared to the reference data for Egyptian boys, 2 to 21 years. The results of comparisons showed that FA's weight for age fell between the 10th & 25th percentile curves for the 13 years boys. The comparison was made by plotting his weight on the Weight-for-Age Percentiles growth charts for Egyptian boys 2 to 21 years.

Percentage of FA's weight change was also calculated and results confirmed an unintentional weight loss of 12% in the last 6 months, which indicated severe weight loss. The pubertal stage was also assessed to estimate if the patient's UC was associated with delayed pubertal development (Table 1 and 2).

Nutritional Problems

Based on laboratory tests, protein loss was noticed at the time of diagnosis, which was evidenced by the protinuria. This is because of the inflammation, diarrhea and decreased food intake.

The patient iron (Fe) and hemoglobin levels were low. Hemoglobin concentration was less than 10 g/dl. To evaluate the clinical significance of anemia, reference values for hemoglobin concentration (in g/dl) was compared to the German KiGGS[3] cutoff (Thierfelder et al., 2008).

Demographics

- Education: Intermediate school (grade 7)
- Occupation: student
- Ethnicity and religion: African Muslim

Table 1. Comparison of BMI-for-Age status for FA using the WHO L, M, and S parameters and percentiles for body mass index for age for boys (FA Case).

Who Reference	
13:0	Age (y)
-1.7168	L
18.2330	M
0.11898	S
14.5	1st
15.1	3rd
15.4	5th
16.3	15th*
16.9	25th
18.2	50th
19.9	75th
20.9	85th
23.1	95th
24.2	97th
26.5	99th

*Source: Aljaaly E, 2020

Table 2. Comparison of Height-for-Age status for FA using the WHO L, M, and S parameters and percentiles for HT-for-age for boys (FA Case).

Who Reference	
13:0	Age (y)
1	L
156.0426	M
0.04760	S
7.4276	SD
138.8	1st
142.1	3rd
143.8	5th
148.3	15th*
151.0	25th
156.0	50th
161.1	75th
163.7	85th
168.3	95th
170.0	97th
173.3	99th

*Source: Aljaaly E, 2020

- Routine vaccinations were given including; poliomyelitis, tuberculosis, diphtheria, tetanus, hepatitis B, measles, mumps, German measles (Rubella) and chicken pox.

Anthropometry

- Usual weight: 42
- Current weight: 39 kg
- Admission weight: 37kg
- Height: 144 cm
- Body Mass Index (BMI): 17.87 Kg/m^2 above the 25th percentile, which indicates that the weight status is within normal range.
- Percentage of weight change: Unintentional weight loss of 12% in 6 months.

Biochemical Data

Conducted laboratory data showed results as follows:

- The patient has microcytic hypochromic anemia with low iron and low ferritin levels due to occult blood loss in stool, a significant manifestation of UC.
- Mild leukocytosis owing to the inflammatory nature of UC.
- Minimal proteinuria, likely due to malnutrition rather than nephropathy. Renal functions are normal.
- Vitamin D insufficiency with a mild decrease in total calcium level.
- Normal thyroid function tests.

Figure 1. Growth Charts for Egyptian boys 2 to 21 years[2]

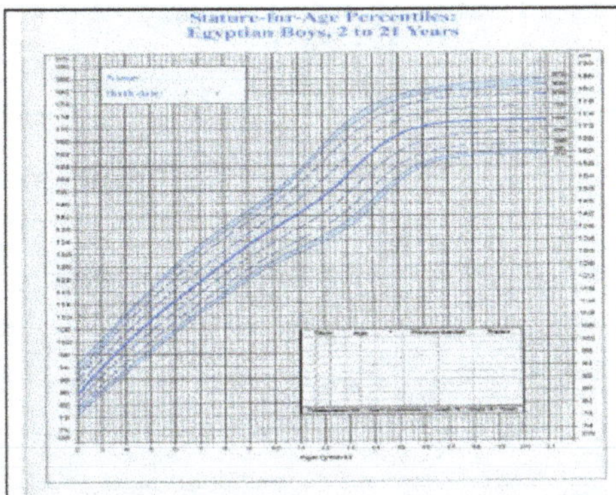

Stature-for-Age for Egyptian boys 2 to 21 years

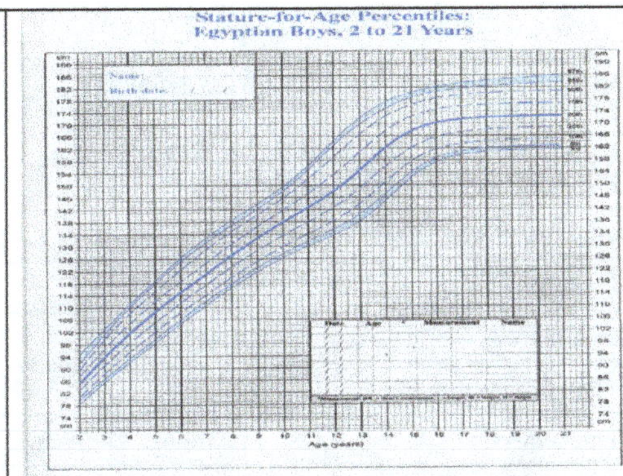

Weight-for-Age for Egyptian boys 2 to 21 years

Nutritional-Focused Physical Examination

- General appearance: pallor.
- Skin: Pale and mildly dry
- Heart: Regular heart rate and normal sound
- HEENT: head, eyes, ears, nose, and throat are free of any medical problem
- Neurologic: well oriented and alert
- Extremities: Normal and no edema
- Chest/lungs: Lungs and chest are clear
- Abdomen: colonic distension
- The review of other systems was unremarkable

Table 3. Biochemical Results

Parameter	Patients Results	Reference
CBC		
HB level	9.8 g/dL	12.1 – 16.6 g/dL
RBC	3.9 (x10^6/uL)	4.5 -5.6 (x10^6/uL)
HCT	31.1%	37 -49%
MCV	65 fl	77-92 fl
MCH	23.8 pg	26-32 pg
MCHC	31%	33-37%
Platlets	230 (x10^3 /uL)	150 - 430 (x10^3 /uL)
WBC	4.5 (x10^3/uL)	4.5-13 (x10^3/uL)
Neutrophils	65.5 (x10^3/uL)	1.8-8 (x10^3 /uL)
Lymphocytes	15%	25-45% (x10^3/uL)
Monocytes	1.8%	3-6%
Basophils	0.3%	0-1%
Eosinophils	1.5%	0-3%
Serum iron	38 mcg/dL	50-120 mcg/dL
Ferritin	6 ng/mL	7-140 ng/mL
Total serum calcium	8 mg/dL	8.8-10.8 mg/dL
25(OH)D,25-hydroxyvitamin D	23 ng/ml	30 ng/ml
Auto antibodies	-ve	-ve
Rheumatoid factor	-ve	-ve
Renal functions	Normal	Normal
Liver enzymes	Normal	Normal
Stool analysis	Normal	Normal
Occult blood in stool	+ve	-ve
Urine analysis	Minimal proteinuria	Nill

* -ve is means negative or normal findings was found when conducting the test.

** +ve Positive or abnormal findings was found when conducting the test.

Medical Management

The aim of this treatment plan is to reduce symptoms or as known by inducing remission of UC. This could allow the patient to have periods without symptoms and to maintain his remission. Some medicine was provided to increase the efficiency of therapy and to reduce the risk of complications and recurrence.

The therapeutic approach for the present case relied on the use of several medicines, which help to control inflammation in both the joints and intestines. Medical treatment included a local steroid injection (via rectal enema) to reduce the inflammation locally. Sulfasalazine and the biologic drug, the anti-tumor necrosis factor therapy (infliximab) used as specific treatments for UC. Symptomatic treatment of knee arthritis was done using the Nonsteroidal anti-inflammatory drugs (NSAIDs).

NSAID is a medicine that reduces pain, decreases fever, and prevents blood clots. It also reduces inflammation when taken in high doses. Physiotherapy sessions and MNT was prescribed in addition to the medications.

Doses of medications were as follows:

- Sulfasalazine: Initial dose 40: 60 mg/kg/day and was given orally. Doses divided into 3:6 doses then a maintenance dose of 30mg/kg/day was divided into 4 doses.
- Infliximab: Induction dose 5mg/kg as intravenous (IV) and was given at 0.2 and 6 weeks and then a maintenance dose of 5 mg/kg was given through IV every 8 weeks.
- NSAID was given according to the severity of arthritis.

Nutritional Management

Aims of the Nutrition Therapy

Nutrition management for this pediatric UC patient was aiming to counter the inflammation, alleviate symptoms and correct nutrient deficiency, prevent and manage malnutrition. As the patient's growth was affected, with nutrition management, we also aimed to promote optimal nutritional status for the patient.

The disease is in remission. Therefore, the approach used was a high-protein and nutrient-dense diet. This is in order to delay nutritional problems between exacerbations (Width & Reinhard, 2018).

Diet in the Maintenance of Remission in Ulcerative Colitis

Strategies that may have a role in maintaining remission in UC disease was prescribed to the patient and his family as follows:

1. Eat a nutrient-dense diet with sufficient protein and energy.
2. Increase the consumption of fruits and vegetables, which might be protective for disease progression.
3. Avoid food high in oxalate.
4. Avoid lactose, wheat, and gluten if the patient is not tolerating them.
5. Increase the intake of foods that are high in antioxidants.
6. Consider oral supplementation for deficient nutrients such as iron.

ADIME Note

Assessment: In order to detect nutrition-related problems, the RD immediately initiated the nutrition assessment and obtained data of the patient after the referral by his physician. Data was collected based on the referral information, the interdisciplinary records and her interview with the patient and his parents. Data collected included dietary history and nutrient intake, health status using anthropometric, biochemical measurements, physical and clinical conditions. Data on social, psychological status was also considered. All data were verified and interpreted to help making the decisions about the nutrition-related problems and its causes. The RD documented data as follows:

In summary, the patient is 13 years old Egyptian male with UC and extra intestinal manifestations in the form of right knee arthritis. Other conditions include iron deficiency anemia, diarrhea, and significant weight loss in the last 6 months.

- Anthropometry:
    - Usual weight: 42 kg.
    - Current weight: 39 kg
    - Admission weight: 37kg
    - Height: 144 cm
    - BMI = Body Mass Index (BMI): 17.87 Kg/m2. The weight status is in the normal range (^{3} 5th percentile), when compared to the WHO reference data. However, in comparison to national healthy peers, the child's weight for his age falls between the 10th & 25th percentile curves for the 13 years Egyptian boys.
    - The patient is short when compared to his healthy international peers, as his height falls between the 5th & 15th percentile curves for 13 years of age boys based on comparison with the WHO reference data. On the other hand, when plotted on the growth charts for Stature-for-Age for Egyptian boys 2 to 21 years, his height is slightly above the 10th percentile
    - Unintentional weight loss (UWL) of >10% in 6 months (significant weight loss).
- Biochemical:
    - Hemoglobin (¯)
    - Serum protein (¯)
    - Iron (Fe) level (¯)
    - Serum ferritin (¯)
    - Total calcium (¯)
    - Vitamin D (¯)

- Clinical:
    - Abdominal pain.
    - Nausea
    - Diarrhea
    - Weight loss
    - Painful right knee joints
    - GI bleeding

Dietary

Based on the reviewed dietary intake to assess nutritional adequacy, collected data showed inadequate intake concerning energy and protein intake. Energy intake was ranging from **800 to 900** kcal/**day** and protein intake was about **24 g/day**, which is less than the required energy, which meets only 49-54% of the required energy and protein, which is only meets 65% of the required protein intake for his age (Width & Reinhard, 2018).

- Patient dietary intake was reduced in the last six months. This was due to his poor appetite, which was combined with diarrhea and abdominal pain.
- Food-related patterns included showed a high consumption of fats and processed meats. The patient used to consume fast food 3-4 times/week.

Nutrition Diagnosis

Three Nutrition diagnosis statements were developed to establish critical links between the above conducted nutrition assessment for the patient and RD's plans for nutrition intervention. PES statements included the etiologies (E), signs or symptoms (S))

- Inadequate oral intake related to loss of appetite and abdominal pain as a result of UC, as evidenced by energy intake of 800 to 900 kcal/day and 24 g of protein/day.
- Unintentional weight loss related to inadequate oral food/beverage intake and altered GI function as evidenced by weight loss of 12% over 6 months and current BMI of 17.87.
- Altered GI function related to GI bleeding and blood loss, as evidenced by anemia.

Intervention: Nutrition interventions was planned to target and address the identified nutrition diagnoses and problem.

Dietary Prescription

The aims of treatment included induction and maintenance of disease remission in a hope to prevent cancer of the affected bowel, improvement in quality of life, and facilitation of normal growth and development. This was achieved by a cooperation of the pediatric gastroenterologist, along with the clinical dietitian.

- Energy and Protein Needs (Estimated for boys 12-13 years) (See Table 4)

Table 4.

Reference Weight	DRI (kcal/kg)	Protein (g/kg)
37	40 x 37 = 1480 kcal	0.92 x 37 = 34.04 g

***Source**: Width & Reinhard (2018).

Since the patient is in the stage of active disease and he experienced significant weight loss in the last 6 months period, in addition to his growth retardation, we planned diet to increase protein intake by 25% initially to help improve linear growth.

For micronutrients, an intravenous (IV) iron supplementation was recommended for the patient because he was clinically active with the disease. Additionally, and as per ESPEN notes for practitioners in 2018 that oral iron replacement is found to be connected with high levels of intolerance and resulting in a lack of compliance by patients. Therefore, they recommended the IV ferric carboxymaltose supplementation as an alternative and better to be tolerated than the oral supplementation, particularly in case of active disease with low hemoglobin<10 g/dL and the patient HG was 9.8 g/dL (Miele et al., 2018).

Dietary Recommendations

- Progress to low-fat, low-fiber, high-protein, high-kilocalories, small frequent meals as tolerated to avoid GI irritation.
- Gradually increase kcal until the requirement is reached.
- Encourage consumption of nutrient-dense diet to prevent nutrient deficiencies.
- Low or normal residue diet, by limiting high fiber, whole grains, nuts, seeds, raw or dried fruits and vegetables to minimize bowel motion to control diarrhea.
- Consume refined carbohydrates such as white pasta, rice, and bread to help to control the disease.

- Avoid high fatty and spicy food, carbonated and caffeinated beverages.
- Vitamin/mineral supplements: e.g. Vitamin D, folate, iron as required.
- Avoid dehydration and maintain good hydration.
- Supplement with omega 3 and prebiotic/probiotic.
- Encourage social support and family engagement to improve the patient's psychological status.

Monitoring and Re-Evaluation

Growth failure was one of the present case outcomes in the last period because of his poor nutritional status, which could affect his disease management. Therefore, it should be monitored closely at monthly bases. This is in order to ensure appropriate referral and treatment. The Physical examination will include anthropometric assessment of growth patterns along with recordings of sexual maturation. All growth parameters will be routinely collected and graphically documented on the appropriate standardized charts for age and gender. Anthropometric measures to be plotted into the appropriate growth charts and since the national growth charts are available, it will be used. The pubertal stage will be assessed every twelve months throughout follow-up visits until puberty is completed. Family growth patterns will also be considered, particularly for his parents' heights.

- Evaluate weight and weight change will be considered regularly and monitored every 3 months.
- Monitor diarrhea and abdominal pain and ask parents to record daily bowel movements
- Monitor intake, appetite and reduced oral intake, altered energy/nutrient metabolism, macronutrients, particularly protein. Regular dietary consulting will be well thought-out, caloric density will be increased and protein supplements will be considered.
- Food Records to assess quality and quantity of food will be repeated for 3 days once a year for this adolescent patient in the following-up period.
- Laboratory values for the related nutrient (e.g. iron, protein) to be observed and samples to be collected every 3 months and before a follow up visit.
- Control of GI symptoms.
- Annual colonoscopy and biopsy will be done after 8-10 years from the start of the disease to rule out any abnormal dysplasia before the development of cancer colon. total colectomy will be the only treatment plan in case of abnormal dysplasia

Other Managements and Referrals to Additional Professionals

Further referrals were to the social worker, the health educator, physiotherapist and psychological therapist. Referrals to these specialists were to evaluate issues related to patient's perceptions, beliefs, and motivations related to his disease and associated problems. Additionally, referrals to other specialists were supportive to assess the patient and parents' level of understanding of disease, the required management, to give detailed instructions about the provided treatment. For example, some referral aimed to train the patient on some techniques and exercises for relaxation and to prevent symptoms such as joint pain.

CONCLUSION

The authors used a number of evidenced-based guidelines in the stage of assessment, diagnosis, planning, treatment and monitoring of the present case. All relevant collected data were compared with standards. The ESPEN and ASPEN guidelines were used in the medical nutrition therapy of the present case study. The patient was presented to the outpatient pediatric clinic with symptoms of ulcerative colitis including diarrhea and abdominal pain. Patient's UC was associated with weight loss, joints pain and anemia. Social support and family engagements was highly encouraged. Patient's perceptions, beliefs, and motivation related to his disease and associated problem were highly considered. Changes in patient and his parents' level of understanding of his disease and the followed management approach was highly achieved, this was evidenced by his exceptional compliance to medical and nutritional treatment and continuous improvement of patient's health status and the control of his disease. Other management approaches included physiotherapy and psychological therapy.

The Mindmap in Figure 2 presents an illustration that concludes the presented case study including the etiology of UC disease and its pathophysiology, the patient's presented signs and symptoms and the-management used for both medical and nutrition care.

Technology Components

Technology components are based on the electronic patients' archiving system of the hospital, colonoscopy, digital X- ray, laboratory investigations and tissue pathology analysis.

Figure 2. A Mindmap of the presented case study.
Source: Khalifa N, 2020

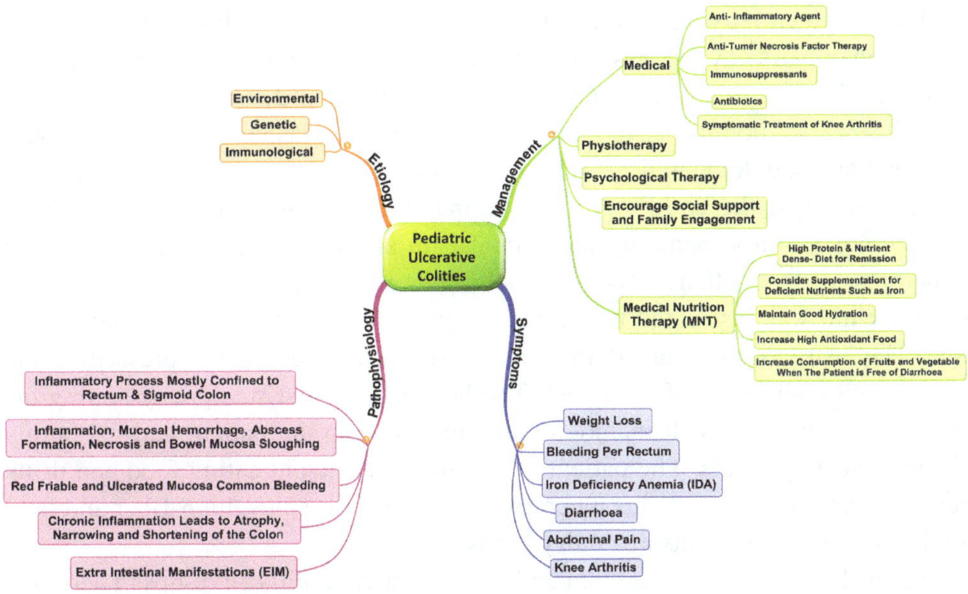

Management and Organizational Concerns

Permissions to conduct this case study included approval from the hospital administration to access patient's data and ethical approval from the parent and the child to report and publish the case. The suggested by book editors' template that include the case evaluation, management and reporting based on the NCP and ADIME note was used.

The treatment provided to the patient involved a range of healthcare professionals, including the pediatric gastroenterologists, the registered dietitian, a specialist nurse, a psychology therapist and a physiotherapist. All care was coordinated by the specialist nurse alongside whole care team. The nurse was the main point of contact for the patient and his family whenever they need help and advice.

More Concerns

In the present case, remission of ulcerative colitis with consequent remission of arthritis was the result after continuous treatment for 4 months. Long-life treatment and follow up were organized including; monitoring of growth, dual energy x-ray absorptiometry (DEXA), to exclude osteoporosis, annual colonoscopy after 8 years from the initial symptoms of UC. As patients with IBD are at risk of vitamin D deficiency and as per recommendations (Pappa et al., 2006), vitamin D was planned, to be routinely measured and supplemented when appropriate.

Anemia potentially leads to a significant reduction in health-related quality of life, which impairs physiological development, growth, and psychosocial processes (Laffolie, 2017), and poses a significant economic burden on health systems. Therefore, close monitoring to patient's anemia status was considered and proper treatment and supplementations were important.

In addition to the child's gastrointestinal (GI) symptoms that are related to his ulcerative colitis including abdominal pain and diarrhea, the child's non-GI symptoms i.e. the swollen and painful knee joint was planned to be closely monitored and the child was instructed to follow a regimen to help him prevent more joint pain. The instructions included an emphasis on taking medicine as prescribed and in consuming all doses of medicine. The healthy diet that was prescribed by the registered dietitian, which included guidelines to help the patient and his family planning healthy meals. The patient is encouraged to avoid eating food and drink items that could exacerbate his ulcerative colitis such as spicy, high-fiber and fatty food, and to carefully consume dairy foods.

It is well known that stress can activate ulcerative colitis flare-ups. Therefore, the medical team emphasized to the patient and family to avoid stress to deactivate ulcerative subsidence, and the psychology therapist trained the patient about some relaxation techniques to practice at home e.g. deep breathing to reduce stress and prevent symptoms such as joint pain.

The patient was also referred to a physical therapist who advised him and his family about the correct technique to decrease pain like applying warm, wet compresses or heating pads on the painful joints, to stretch the affected joints and do range-of-motion exercises. Patient was also instructed to elevate the inflamed swollen joint during active inflammation.

Drug–nutrient interactions were also evaluated in this case as numerous drugs that are used to treat IBD, including UC could directly affect patients' nutritional intake or inhibit absorption of some nutrients. They could also influence the metabolism and loss of some nutrients. A good example is the antagonistic interaction of methotrexate with folate metabolism and its inherent side-effect of nausea. Prophylactic supplementation was recommended as part of the management of IBD patients. Similarly, the long-term effects of steroids on calcium excretion, bone restoration, growth, body composition and nutritional intake are all been recognized.

A follow up plan was done including; follow up of medications and monitoring of side effects. Follow up of the patient's growth (weight and height). Annual colonoscopy is planned after 8 years from the onset of the disease to detect any early dysplasia. Screening for osteoporosis is done from the initial time of presentation.

REFERENCES

Abraham, B. P., & Kahn, S. A. (2014). Transition of care in inflammatory bowel disease. *Gastroenterology & Hepatology, 10*(10), 633. PMID:27540335

Bain, B. J., Lewis, S. M., & Bates, I. (2006). Basic haematological techniques. *Dacie and Lewis Practical Haematology, 4*, 19-46.

Beaugerie, L., & Itzkowitz, S. H. (2015). Cancers complicating inflammatory bowel disease. *The New England Journal of Medicine, 372*(15), 1441–1452. doi:10.1056/NEJMra1403718 PMID:25853748

Bernstein, C. N., Blanchard, J. F., Rawsthorne, P., & Yu, N. (2001). The prevalence of extraintestinal diseases in inflammatory bowel disease: A population-based study. *The American Journal of Gastroenterology, 96*(4), 1116–1122. doi:10.1111/j.1572-0241.2001.03756.x PMID:11316157

Bradley, G. M., & Oliva-Hemker, M. (2012). Pediatric ulcerative colitis: Current treatment approaches including role of infliximab Biologics. *Targets and Therapy, 6*, 125–134. PMID:22740771

Cardile, S., & Romano, C. (2014, January 7). Current issues in pediatric inflammatory bowel disease-associated arthropathies. *World Journal of Gastroenterology, 20*(1), 45–52. doi:10.3748/wjg.v20.i1.45 PMID:24415857

Cole, T. J. (1990). The LMS method for constructing normalized growth standards. *European Journal of Clinical Nutrition, 44*(1), 45–60. PMID:2354692

Conrad, M. A., & Rosh, J. R. (2017). Pediatric inflammatory bowel disease. *Pediatric Clinics, 64*(3), 577–591. PMID:28502439

D'Haens, G., Geboes, K., Peeters, M., Baert, F., Ectors, N., & Rutgeerts, P. (1997). Patchy cecal inflammation associated with distal ulcerative colitis: A prospective endoscopic study. *The American Journal of Gastroenterology, 92*, 1275–1279. PMID:9260788

de Bie, C. I., Buderus, S., Sandhu, B. K., de Ridder, L., Paerregaard, A., & Veres, G. (2005). Inflammatory bowel disease in children and adolescents. Recommendations for diagnosis: the Porto criteria. Medical position paper: IBD working group of the European Society for Paediatric Gastroenterology, Hepatology and Nutrition (ESPGHAN). *Journal of Pediatric Gastroenterology and Nutrition, 41*, 1–7. doi:10.1097/01.MPG.0000163736.30261.82 PMID:15990620 de Onis, M., & ... . (2007). Development of a WHO growth reference for school-aged children and adolescents. *Bulletin of the World Health Organization*, *85*(09), 660–667. doi:10.2471/BLT.07.043497 PMID:18026621

Evon, G. P., & Ravikumara, M. (2010, March). Endoscopic and Histologic Findings in Pediatric Inflammatory Bowel Disease. *Gastroenterology & Hepatology*, *6*(3). PMID:20567564

Forbes, A., Escher, J., Hébuterne, X., Kłęk, S., Krznaric, Z., Schneider, S., Shamir, R., Stardelova, K., Wierdsma, N., Wiskin, A. E., & Bischoff, S. C. (2017). ESPEN guideline: Clinical nutrition in inflammatory bowel disease. *Clinical Nutrition (Edinburgh, Lothian)*, *36*(2), 321–347. doi:10.1016/j.clnu.2016.12.027 PMID:28131521

Glickman, J. N., Bousvaros, A., Farraye, F. A., Zholudev, A., Friedman, S., Wang, H. H., Leichtner, A. M., & Odze, R. D. (2004). Pediatric patients with untreated ulcerative colitis may present initially with unusual morphologic findings. *The American Journal of Surgical Pathology*, *28*(2), 190–197. doi:10.1097/00000478-200402000-00006 PMID:15043308

Hyams, J. S. (2005). Inflammatory bowel disease. *Pediatrics in Review*, *26*(9), 314–320. doi:10.1542/pir.26-9-314 PMID:16140873

Johnson-Wimbley, T. D., & Graham, D. Y. (2011). Diagnosis and management of iron deficiency anemia in the 21st century. *Therapeutic Advances in Gastroenterology*, *4*(3), 177–184. doi:10.1177/1756283X11398736 PMID:21694802

Kugathasan, S., Judd, R. H., Hoffmann, R. G., Heikenen, J., Telega, G., Khan, F., ... Yaffe, M. (2003). Epidemiologic and clinical characteristics of children with newly diagnosed inflammatory bowel disease in Wisconsin: A statewide population-based study. *The Journal of Pediatrics*, *143*(4), 525–531. doi:10.1067/S0022-3476(03)00444-X PMID:14571234

Laffolie, J. D., Laass, M. W., Scholz, D., Zimmer, K. P., & Buderus, S.CEDATA-GPGE Study Group. (2017). Prevalence of anemia in pediatric IBD patients and impact on disease severity: Results of the pediatric IBD-registry CEDATA-GPGE®. *Gastroenterology Research and Practice*, 2017. PMID:29358946

Laharie, D. (2017). Towards therapeutic choices in ulcerative colitis. *Lancet*, *390*(10090), 98–99. doi:10.1016/S0140-6736(17)31263-1 PMID:28527707

Lee, J. J., Escher, J. C., Shuman, M. J., Forbes, P. W., Delemarre, L. C., Harr, B. W., Kruijer, M., Moret, M., Allende-Richter, S., & Grand, R. J. (2010). Final adult height of children with inflammatory bowel disease is predicted by parental height and patient minimum height Z-score. *Inflammatory Bowel Diseases*, *16*(10), 1669–1677. doi:10.1002/ibd.21214 PMID:20127995

Levesque, B. G., & Sandborn, W. J. (2012). Infliximab versus ciclosporin in severe ulcerative colitis. *Lancet*, *380*(9857), 1887–1888. doi:10.1016/S0140-6736(12)61259-8 PMID:23063315

Levine, J.S., & Burakoff, R. (2011). Extraintestinal Manifestations of Inflammatory Bowel Disease. *Gastroenterology & Hepatology*, *7*(4).

Mahan, L. K., & Raymond, J. L. (2016). *Krause's food & the nutrition care process-e-book*. Elsevier Health Sciences.

Mamula, P., Markowitz, J. E., & Baldassano, R. N. (2013). *Pediatric inflammatory bowel disease* (2nd ed.). Springer Science of Business Media. doi:10.1007/978-1-4614-5061-0

Miele, E., Shamir, R., Aloi, M., Assa, A., Braegger, C., Bronsky, J., ... Koletzko, S. (2018). Nutrition in pediatric inflammatory bowel disease: A position paper on behalf of the Porto Inflammatory Bowel Disease Group of the European Society of Pediatric Gastroenterology, Hepatology and Nutrition. *Journal of Pediatric Gastroenterology and Nutrition*, *66*(4), 687–708. doi:10.1097/MPG.0000000000001896 PMID:29570147

Pappa, H. M., Gordon, C. M., Saslowsky, T. M., Zholudev, A., Horr, B., Shih, M. C., & Grand, R. J. (2006). Vitamin D status in children and young adults with inflammatory bowel disease. *Pediatrics*, *118*(5), 1950–1961. doi:10.1542/peds.2006-0841 PMID:17079566

Sawczenko, A., & Sandhu, B. K. (2003). Presenting features of inflammatory bowel disease in Great Britain and Ireland. *Archives of Disease in Childhood*, *88*(11), 995–1000. doi:10.1136/adc.88.11.995 PMID:14612366

Schorr-Lesnick, B., & Brandt, L. J. (1988). Selected rheumatologic and dermatologic manifestations of inflammatory bowel disease. *The American Journal of Gastroenterology*, *83*, 216–223. PMID:3278591

Soda, A., Midha, V., Sood, N., & Bhatia, A. S. (2003). Incidence and prevalence of ulcerative colitis in Punjab, North India. *Gut*, *52*(11), 1587–1590. doi:10.1136/gut.52.11.1587 PMID:14570727

Stringer, D. A. (1987). Imaging inflammatory bowel disease in the pediatric patient. *Radiologic Clinics of North America*, *25*, 93–113. PMID:3823396

Thierfelder, W., Dortschy, R., Hintzpeter, B., Kahl, H., & Scheidt-Nave, C. (2008). Biochemical measures in the German Health Interview and Examination Survey for Children and Adolescents (KiGGS) 1. *Laboratoriumsmedizin (Berlin)*, *32*(2), -. doi:10.1515/JLM.2008.010et

Trost, L. B., Bergfeld, W. F., & Calogeras, E. (2006). The diagnosis and treatment of iron deficiency and its potential relationship to hair loss. *Journal of the American Academy of Dermatology*, *54*(5), 824–844. doi:10.1016/j.jaad.2005.11.1104 PMID:16635664

Van Limbergen, J., Russell, R. K., Drummond, H. E., Aldhous, M. C., Round, N. K., Nimmo, E. R., Smith, L., Gillett, P. M., McGrogan, P., Weaver, L. T., Bisset, W. M., Mahdi, G., Arnott, I. D., Satsangi, J., & Wilson, D. C. (2008). Definition of phenotypic characteristics of childhood-onset inflammatory bowel disease. *Gastroenterology*, *135*(4), 1114–1122. doi:10.1053/j.gastro.2008.06.081 PMID:18725221

Width, M., & Reinhard, T. (2018). *The Essential Pocket Guide for Clinical Nutrition*. Wolters Kluwer Health.

Williams, C. B., & Nicholls, S. (1994). Endoscopic features of chronic inflammatory bowel disease in childhood. *Bailliere's Clinical Gastroenterology*, *8*(1), 121–131. doi:10.1016/S0950-3528(06)80022-9 PMID:8003739

KEY TERMS AND DEFINITIONS

KiGGS: The German Health Interview and Examination Survey for Children and Adolescents (KiGGS). Is the first nationwide comprehensive study on the health of children and adolescents living in Germany.

LMS Parameters: L means Lambda for the skew, Mu for the median, and S for Sigma for the generalized coefficient of variation. The method was established by Cole, T in 1990 to calculate percentiles and z-scores by health professionals.

ENDNOTES

1. The LMS parameters: L means Lambda for the skew, Mu for the median, and S for Sigma for the generalized coefficient of variation. The method was established by Cole, T in 1990 to calculate percentiles and z-scores by health professionals.
2. http://dempuegypt.blogspot.com/2008/11/egyptian-gorwth-curves-boys-2-21-years.html
3. The German Health Interview and Examination Survey for Children and Adolescents (KiGGS). Is the first nationwide comprehensive study on the health of children and adolescents living in Germany

Chapter 9
Irritable Bowel Syndrome (IBS)

Eram Albajri
King Abdulaziz University, Saudi Arabia

Manal Naseeb
King Abdulaziz University, Saudi Arabia

EXECUTIVE SUMMARY

The proposed case will discuss irritable bowel syndrome. Individualized medical nutrition therapy is critical in the disease management. In this case, the learner will be provided with details to conceptualize the case and will be able to conduct a comprehensive nutrition assessment to evaluate the nutritional status. After identifying and prioritizing nutrition problems, the learner will determine the nutrition diagnoses and write proper statements. Based on the collected data, the learner will develop a nutrition care plan with appropriate goals, interventions, and strategies for monitoring and evaluation. Unspecified-IBS encounter challenges with food as it triggers the symptoms. Thus, the learner will evaluate the nutrient composition of dietary history and provide a substitute considering individual tolerance and severity of the symptoms. In addition, FODMAP will be applied. It also teaches patients what foods or eating patterns would be best (or best to avoid) for their day-to-day activities through self-awareness of symptoms and dietary food log.

INTRODUCTION

Irritable bowel syndrome (IBS) is the most common of the functional gastrointestinal (GI) disorders that affect the large intestine. IBS is considered a chronic disorder characterized by intermittent abdominal pain or discomfort associated with altered bowel movement for at least three months. IBS is also considered a disorder of

DOI: 10.4018/978-1-7998-3802-9.ch009

gut-brain interactions as it is related to how the brain and gut work together. The gut becomes more sensitive and changes how the bowel muscle contract leading to abdominal pain, bloating, diarrhea, constipation, or a combination of diarrhea and constipation. Even with these troublesome symptoms, IBS is not a life-threatening condition, however; it could intensely change the quality of life and work productivity. The prevalence of IBS varies throughout the world. It ranges from 10% to 23% in the general population worldwide, with the highest prevalence of 21% in South America and the lowest prevalence of 4.2% in South Africa. In the Arab region, the prevalence of IBS is ranged from 8.9% to 31.8%. In Saudi Arabia, the prevalence of IBS was 22.9% (Alosaim M., Ali A., & H., 2016). The prevalence of IBS is higher in women than men by a 2:1 ratio. Younger people are more likely to develop IBS than people older than 50 years. This disorder is classified into four subtypes, each with slightly different symptoms, depending on the bowel habits (stool type and frequency). These subtypes include irritable bowel syndrome constipation-predominant (IBS-C), irritable bowel syndrome diarrhea-predominant (IBS-D), irritable bowel syndrome mixed (IBS-M), and irritable bowel syndrome unspecified (IBS-U). To distingue between these classifications of IBS, health care provider would investigate how stool type (watery vs. solid) and frequency (number of times) change in response of abdominal pain (a common symptom in this disorder). (Chey, Kurlander, & Eswaran, 2015; Lacy et al., 2016; Moayyedi et al., 2017).

The precise cause of IBS remains unknown; however, several factors have been linked to increasing the risk of IBS. These include lifestyle factors such as diet, smoking, and alcohol consumption; psychological factors such as stress and anxiety; genetic factors; small intestinal bacterial overgrowth; food intolerance as well as severe infection in the GI system. Although the pathophysiology is not entirely recognized, understanding the pathogenesis of IBS is vital in developing newer pharmacotherapy agents to target the known pathophysiologic mechanisms. The pathogenesis of the IBS is complex and multifactorial. Several pathophysiological abnormalities have been described, including altered gastrointestinal motility, increased sensitivity of the GI tract to internal and external stimuli, disturbances of brain-gut interactions, food intolerance, bacterial overgrowth, post-infectious reactivity, dysregulation of serotonin concentrations in the GI tact, genetic susceptibility, and psychosocial stress factors. Nervous system alterations can result in abnormal gastrointestinal motility and visceral hypersensitivity. Researchers found that concentrations of serotonin are associated with IBS. Low serotonin concentrations are associated with constipation whereas higher serotonin concentrations are associated with diarrhea (Academy of Nutrition and Dietetics, 2020; Alharbi, 2018; Canadian Society of Intestinal Research, 2018; Cedars-Sinai, 2020; Chey et al., 2015; Lacy et al., 2016; Lehrer, J. K., 2019; Mayo Clinic, 2018; Peyton & Greene, 2014; WebMD, 2020).

There is no specific diagnostic test or marker for IBS. Generally, IBS is diagnosed solely on symptoms. However, symptoms of IBS may be mistaken with inflammatory bowel disease (IBD), celiac disease, intolerance for carbohydrates such as fructose and lactose, etc., and may not be explained by structural abnormalities, which make it challenging for the physicians to diagnose. A careful history and physical exams are the most critical steps for the initial diagnosis. In general, symptoms of IBS are often recurrent and vary from patient to patient. Signs and symptoms range from lower abdominal pain or discomfort, bloating, diarrhea, constipation, nausea, mucus in the stool, and incomplete evacuation; however, not all the symptoms are gastrointestinal. Common non-gastrointestinal symptoms are fatigue, chest discomfort, and headaches. ROME III identify criteria for diagnosing IBS, these include recurrent abdominal pain or discomfort three days per month in the last three months and association with two more of the following: improvement with defecation, onset associated with a change in the frequency of stool and/or onset associated with a change in form of stool. The American College of Gastroenterology (ACG) also develops a definition for IBS, which states that IBS is diagnosed when abdominal pain or discomfort that occurs in association with altered bowel habits for at least three months. Patients often experience a relapse of symptoms over time. Individuals with IBS may alternate between classifications and the actual distinction may depend on when the history was taken regarding bowel habits. Due to these symptoms, patients with IBS often suffer from decease quality of life, decreased productivity, increased missed work and school days, and increased health burden (Academy of Nutrition and Dietetics, 2020; Cedars-Sinai, 2020; Chey et al., 2015; Ford et al., 2018; Moayyedi et al., 2017; National Institute of Health,2020).

A common valid and reliable tool used for assessing bowel habit is the Bristol Stool Form Scale (BSFS). This self-diagnostic chart has seven different pictures on a chart and each representing a specific pattern of stool. The samples capture the range between the two extreme ends of stool type spectrum. At one end of the spectrum is hard stool representing constipation while on the other end of the spectrum is watery stool representing diarrhea. For example, Type 1 (starting form the top of the chart) has few brown circles that has this descriptive next to it “separate hard lumps, like nuts, hard to pass” while Type 2 is described as “sausage-like but lumpy”. These two types indicate constipation. Type 3 is “like a sausage but with cracks in the surface” while Type 4 is “like a sausage or snake, smooth and soft”. Types 3 and 4 indicate ideal stools which are easy to pass. The last three types indicate diarrhea and urgency and they include soft blobs with clear-cut edges. Type 5 is considered as “fluffy pieces with ragged edges”, while “a mushy stool” can best describe type 6, and “watery, no solid pieces” can describe type 7 (Continence Foundation of Australia, 2020).

Management of IBS should mainly focus on alleviating symptoms and reassuring the patient that IBS is not a severe illness. Effective patient, gastroenterologist, and dietitian relationship is a critical component to establish the most appropriate management option. Management is often symptom-specific, involving medical, lifestyle, psychological, and nutritional components. All these components share the same goal, which is to minimize and improve symptoms and improve the quality of life. The medical components include medications, which focused on reducing or treating the symptoms and stress reduction such as antidiarrheal, antispasmodic, pain medication, and antidepressants. The lifestyle components include smoke cession, regular exercise, and adequate sleep. The psychological components include cognitive-behavioral therapy, stress management, and hypnotherapy. Complementary and Alternative Medicine (CAM) therapies are new under investigating management approaches used in alleviating IBS symptoms. These may involve herbal therapies, acupuncture, yoga, relaxation, and other mindfulness activities. Of interest, acupuncture has been found to cause physiological changes that may affect various endogenous neurotransmitter systems, thus minimize the severity of the symptoms. Currently, many questions about the efficacy and safety of CAM therapies still exist; however, the collaboration between CAM practitioners, primary care doctors, and gastroenterologists with their patients could help to find the appropriate treatment. Further research in this area is still required to determine the definite recommendations that can be made.

Nutrients presence in the GI tract affects GI motility, sensitivity, barrier function, and gut microbiota, making dietary management an important tool in the treatment of IBS. The first line approach in dietary management is healthy eating which include adhering to regular meal pattern, small frequent meals, avoid skipping meals, chew food thoroughly, reduce intake of caffeine, spicy and high fat foods, avoid or reduce intake of alcohol, as well as regular physical activity, and adequate hydration. Caffeine consumption is known to increase gastric acid secretion and colonic motor activity as it is known as a colonic stimulant. Moreover, ingestion of spicy foods triggers GI symptoms such as abdominal pain and gastroesophageal reflux, which are common symptoms in IBS symptoms due to the presence of Capsaicin, an active component of chilli peppers. High fat intake can result in gas retention and bloating. Limit or avoid alcohol consumption is recommended as it affects gastrointestinal motility, absorption, and permeability. Moderate physical activity such as yoga, walking, and cycling are preferred compared to strenuous exercise. It increases GI motility, decreases neuroimmuno-endocrine alterations, and splanchnic blood flow. Additionally, physical activity improves psychological symptoms. The main aims of the nutrition management are to adjust foods to improve symptoms through diet modification such as diet low in Fermentable Oligo-, Di-, Mono-saccharides and Polyols (FODMAPs), to ensure adequate nutrient intake, to normalized eating pattern, to identify food allergies and intolerance, to avoid food that increase gas and abdominal distention, to consider use of prebiotics and probiotics as it may effect IBS through various mechanism such as GI dysregulation, intestinal microbiota, intestinal immune function, and increase the tolerance for FODMAPS rich foods. However, researchers are still studying the use of probiotics to treat IBS (Academy of Nutrition and Dietetics, 2020; Chey et al., 2015; Lacy et al., 2016; Moayyedi et al., 2017; Peyton & Greene, 2014). Implementation of nutrition intervention should start from a simple approach to the complex. A registered dietitian, counseling patients with IBS should include assessment of patient's current food intake to determine food triggers, assess nutritional status, review all medications used, review GI symptoms, review supplementation used, and review behavioral therapy.

FODMAP is a dietary intervention that aims to reduced symptoms of IBS. The diet can be adjusted to trial elimination of foods that are not tolerated, while monitoring the symptoms of IBS. The acronym stands for specific fermentable short chain carbohydrates, which are poorly absorbed in the intestine including oligosaccharides (fructan and galacto-oligosaccharides), disaccharides (lactose), monosaccharides (fructose) and polyols (sugar alcohol). Fructan is oligosaccharides that is found in wheat products, rye, garlic, onion, leeks, and artichokes. Due to the lack of enzymes to fully hydrolyze fructan, the unabsorbed particles reach the colon goes under fermentation and results in bloating and diarrhea. Another type of oligosaccharides is galacto-oligosaccharides that causes flatulence and gas. It is found in foods such as dairy products, beans, lentils, soybeans, and nuts. Lactose is a type of disaccharides that is found in dairy products. Fructose is a type of monosaccharides that is found mostly in fruits, honey, and high-fructose corn syrup. Polyols are sugar alcohols such as sorbitol, mannitol, maltitol, erythritol, xylitol, and isomalt. These are used in producing low caloric and sugar-free products. Polyols are also found in apricots, avocados, cherries, nectarines, peaches, and plums and mushrooms. High FODMAP foods and alternative low FODMAP foods are displayed in Table 1. Researches have shown that patients who stick with the low FODMAP diet had improves their quality of life (Academy of Nutrition and Dietetics, 2020; Fedewa, A., & Rao, S. S. 2014)

The primary mechanism of action of FODMAP, which are short-chain carbohydrates, has two components 1) gas production and 2) osmotic effect. Increase gas production, which results from the rapid fermentation of these food items by gut bacteria. On the other hand, the osmotic effect is exerted by drawing more fluid into the gut. The increase in gas production and fluid in the luminal leads to distention and increase visceral hypersensitivity; thus, development of the symptoms including pain, bloating, diarrhea and/or constipation. It had been suggested that high FODMAP foods affect gastrointestinal endocrine cells, which responsible to regulate gastrointestinal sensation, motility, secretion, absorption, and immune defense and food consumption (Academy of Nutrition and Dietetics, 2020, Johns Hopkins medicine, 2020; Stanford Health Care, 2020).

A registered dietitian should be supervising the administering of FODMAP diet as the cutoff value for acceptable amounts is individualized. FODMAP diet involves three main phases. The first phase is restricting all foods high in FODMAP. The aim here is to understand how these food components may exacerbate the symptoms. In addition, providing the patient with knowledge about these food items and where they are in food. The duration of this phase may range from 2 to 6 weeks depends on the severity of the condition. If symptoms did not improve, the diet should be terminated; however, if symptoms improved, the second phase should be initiated. The aim of the re-challenge phase, "the second phase," is to slow, controlled reintroduce high FODMAP foods by food group, one item at a time to test patients' tolerance and specify the components in FODMAP that are the cause of the symptoms. There are two approaches to proceed in this phase which are the slow approach or the faster approach. The only difference between these two approaches is the frequency, wherein the slow approach, patients will wait a couple of days between introducing a new food item. On the other hand, in the faster approach, patients will add a new item each day. The second phase helps to improve nutritional adequacy and food variety. The last phase is the personalized FODMAP diet, which aims to improve food quality by mildly limiting food restriction and providing substitutions. One of the suggested reasons for personalized FODMAP is that probably due to the intestinal microbiota differing between individuals. In this phase, patients are self-empowered as they increase and decrease restriction as IBS fluctuates in severity. Patients will understand their bodies and how diet may impact them. This will help them by minimizing stress about the unknown cause of their symptoms and what they can do to help relieve pain. Implementation of low FODMAP diet is challenging especially for adequate intake of fibers and calcium as well as restricting intake of prebiotic fructans and galacto-oligosaccharides could alter luminal microbiota. Dietitians who specialized in GI are a key towards success of this complex approach. Nutritional deficiencies could arise with low FODMAPs diet include folate, thiamin, vitamin B6, calcium, as well as vitamin D; however, the goal is to minimize or eliminate GI symptoms with most tolerable intake level of FODMAPs foods. Registered dietitian should provide a number of resources including mobile apps, cookbooks, and websites to facilitate adherence to the diet. (Academy of Nutrition and Dietetics, 2020).

There are several complications form IBS; however, none of them are life-threatening. IBS does not lead to cancer or other serious bowel-related conditions. Long time constipation could lead to fecal impaction, which causes headaches, nausea, and vomiting. Malnutrition is another complication that could result from cutting back on some foods without working with a registered dietitian to ensure adequate nutrients intake. In addition, chronic constipation or diarrhea can cause hemorrhoids. People with IBS may also suffer from poor quality of life due to severe symptoms. The signs and symptoms of IBS can lead to mood disorders such as depression and anxiety, which can make IBS worse. The prognosis of the IBS is not known. The IBS does not affect life expectancy or lead to other serious diseases. There is no cure for IBS; however, care should be tailored to help patients to deal with their symptoms. The symptoms can be minimized by dietary changes, reduce stress, and medication. Irritable bowel syndrome unspecified (IBS-U) is the focus of this case and will be discussed in detail.

CASE DESCRIPTION

Patient's Details

- Age: 34
- Gender: Female

Case History

Stephanie is a 34-years old female who was diagnosed with IBS Unspecified (IBS-U) three months ago by her primary care physician. Her doctor requested a complete checkup, including lab test, physical examination, and abdominal x-ray. The results were normal, but the symptoms persisted. The doctor requested colonoscopy and endoscopy, which also turned normal except for signs of gastritis.

She followed a gluten-free diet for a month per her physician's suggestion, but her symptoms did not improve. She had an intermittent episode of abdominal cramping and bloating associated with 4-6 loose, watery stool and hard stool occurring ~2 days per week. Her abdominal cramp seems to occur shortly after meals or at times of increased stress and subsides after a bowel movement. She feels abdominal fullness quickly after she starts eating.

The patient mentioned that symptoms started when she was accepted to the PhD program. She admitted to feeling stressed and anxious all the time because of the tremendous amount of pressure. In addition to her study, she works two jobs. The doctor referred patient to a registered dietitian to help her manage her abdominal symptoms through adjustment of her diet pattern by providing the proper nutrition education specific to her needs and case. With the help of the registered dietitian, Stephanie would be self-empower to identify specific foods that cause or worse her symptoms.

- Medical history (Hx): Gastroesophageal reflux disease (GERD), anemia, gastritis
- Surgical history: None
- Smoking: No

Family history: patient's family history is remarkable for type 2 diabetes and cardiovascular disease (CVD). Her father (age 50) has type 2 diabetes and cardiovascular disease. Her paternal grandfather (deceased at the age of 80) had the same condition. No other family history of any GI disorders or malignancies.

Main Medical Diagnosis

Irritable bowel syndrome unspecified (IBS-U)

Demographics

- Marital status: Single
- Education: Graduate student
- Occupation: Full time PhD student, works as research assistant and project manager.
- Ethnicity and religion: American Muslim

Social History: Stephanie lives alone in the one-bedroom, one-story apartment she has occupied for the last five years ago. Her parents helped her financially to finish her master's program, and after graduation, she did not find a job and decided to get a Ph.D. degree to increase her chance for hiring. Her scholarship was denied, and she had to work two jobs to cover the cost of her Ph.D. program. She never experienced such challenging circumstances. When asked about her social life, she admitted that since she started her Ph.D., she didn't have time to contact or go out with anyone.

Anthropometry

- Usual weight (Wt): 51 kg
- Current weight: 50 kg
- Height (Ht): 1.59 m

Table 1. Biochemical Data

Parameter	Patients Results	Reference
White Blood Cells	4.9 THO/uL	4.0 - 11.0 THO/uL
Red Blood Cells	4.57 MIL/uL	3.80 - 5.30 MIL/uL
Hemoglobin	13.0 g/dL	12.0 - 16.0 g/dL
Hematocrit	40%	36 - 46%
RDW	21.0%	11.5 - 14.5%
MCH	29 pg	27 - 33 pg
MCHC	33 g/dL	31 - 36 g/dL
MCV	88 fL	80 - 100 fL
Platelets	201 THO/uL	150 - 400 THO/uL
Ferritin	198.3 ng/mL	13.0 - 150.0 ng/mL
Urea Nitrogen	11 mg/dL	8 - 20 mg/dL
Sodium	142 mmol/L	136 - 144 mmol/L
Potassium	4.6 mmol/L	3.6 - 5.1 mmol/L
Calcium	9.5 mg/dL	8.9 - 10.3 mg/dL
Total Protein	7.3 g/dL	6.1 - 7.9 g/dL
Albumin	4.3 g/dL	3.5 - 5.1 g/dL

Nutritional-Focused Physical Examination

- General appearance: 34-year-old female with healthy appearance, no acute distress
- Heart: Regular rate and rhythm, heart sounds normal
- HEENT:
  - *Eyes:* Clear
  - *Ears:* Clear
  - *Nose:* Within Normal Limits (WNL)
  - *Throat:* Pharynx clear
- Genitalia: Normal
- Neurologic: Alert and oriented
- Extremities: No edema
- Skin: Skin pale without rash
- Chest/lungs: Lungs clear to auscultation and percussion
- Abdomen: Distension with moderate pain

Vital Signs

- Pulse:82 bpm
- Temp: 36.5°C
- Blood pressure: 115/75 mm Hg
- Resp rate: 18 bpm

Food/Nutrition-Related History

Patient states she has been following gluten-free diet for a month. She mentioned that her symptoms did not improve, and she stopped it. She had lost 1 kg since she was diagnosed. She likes to drink coffee and chew gum regularly. She loves cooking for her herself. She rarely eats outside.

Table 2. 24-Hour Recall

Meal	Food Items and Quantities
Meal 1 "Breakfast"	Coffee (1 cup) with whole milk (3 tbsp), bagel (2)
Meal 2	Apple (1)
Meal 3 "Lunch"	Sandwich (turkey), Mushroom soup (1 cup) from home
Meal 4	Mixed dried fruits (1 cup), yoghurt, Coffee (1 cup)
Meal 5 "Dinner"	Pasta with ground beef (1 piece) and salad (cabbages, cauliflower, and broccoli)
Meal 6	Chamomile tea (1 cup)

- Food allergies/intolerances: None
- Food purchase/preparations: Self
- Vitamin and mineral supplementation: Vitamin D 800 International Units (IU), and Multivitamin daily

Medications

Pantoprazole 40mg (as needed), BENTYL (20mg)

Solutions and Recommendations

Based on the information above, dietary component and stress are the main triggers of stephanie's symptoms.

Her case can be controlled by managing stress and by making changes in your diet and lifestyle. This section will focus mainly on the dietary intervention. General guidelines for people with IBS involve the following:

- Set goals by the patient and registered dietitian with consistent follow-up for additional interventions as required
- Identifying food intolerances and providing substitutions to maximize nutritional status and assist in controlling the symptoms
- Normalize eating patterns and ensure adequacy of all nutrients
- Avoid foods that exacerbate symptoms
- Avoid food that increase gas production and abdominal bloating such as caffeine, carrots, celery, onions
- Follow Low FODMAPS (fermentable oligosaccharides, disaccharides, monosaccharides and polyols) diet
- Follow Low lactose diet, if lactose intolerance
- Eat high-fiber foods, may change depend on the bowel movement
- Drink plenty of fluids to compensate for fluid loss
- Exercise regularly to maintain GI function and minimize stress and anxiety
- Avoid or limit caffeine to 400 mg to limit anxiety and bowel movement
- Takes vitamin and mineral supplements, in case of deficiencies
- Consider use of probiotic

Disease Pathophysiology Mind Map (Figure 1)

Main Aim of the Nutrition Therapy

- Adjust foods to improve symptoms
- Diet modification (Diet low in FODMAPs)
- Identify food allergies and intolerances
- Avoid foods that increase gas and flatulence
- Normalize eating patterns
- Ensure adequate nutrient and fluid intake
- Consider use of prebiotics and probiotics
- Avoid or limit caffeine
- Educate about the effectiveness of herbal therapies

Figure 1. unspecified irritable bowel syndrome (IBS-U) etiology, pathophysiology, sign and symptoms and case management

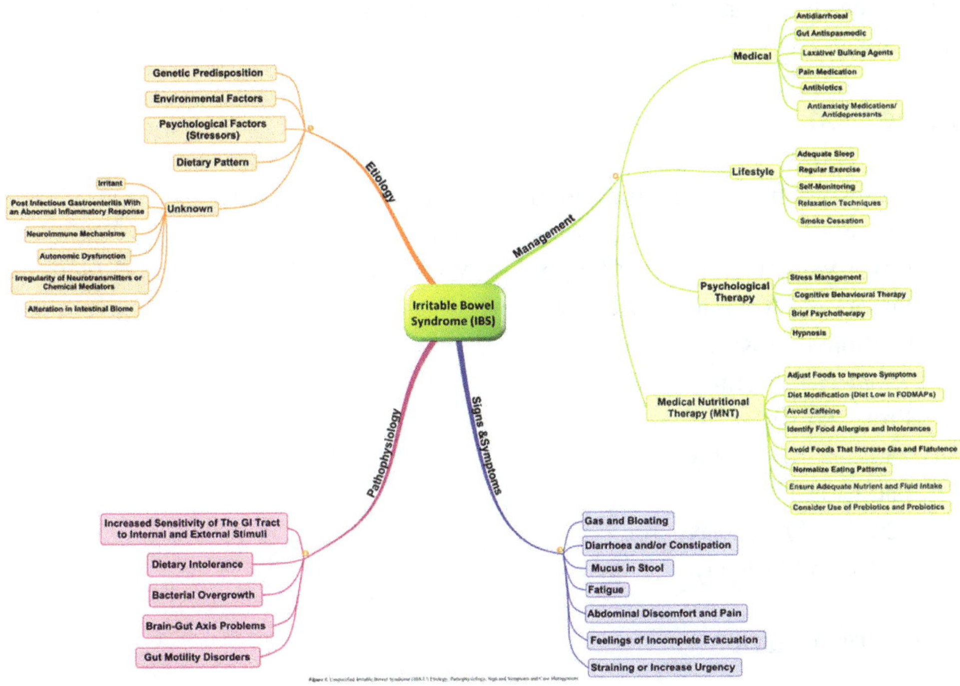

ADIME Note

Assessment: 34 y.o American female s/p IBS-U with history of GERD, anemia, gastritis; patient c/o intermittent episode of abdominal cramping and bloating associated with 4-6 loose watery stool and hard stool occurring twice a week; pt. Reported high stress level; physical activity: inactive

- Labs: WNL
- Ht: 1.59 cm; Wt: 50 kg; Body Mass Index (BMI):19.8 (normal); %weight change: 1.96 in 3 months (WNL)
- Clinical: pale skin may be sign of dehydration
- Food drug interaction: Pantoprazole (↓ Fe and vitamin B12 absorption; avoid gingko or St John's Wort "SJW"), BENTYL (↓ taste acuity)
- Diet Hx: reveals consumption of high gas producing foods and foods may trigger symptoms

Diagnosis: Food- and nutrition-related knowledge deficit (NB-1.1) related to lack of nutrition educations evidenced by the 24-hour food recall that shows inappropriate food choices (high amounts of fructose and oligosaccharides) and exacerbation of symptoms

Intervention

- Prescription: Carbohydrate-modified diet (low FODMAP)
- Energy: Using Mifflin St. Jeor equation for females;
- $(10 \times \text{weight}) + (6.25 \times \text{height}) - (5 \times \text{age}) - 161 = 1164 \times 1.2$ (activity factor) = 1400 kilocalorie(kcal)/day
- Carbohydrates: (50%)
- 700/4 = 175 grams (gm)/day
- Protein: (20%)
- 280/4 = 70 gm/day
- Fat: (30%)
- 420/9 = 47 gm/day
- Fluids: 3 liters/day

Recommendations

- Diet modified for specific foods or ingredients (ND-1.2.8) (Gas and flatulence-producing foods)
- Nutrition education on the low FODMAP diet:
  - Implement appropriate restriction (phase 1)
  - Provide a list of high and low foods content of these nutrients, provide sample menu and tips to alter diet
- Have patient keep diet and symptom records to check adherence
- Limit caffeine consumption from coffee or other sources of caffeine
- Educate her about the use of herbal therapy and explain that chamomile can aggravate symptoms of grass allergies
- Ensure adequate fluid intake
- Regular moderate physical activity for at least 150 min per week to decrease stress and improve overall health
- Referral to psychotherapist

Monitoring/Evaluation

- Assess food and symptoms records
- Monitor bowel movement

- Monitor fluid intake
- Monitor weight change

Table 3. Client Education Materials for Food Substitutions

Food Items	Reason for Substitution	Substitutions
Whole milk	Lactose intolerance is common in people with IBS Feeling discomfort	Evaporated, skim, and low-fat milk Soy milk Almond Milk Powdered milk
Coffee (caffeine)	May cause osmotic effect leading to diarrhea To limit anxiety	Decaffeinated coffee Caffeine-free teas Soft drinks without caffeine Rehydration beverages
Gum	Contains artificial sweeteners such as sorbitol and xylitol which are polyols that leads	Omit
Mushroom soup	Mushroom contains polyols may cause gas	Potato soup
Mixed dried fruits Apple	High in fructose	Banana Orange Berries
salad (cabbages, cauliflower, and broccoli)	All food items may cause gas	Cucumber Lettuce Tomato Bell pepper
Yogurt	If lactose intolerance	lactose-free yogurt with live active cultures and added probiotics
Chamomile tea	High in FODMAP affecting bowel movement	Peppermint tea Green tea

Follow-Up Visit (After a Month)

ADIME Note

Assessment 34 y.o American female s/p gases with IBS-U with history of GERD, anemia, gastritis; patient visit the clinic for follow-up after 1 month of starting low FODMAP diet; pt. reported symptoms improved except gases; pt. still reported high stress level; physical activity: active

- Labs: WNL
- Ht: 1.59 cm; Wt: 50 kg; Body Mass Index (BMI):19.8 (normal)

- Diet Hx: Based on the food diary, consumption of high gas producing food as a substitute was identified, which trigger the symptoms

Diagnosis: Inappropriate intake of types of carbohydrate (oligosaccharides) (NB-1.7) related to limited understanding of appropriate food intake for reported IBS symptoms as evidenced by reports of excessive gases associated with consumption of foods with high amounts of oligosaccharides (soy milk).

Intervention

- Prescription: Continue on Carbohydrate-modified diet (low FODMAP)
- Recommendations:
    - Diet modified for specific foods or ingredients (ND-1.2.8) (Gas and flatulence-producing foods)
    - Re-educate with more detailed nutrition explanation on the diet, provide a list of high and low foods content of these nutrients, provide sample menu and tips to alter diet
    - Emphasis on healthy dietary habits (regular meal pattern, avoid high fat and spicy food, and limit caffeine consumption)
    - Continue recording diet and symptom to check adherence
    - Address nutrient deficiencies, if necessary
    - Ensure adequate fluid intake
    - Emphasis on regular exercise (150 min /week) to reduce stress

Monitoring/Evaluation

- Assess food and symptoms records, if symptoms improved, processed to the next phase (re-challenge) of low FODMAP diet
- Adjust foods eliminated from diet based on their association with symptoms of IBS.
- Monitor bowel movement
- Monitor fluid intake
- Monitor weight change
- Follow-up after 2 weeks to assess readiness to the next phase

CONCLUSION

Overall, dietary management has shown as a key tool in the management of IBS. Detailed dietary history in IBS patients is the most important step to rule out the effect of certain foods or dietary components in aggravating the symptoms. Detailed dietary history includes meal pattern, amount and type of food, ability to complete meal preparation, previous diet or food restrictions, The anxiety of patients with IBS and obsessive eating behaviors associated with GI distress could lead to unnecessarily self-restrictive diets, which could result in nutritional deficiencies. Therefore, it is of the utmost important for registered dietitian to provide detailed dietary recommendations for patients with IBS. Furthermore, nutrition therapy for IBS is highly individualized and require goals set by the patient and registered dietitian with consistent follow-up for additional interventions as needed for successful nutritional management of the symptoms and improve quality of life. The main approach for medical nutrition therapy includes detailed dietary education while focusing on the food responsible for the onset and worsening the symptoms of IBS. Moreover, avoidance and gradually re-introduction of specific food components is one of the keys for management of IBS.

Table 4. High FODMAP Foods and Low FODMAPS Foods (Alternative)

FODMAP	High FODMAP Foods	Low FODMAP Foods
Oligosaccharides: fructans and/ or galacto-oligosaccharides	Vegetables: artichokes, asparagus, beetroot, Brussels sprouts, broccoli, cabbage, fennel, garlic, leeks, shallots, okra, onions, peas Cereals: wheat & rye when eaten in large amounts (e.g., bread, pasta, crackers) Legumes: Chickpeas, lentils, red kidney beans, baked beans Fruits: watermelon, custard apple, white peaches, rambutan, kaki	Vegetables: carrot, cucumber, potato, bell pepper, eggplant, green beams, lettuce, spinach, chives, parsnip, pumpkin, silverbeet, spring onion (green only), tomato, zucchini, bamboo shoots, bok choy, choko, choy sum Cereals: wheat-free flour and products made with these (e.g., bread, pasta, crackers), spelt and spelt products, oats, corn, rice, quinoa Legumes: canned chickpeas
Disaccharides: Lactose	Milk (cow, goat, sheep), yoghurt, soft & fresh cheeses (e.g., Ricotta, Cottage), ice cream	Lactose-free milk, rice milk, lactose-free yoghurt, hard cheeses (e.g., Cheddar, Parmesan, Swiss, Brie, Camembert), butter, ice-cream substitutes (e.g., dairy-free gelato, sorbet)
Monosaccharides: Fructose	Fruits: apple, pears, nashi pears, clingstone, peaches, mango, sugar snap peas, watermelon, tinned fruit in natural juice, dried fruits Honey Sweeteners: fructose, high fructose corn syrup	Fruits: banana, blueberry, grapefruit, grape, honeydew melon, kiwifruit, lemon, lime, mandarin, orange, raspberry, pawpaw, star fruit, passion fruit, rockmelon, carambola, durian Honey substitutes: maple syrup Sweeteners: sugar, glucose, artificial sweeteners not ending in "-ol"
Polyols	Fruits: apple, apricots, cherries, longon, lychee, nashi pears, nectarines, pears, peaches, plums, prunes, watermelon Vegetables: avocado, cauliflower, mushrooms, snow peas Sweeteners: sorbitol, mannitol, xylitol & others ending in "-ol", isomalt	Fruits: banana, blueberry, grapefruit, grape, honeydew melon, kiwifruit, lemon, lime, mandarin, orange, raspberry, pawpaw, star fruit, passion fruit, rockmelon, carambola, durian Sweeteners: sugar, glucose, artificial sweeteners not ending in "-ol" (e.g., sucralose, aspartame)

Adapted from: Diet in Irritable Bowel Syndrome: What to Recommend, Not What to Forbid to Patients

CONFLICT OF INTEREST

Eram Albajri and Manal Naseeb declare that they have no conflict of interest.

REFERENCES

Academy of Nutrition and Dietetics. (2020). *Nutrition care manual*. Retrieved from https://www.nutritioncaremanual.org/?err=NLI

Alharbi, S. H. (2018). Epidemiology of Irritable Bowel Syndrome in Saudi Arabia. *American Journal of Medicine and Medical Sciences*.

Alosaim, M., & Ali, A., & H., R. (2016). Epidemiology of Irritable Bowel Syndrome; A Systematic Review of Literature. *Journal of Health Informatics in Developing Countries*, *10*(1).

Canadian Society of Intestinal Research. (2018). *IBS global impact report 2018*. Retrieved from https://badgut.org/ibs-global-impact-report-2018/

Chey, W. D., Kurlander, J., & Eswaran, S. (2015). Irritable bowel syndrome: A clinical review. *Journal of the American Medical Association*, *313*(9), 949–958. doi:10.1001/jama.2015.0954 PMID:25734736

Continence Foundation of Australia. (2020). *Irritable bowel syndrome (IBS)*. Retrieved from https://www.cedars-sinai.org/health-library/diseases-and-conditions/i/irritable-bowel-syndrome-ibs.html

Cozma-Petruţ, A., Loghin, F., Miere, D., & Dumitraşcu, D. L. (2017). Diet in irritable bowel syndrome: What to recommend, not what to forbid to patients. *World Journal of Gastroenterology*, *23*(21), 3771–3783. doi:10.3748/wjg.v23.i21.3771 PMID:28638217

Fedewa, A., & Rao, S. S. (2014). Dietary fructose intolerance, fructan intolerance and FODMAPs. *Current Gastroenterology Reports*, *16*(1), 370. doi:10.100711894-013-0370-0

Ford, A. C., Moayyedi, P., Chey, W. D., Harris, L. A., Lacy, B. E., Saito, Y. A., ... Syndrome, A. T. F. M. I. B. (2018). American College of Gastroenterology Monograph on Management of Irritable Bowel Syndrome. *The American Journal of Gastroenterology*, *113*, 1–18. doi:10.103841395-018-0084-x PMID:29950604

John Hopkins Medicine. (2020). *Irritable bowel syndrome (IBS)*. Retrieved from https://www.hopkinsmedicine.org/health/conditions-and-diseases/irritable-bowel-syndrome-ibs

Lacy, B. E., Mearin, F., Chang, L., Chey, W. D., Lembo, A. J., Simren, M., & Spiller, R. (2016). Bowel Disorders. *Gastroenterology, 150*(6), 1393–1407.e1395. doi:10.1053/j.gastro.2016.02.031 PMID:27144627

Lehrer, J. K. (2019). *Irritable bowel syndrome (IBS): practice essentials, background, pathophysiology*. Retrieved from https://emedicine.medscape.com/article/180389-overview

Mayo Clinic. (2018). *Irritable bowel syndrome - symptoms and causes*. Retrieved from https://www.mayoclinic.org/diseases-conditions/irritable-bowel-syndrome/symptoms-causes/syc-20360016

Moayyedi, P., Mearin, F., Azpiroz, F., Andresen, V., Barbara, G., Corsetti, M., Emmanuel, A., Hungin, A. P. S., Layer, P., Stanghellini, V., Whorwell, P., Zerbib, F., & Tack, J. (2017). Irritable bowel syndrome diagnosis and management: A simplified algorithm for clinical practice. *United European Gastroenterology Journal, 5*(6), 773–788. doi:10.1177/2050640617731968 PMID:29026591

National Institute of Health. (2020). *Irritable bowel syndrome (IBS)*. Retrieved from https://www.niddk.nih.gov/health-information/digestive-diseases/irritable-bowel-syndrome

Peyton, L., & Greene, J. (2014). Irritable bowel syndrome: current and emerging treatment options. *P & T: A Peer-Reviewed Journal for Formulary Management, 39*(8), 567-578.

Stanford Health Care. (2020) *Low FODMAP diet*. Retrieved from https://stanfordhealthcare.org/medical-treatments/l/low-fodmap-diet.html

Web, M. D. (2020). *Irritable bowel syndrome*. Retrieved from https://www.webmd.com/ibs/guide/digestive-diseases-irritable-bowel-syndrome#3

KEY TERMS AND DEFINITIONS

Abdominal Bloating: Is buildup of gas in the stomach and intestines and feels full and tight.

Antidepressants: Medications used to treat major depressive disorder, some anxiety disorders, some chronic pain conditions, and to help manage some addictions.

Antispasmodic: Medication used to relieve spasm of involuntary muscle.

Cognitive Behavioral Therapy: Is a form of psychological treatment that has been demonstrated to be effective for a range of problems including depression, anxiety disorders, alcohol and drug use problems, marital problems, eating disorders and severe mental illness.

Constipation: Is a condition in which there is difficulty in emptying the bowels, usually associated with hardened feces.

Diarrhea: Is a condition in which loose, watery bowel movements that may occur frequently and with a sense of urgency.

Food Intolerance: Is digestive problems that occur after a certain food is eaten.

Hemorrhoids: Swollen blood vessels around your anus, the opening where stool comes out, can hurt and bleed.

Inflammatory Bowel Disease: Is a term for two conditions (Crohn's disease and ulcerative colitis) that are characterized by chronic inflammation of the gastrointestinal (GI) tract. Prolonged inflammation results in damage to the GI tract.

Hypnotherapy: Is a type of complementary medicine in which hypnosis is used to create a state of focused attention and increased suggestibility during which positive suggestions and guided imagery are used to help individuals deal with a variety of concerns and issues.

Probiotics: Microorganism introduced into the body for its beneficial qualities.

APPENDIX: ABBREVIATIONS

BMI: Body mass index
BPM: Beat per minute
HEENT: Head, eyes, ears, nose, throat
MNT: Medical nutrition therapy
IBS: Irritable Bowel Syndrome
IBS-C: Irritable Bowel Syndrome, predominant constipation
IBS-D: Irritable Bowel Syndrome, predominant diarrhea
IBS-M: Irritable Bowel Syndrome, predominant Mixed
IBS-U: Irritable Bowel Syndrome, unspecified
GI: Gastrointestinal
IBD: Inflammatory bowel disease
ACG: American College of Gastroenterology
CAM: Complementary and Alternative Medicine
FODMAPs: Fermentable Oligo-, Di-, Mono-saccharides And Polyols
GERD: Gastroesophageal reflux disease
CVD: Cardiovascular disease
RDW: Red cell distribution
MCV: Mean corpuscular volume
MCH: Mean corpuscular hemoglobin
MCHC: Mean corpuscular hemoglobin concentration
WNL: Within normal limit
S/p: Status post
C/o: Complain of
SJW: St John’s Wort

Chapter 10
The Positive Impact of Weight Management on Liver Cirrhosis

Heba Abdulkarim Sanousi
Doctor Soliman Fakeeh Hospital, Saudi Arabia

Almoutaz Hashim
Doctor Soliman Fakeeh Hospital, Saudi Arabia

EXECUTIVE SUMMARY

Weight management offers patients with liver cirrhosis significant health benefits. This case study describes the treatment of liver cirrhosis through dietary interventions. A 48-year-old male presented at Doctor Soliman Fakeeh Hospital in Saudi Arabia, Jeddah. The patient was suffering from morbid obesity (BMI= 43.76 kg/ m^2), non-alcoholic steatohepatitis, and chronic hepatitis B viral infection. Sleeve gastrectomy surgery was not possible due to the patient having liver fibrosis (stage 4). Alternatively, he was offered a healthy lifestyle intervention involving advisement regarding dietary habits and the initiation of a regular exercise routine. FibroScan was repeated seven months after the dietary intervention, where it was observed that the liver fibrosis improved from stage 4 to stage 3 post-treatment. Additionally, the patient lost almost 29% of his original body weight. In this case, weight management through following a healthy, balanced diet and increasing physical activity for one year produced remarkable improvement in the patient's liver cirrhosis related to non-alcoholic steatohepatitis.

DOI: 10.4018/978-1-7998-3802-9.ch010

INTRODUCTION

The liver is the largest organ in the human body. It has several essential functions, such as detoxification, protein synthesis, red blood cell decomposition, and the production of biochemical substances such as bile, cholesterol, enzymes, and hormones. The hormone cholecystokinin (CCK) stimulates the release of pancreatic lipase and the contraction of the gallbladder that enables it to release bile salts. Together, the pancreatic lipase and bile salts metabolize triglycerides into free fatty acids for easy transportation across the intestinal membrane. Once they cross the membrane, they convert back into triglycerides that combine with cholesterol within chylomicron vesicles. This enables the circulation of these fat molecules throughout the circulatory system, so that they can be delivered to the liver or become stored as fat in adipose tissue throughout the body. Additionally, the liver activates the storage of glycogen energy molecules, fat-soluble vitamins (A, E, D, K, and B_{12}), and minerals (iron and copper) (Arjun Kalra & Faiz Tuma, 2018).

The following case study demonstrates how adhering to a healthy, balanced diet helped a patient improve their liver cirrhosis through weight management and motivation. According to Anand (1999), liver cirrhosis is the most common disease in the world. The number of deaths from cirrhosis in the United States ranges from 12 to 15 per 100,000 within the general American population (Anand, 1999). Additionally, approximately 500,000 people globally die each year from hepatitis B virus (HBV)-related liver disease (Marugán & Garzóno, 2009). In terms of obesity, the World Health Organization (2020) has defined it as excessive fat accumulation that could negatively affect a person's health. According to Schiavo et al. (2018), there is a strong parallel between obesity and non-alcoholic fatty liver disease that may lead to the development of cirrhosis. Many studies have found that morbid obesity may lead to liver diseases such as cirrhosis, which is also demonstrated in this case study. This case study reflects the extent to which a patient's success in overcoming obesity and treating fibrosis (through dietary change and lifestyle modification) has the potential to substantially impact their overall prognosis.

Following a healthy balanced diet can be used as a therapy to reduce the risk of developing many health conditions, such as diabetes, fatty liver, and cardiovascular diseases. According to previous studies up to the present time, a strong correlation has been established between consuming a healthy diet and having a functional health status. For example, following a well-balanced diet, together with increased physical activity or undergoing a surgical intervention, such as gastric sleeve, gastric bypass, or gastric band, has been proven to be a successful method of treatment. Bray, Frühbeck, Ryan, and Wilding (2016) found that different types of bariatric surgeries among obese patients produced remarkable results in terms of weight loss. Each of these options can lead to significant consequences regarding weight loss to treat specific conditions, including type two diabetes mellitus, non-alcoholic fatty liver disease (NAFLD), and high blood pressure. According to Riazi et al. (2019), losing weight by bariatric surgery can cure NAFLD. Non-alcoholic fatty liver disease, commonly known as fatty liver, is caused by excessive food intake or insulin resistance. Most people who suffer from obesity or who are overweight are more susceptible to developing fatty liver (Riazi et al., 2019). Untreated NAFLD may lead to inflammation of the liver in the form of a condition known as non-alcoholic steatohepatitis (NASH), which eventually causes fibrosis. Non-alcoholic steatohepatitis is characterized by liver inflammation and fibrosis progression (Wong et al., 2016).

In the following case study, the patient had unhealthy dietary habits. He was addicted to sugary foods and soft drinks, especially Pepsi, where he drank excessive amounts of almost two to three cans (660-990ml) per day. Through a dietary intervention, which included the avoidance of white sugar, soft drinks, and all junk foods, this patient was gradually able to lose weight. There was also a rapid response in terms of the treatment of HBV. Therefore, this patient's lifestyle change, where they became more physically active in addition to following a balanced diet, helped to improve their liver function. Riazi et al. (2019) found that weight management, through adhering to a healthy diet and exercising, had a significant positive influence on NAFLD. Liver cirrhosis is divided into four well-defined stages (F1 to F4) (Nall, 2018). Each phase differs from the others in terms of the severity of the fibrosis. If the patient reaches F4, they have liver cirrhosis, as was the case in this case study. It has been found that while liver cirrhosis may not heal, taking medication and following a healthy balanced diet has the potential to help cure or improve this condition (Nall, 2018). As this study progressed, it was observed using the FibroScan that after seven months of following a healthy diet, exercising, and receiving medical treatment, the patient's liver cirrhosis reverted from stage 4 to stage 3, marking a clear improvement of his condition. The FibroScan was used to determine the stage of the fibrosis rather than the ultrasound because it is more accurate.

ORGANIZATION BACKGROUND

This case study demonstrates that liver cirrhosis can be improved by weight reduction produced through a healthy diet, although the patient initially attempted to undergo bariatric surgery. Although he was eligible for the gastric sleeve procedure due to his high body mass index (BMI; 43.76 kg/m^2), he was not a candidate since he had advanced liver cirrhosis. Treatment was conducted at Doctor Soliman Fakeeh Hospital in Jeddah. The patient was referred to the dietetics clinic from another hospital after a failed attempt to undergo a gastrectomy sleeve surgical procedure.

The gastroenterologist advised the patient to meet with the nutritionist to explore weight reduction management. Monthly consultations at the nutrition clinic were scheduled; however, the patient did not attend all sessions due to several personal circumstances, as described below. Permission was granted by the patient via telephone consent to publish this case study.

SETTING THE STAGE

The nutritional care process has been implemented as a policy at the Doctor Soliman Fakeeh Hospital. The nutrition assessment collected data regarding all of the following: anthropometric measurements, biochemical parameters, clinical information, dietary data, nutritional status, nutritional intervention, and nutritional education.

CASE DESCRIPTION

Case Concerns

There were several concerns about this case study in terms of the patient, including his ability to maintain regular follow-up sessions throughout the entire treatment schedule. Initially, the patient's willingness to lose weight was very weak due to his disappointment from his failed attempt to undergo the gastrectomy sleeve surgery, as well as being newly diagnosed with HBV. Psychologically, he suffered from anxiety and depression. However, after the initial sessions of his nutritional education, the patient's negative feelings and emotions started to gradually improve because he was advised to change his eating habits rather than having to follow a diet. For example, he was told to reduce his daily intake of soft drinks, avoid eating junk food, and increase his daily consumption of water. Interestingly, he accepted the concept of changing his lifestyle and eating habits, and successfully followed these instructions for one month. The immediate result in the first month was weight loss of 10 kg directly from changing his eating habits and lifestyle. Over time, the patient followed all of the instructions about his diet, and he was quite successful in responding to the challenge to lose weight. According to the patient, this fundamental change to his lifestyle had a positive impact on his family as well, since they also adopted his new eating habits. However, regarding patient follow-up, he was unable to attend all of the scheduled monthly sessions due to various personal circumstances, including his distant geographical location. He lived in another city, which was far from the hospital. Additionally, the patient did not bring reports, such as blood test results, to each visit, which made it difficult to monitor his progress.

Case Components

In this case study, information related to dietary habits, past medical history, and all issues connected to the case are presented. Additionally, there is a strategy brief outlining how the patient overcame each health issue through either medication or a nutrition intervention. The nutritional care process in this case study included the following: nutrition assessment and reassessment of each visit, nutrition diagnosis, nutrition intervention, and, finally, nutrition monitoring and evaluation. Significant improvements were observed in terms of the patient's nutritional status and psychological well-being at each clinical visit.

Management and Organizational Concerns

This case study was conducted over a one-year period that included consultations and follow-up visits at both the nutrition and gastroenterology clinics. During this time, the patient took a medication (entecavir) prescribed by his physician and followed a diet plan provided by a clinical dietician. The diet therapy in this case study was based on the American dietary program MyPlate. According to the United States Department of Agriculture (USDA, 2019), MyPlate was designed to promote a healthy eating style for everyone whereby it helps them to choose exact quantities and qualities of foods from each of the food groups. The central reason for choosing USDA guidelines was to allow the patient to consume foods from all food groups, enabling him to meet his nutritional needs without feeling deprived. Total caloric intake was gradually decreased each month to help him lose weight in a healthy fashion, by losing fat while maintaining the fat free mass that he had before beginning the diet therapy. Additionally, he exercised five times per week by himself, either walking, running, or jogging for around one hour daily, which also helped him to reduce his weight. The patient's overall response to this intervention provides insights that might be helpful for future investigations involving patients with similar conditions. It was observed that this patient became increasingly motivated with each clinical visit, due to the positive results he achieved in terms of reaching his goal to lose weight. Such positive reinforcement encouraged him to maintain the newly-adopted lifestyle changes that he developed through this nutrition education program. Moreover, he experienced significant improvements in sleep, mood, and his overall psychological status. No follow-up meeting was conducted after the completion of the treatment period.

Current Challenges Facing the Patient

Throughout this one-year case study, which occurred from November 2018 to November 2019, there were some challenges. First, it was not possible to maintain monthly meetings with the patient due to his geographical location. He lived in another city, which made it difficult for him to come to the clinic every month. Second, a monthly blood test was not taken to help monitor and compare results for unknown reasons. Third, there were initially some difficulties with changing and adjusting to new eating habits due to his excessive intake of desserts and soda. However, over time, the patient adapted to his new diet. Fourth, the patient faced some difficulties at the beginning of the intervention regarding exercise, as he had not previously engaged in any physical activity throughout his life, such as walking or running. However, he tried to strictly apply the instructions regarding physical activity, as often as he could. Fifth, the patient was having trouble as he would continuously forget to drink water. Therefore, he did not fully meet his nutritional requirement for water intake, which caused him to experience dehydration and constipation. Finally, a lack of family support was another challenge in this case study. Specifically, the patient's family consumed sweets and chocolate on a daily basis, which he loved. Thus, he found it quite challenging to refrain from eating these sugary foods, even though he was given healthy alternatives.

Patient's Details

- Age: 48 years old
- Gender: Male

Case History

Case Description

A 48-year-old Saudi Arabian male was suffering from morbid obesity with a very high BMI of 43.76 kg/m^2. He attempted to undergo gastric sleeve surgery but was unsuccessful due to his liver cirrhosis, which was discovered during the operation. According to many studies, there is a strong connection between obesity and liver cirrhosis. Patients with NASH who are smokers and obese are more likely to develop liver cirrhosis (Samji, Heda, Kovalic, & Satapathy, 2020). The patient was advised by the surgeon consultant to visit the gastroenterology clinic in order to begin treatment for liver cirrhosis. After completion of a medical examination and blood tests, it was discovered that the patient was positive for HBV. According to Marugán & Garzóno (2009), patients with HBV are at a high risk of developing liver cirrhosis. The first polymerase chain reaction (PCR) quantitative result for HBV was 22,286,783 IU/ml in August 2018. After starting a course of entecavir to treat the HBV, another PCR test was conducted in September 2019. During that time, the level of HBV decreased to 29 IU/ml. For a complete overview of hepatitis B virus DNA pre- and post-treatment, see Table 1. In addition, the patient lost almost 29% of his body weight by changing his lifestyle and following a healthy diet along with exercising.

- Medical History: The patient was suffering from morbid obesity and attempted to undergo gastric sleeve surgery. Liver cirrhosis was discovered during the surgery. After completing a consultation and medical observation, it was found that the patient was positive for HBV and had NASH. Budd and Cusi (2020) have stated that obese and diabetic patients are at the highest risk for NASH. Increased BMI is a predictor of decompensation of the liver (Schiavo et al., 2018).
- Surgical History: No prior surgeries except for the filed bariatric surgery attempt for a sleeve gastrectomy to lose weight.
- Smoking: The patient was a smoker but inconsistently. He smoked two to three packages per week, which was mood-dependent.
- Family History: Both of the patient's parents were deceased. They had suffered from type two diabetes mellitus and hypertension. The father suffered from the hepatitis C virus.

Main Medical Diagnosis

Demographics

- Marital status: The patient was married and had seven children.
- Education: The patient completed intermediate school (a middle school).
- Occupation: The patient was a retired military employee in the government sector.
- Ethnicity and religion: The patient was a Saudi Arabian Islamic Arab.

Anthropometry

- Current weight: 99 kg
- Admission weight: 137 kg
- Height: 177 cm
- Body mass index based on admission weight: 43.76 kg/m^2 (Morbid obesity, class III)

- Body mass index based on current weight post-dietary therapy: 31.62 kg/m^2 (Obesity class I)

Biochemical Data

Since the patient had liver cirrhosis and a family medical history, the gastroenterologist requested testing for both hepatitis B and C viruses. The hepatitis C virus was non-reactive. However, the patient's hepatitis B count was very high in comparison to the reference range, as detected by a quantitative PCR test. The patient responded to anti-HBV therapy. A repeat test (13 months later) indicated that the HBV count had decreased to 29 IU/ml, which is within the normal range. The patient had normal complete blood count (CBC) blood results, which included hemoglobin, white blood cell, and red blood cell counts. His INR level was slightly higher than the normal range. When international normalised ratio (INR) levels are too high, there is a risk of bleeding. Furthermore, alpha-fetoprotein is a protein produced by the liver. Scientifically, liver damage can negatively affect the level of alpha-fetoprotein. In this case study, the patient's alpha-fetoprotein exceeded the normal range due to some liver issues, including HBV, NASH, and liver cirrhosis. Albumin levels were on the lower side of the normal range, which is commonly observed in those with liver disease (Mahan et al., 2011). The results regarding the liver enzymes, which included aspartate aminotransferase (AST), alanine aminotransferase (ALT), and alkaline phosphatase (ALP), were within the normal range. Among patients with liver disease, these enzymes (AST, ALT, and ALP) are usually elevated in the blood due to various issues, such as damage to the liver, obstruction of the bile duct, and bone disorders (Lab Tests Online, 2019). However, in this case study, the results for liver enzymes post and pre-treatment were normal. Finally, the patient's bilirubin level was within the reference range. For a complete overview of blood test results pre-intervention, see Table 2.

After one year of treatment and dietary intervention, blood tests were repeated. There was definite improvement observed in the results. However, some blood test results were missing, such as those for INR and alpha-fetoprotein. For a complete overview of blood test results post-intervention, see Table 3.

Nutritional-Focused Physical Examination

- General appearance: The patient appeared pale and fatigued. He felt tired after engaging in any activity due to his excessive weight.
- Heart: No physical issues with the heart were observed. During each visit, the patient's pulse was normal at approximately 80- 90 beats per minute.

- HEENT: A HEENT examination was conducted regularly. There were no medical issues regarding the head, ear, eyes, nose, or throat.
- Genitalia: The patient disclosed no medical issues.
- Neurologic: Normal.
- Extremities: There was no edema in the upper or lower limbs. Furthermore, there were no amputations of either the upper or lower limbs.
- Skin: The patient's skin was extremely dry due to insufficient water intake.
- Chest/lungs: The patient indicated that he had sleeping difficulties due to his excessive weight. He indicated that he had difficulty breathing, and that these issues were worsened by smoking cigarettes.
- Peripheral vascular: There were no health issues in this regard.
- Abdomen: There were no ascites, and the abdomen usually was flat and soft. The patient was sometimes bothered by the presence of gas.

Vital Signs

- Date of initial visit: 29th November, 2018
- Pulse: 80-90 beats per minute.
- Temp: 37 degrees Celsius.
- Blood pressure: 116/ 79 millimeters of mercury
- Respiratory rate: 14-17 breaths per minute.

Food/Nutrition-Related History

The nutritionist asked the patient to complete a 24-hour dietary recall for the meals that he had eaten within one day before beginning to change his eating behavior. After conducting the nutritional analysis, it was observed that he was consuming many high-calorie foods, such as cookies and junk food, and also showed an excessive intake of soft drinks. In addition, he did not drink a sufficient amount of water. The example of a daily eating pattern included as Table 4, including food quantities and the timing of each meal, may help to explain this patient's morbid obesity and the formation of fat in his liver.

- Food allergies/intolerances: The patient did not have any food allergies or intolerances.
- Food purchase/preparations: The patient lived with his family. His spouse prepared the meals. All family members ate all meals together except for breakfast. While at work, the patient always ate breakfast from a restaurant with his friends.
- Vitamin and Mineral Supplementation:

- The patient took one Centrum multivitamin tablet daily.

Medications

Entecavir was given to the patient to treat HBV. This medication is used as a long-term treatment for hepatitis B infection. The function of this drug is to decrease the quantity of HBV in the human body, not to treat the HBV itself (U.S. National Library of Medicine, n.d.).

Solutions and Recommendations

Disease Pathophysiology Mind Map

The patient was suffering from many different health issues. These conditions included: morbid obesity, NASH, liver cirrhosis, and HBV.

Morbid Obesity

If BMI is higher than 40 kg/m^2, it is defined as morbid obesity. The BMI of the patient in this case study was 43.76 kg/m^2. Since his BMI was very high, he attempted to undergo gastric sleeve surgery. Unfortunately, the procedure could not be completed due to the presence of liver cirrhosis. A change in dietary behavior was implemented through the regular professional guidance of a nutritionist. The patient successfully achieved his goal of losing weight. He lost almost 39 kg in one year by following a well-balanced diet as well as engaging in regular physical activity. He consumed six small meals throughout each day. His final current weight after finishing the nutritional program and medical treatment intervention was 99 kg, and his BMI dropped to 31.62 kg/m^2. During the first month, the total weight loss was 10 kg, mainly resulting from removing soft drinks from his diet and avoiding sweets and desserts. Moreover, on average, his weight loss was 5 to 6 kg per month. For a complete overview of the patient's weight loss curve over one year of nutritional and medical intervention, see Figure 1.

Hepatitis B Virus

The HBV is a widespread health problem. Several studies have found that individuals with HBV are more likely to have liver cirrhosis. Marugán and Garzóno (2009) found that 15% to 40% of patients with a medical history of HBV may experience complications during their lifetimes, such as cirrhosis or hepatocellular carcinoma. This case study supports the validity of previous research that found a connection between HBV and the development of liver cirrhosis, since this patient had both. The first blood test indicated HBV at 22,286,783 IU/ml, which is a very high count that exceeds the reference range. After eleven months of taking medication (entecavir), HBV concentration decreased to 60.9 IU/ml. A repeat test two months later indicated a further decrease in concentration to 29 IU/ml, which is within the normal range.

Non-alcoholic Steatohepatitis

Non-alcoholic steatohepatitis (NASH) is presented in the second stage of untreated fatty liver. When the patient had his first medical assessment, it was discovered that he had NASH. After being treated with medication and following a healthy diet and exercising, his health status significantly improved. According to a previous study (Wong et al., 2016), weight reduction of 10% due to dietary restriction and regular exercise is sufficient to reverse NASH in most patients.

Liver Cirrhosis

There is a strong correlation between obesity and fatty liver. Over time, untreated NASH will lead to fibrosis, as was the case with the patient in this case study. He also suffered from obesity due to the excessive intake of fatty and sugary foods. These poor dietary habits negatively affected his health in terms of causing him to develop a fatty liver, which eventually developed into cirrhosis. This liver cirrhosis was discovered during the unsuccessful attempt at sleeve gastrectomy surgery.

ADIME Note

Nutrition Assessment

- Anthropometry:
    - Weight at the end of study (Current weight): 99 kg (After one year of lifestyle modification)
    - Weight before the nutritional intervention: 137 kg
    - Height: 177 cm
    - Initial body mass index: 43.76 kg/m^2 (Morbid obesity class III)
    - Current body mass index: 31.62 kg/m2 (Obesity class I)
    - Ideal body weight: 72 kg
    - Adjusted body weight: 97 kg
    - Measurements of body circumferences on 29th November, 2018 (first visit):
        - Arm: 44 cm
        - Waist: 141cm (higher than the normal range >102 cm)
        - Hip: 138 cm

- Measurements of body circumferences on 15th November, 2019 (last visit):
    - Arm: 40 cm
    - Waist: 132 cm (higher than the normal range >102 cm)
    - Hip: 130.5 cm
- Biochemical: See Table 2.
- Clinical: The patient was a 48-year-old Saudi Arabian male diagnosed with liver cirrhosis (stage 4), HBV, and morbid obesity. Liver cirrhosis was discovered during a failed sleeve gastrectomy.

Dietary Requirements for Liver Cirrhosis Patient

Nutritional needs for cirrhotic patients vary from person to person, depending on BMI. The energy requirement for obese patients (BMI: > 40 kg/m^2) with liver cirrhosis is not less than 20-25 kcal/kg/day (Amodio et al., 2013). In terms of protein requirements, cirrhotic patients need a sufficient amount of protein, ranging from 1.2-1.5 g/kg/day, in order to sustain adequate muscle mass (Schiavo et al., 2018).

Nutrition Diagnosis

PES Statement

Excessive energy intake related to frequent consumption of fatty foods and sugary beverages, as evidenced by elevated BMI (43.76 kg/m^2), morbid obesity, as well as the 24-dietary recall.

Nutrition Intervention

Prescription

Total Energy Requirement: (Mahan et al., 2011)
(25-40 calories per kilogram of body weight)
Due to the patient being obese, the adjusted body weight was used.
$72 \text{ kg} \times 25 \text{ kcal} = 2425 \text{ kcal}$
$2425 - 500 = 1925$ kcal/day
Protein Requirement: (Mahan et al., 2011)
(1.2-1.5g per kilogram of the ideal body weight)
$1.5\text{g} \times 72 \text{ kg} = 108$ g/day
$108 \times 4 = 432$ kcal/day
23% of total calories should come from protein
Fat Requirements: (Mahan et al., 2011)
(25-40% from the total calories)

$30 \times 1900 \div 100 = 570$ kcal
$570 \div 9 = 63$ g/day
Carbohydrate Requirements:
47% of CHO from the total calories
$47 \times 1900 \div 100 = 893$ kcal/ day
$893 \div 4 = 223$ g/day
Fluid requirement by weight:
20 kg = 1500 + 20ml / kg 20 kg
Actual weight: 137 kg
$137 - 20 = 117$
$117 \times 20 = 2340$
$2340 + 1500 = 3840$ ml/day

Education

The patient was provided with written and verbal instructions on how to prepare healthy meals high in protein. For example, instead of using cream cheese, he was advised to consume low-fat cheese with eggs. He was also educated about how to substitute soft drinks with healthy beverages (such as smoothies with no added sugar), how to reduce his weight by following a healthy diet, how to be more physically active, and how to be more motivated. Instead of drinking soft drinks with meals, dairy products like milk or yogurt were also recommended as healthy choices that are high in protein. The most critical point in a patient's education session was his conviction to select healthy foods for the "cheating" meal that he was allowed on the open day of his meal plan. For example, instead of eating a fried burger, he ate a grilled one. In addition, he was educated about techniques for improving water consumption, such as adding natural flavors in the form of a slice of lemon or orange. Another recommendation was to change the temperature of the water, either trying cold water or water at room temperature to determine his preference. All of these small changes that started in the treatment sessions ultimately helped the patient to manage his weight and improve his health.

It is also notable that the patient was encouraged in his efforts to manage his weight through the nutritionist's motivational interviewing during the treatment sessions. Throughout the intervention, although the focus was on nutrition and medication, a psychological aspect was involved as well. In order to help facilitate the patient's success, the nutritionist listened to the patient carefully to understand his motivation for losing weight, empathized with the patient to let him know he was understood, and also empowered the patient to help him embrace healthier lifestyle practices. While the patient might have been able to manage his weight on his own, it is very likely that having the nutritionist's educational and psychological support helped him to achieve weight management.

Goals

- Lose weight.
- Lower the percentage of fat mass in body composition.
- Monitor muscle mass.
- Reduce liver cirrhosis complications, such as ascites and hepatic encephalopathy, over the long term.
- Improve dietary habits.
- Meet nutritional requirements (macronutrients and micronutrients) without privation or boredom.
- Consume a sufficient amount of water.

Dietary Recommendations

- Follow a high-protein diet.
- Avoid all soft drinks.
- Avoid high-fat, overly sweet foods, including junk food.
- Add vegetables (fresh or cooked) to meals as well as fruits (fresh or fresh juice) to avoid mineral and vitamin deficiency.
- Drink plenty of healthy liquids and water to avoid dehydration and to meet water intake requirements.
- Follow lists of healthy food options provided for each food group.

Monitoring/Evaluation

- Clinical follow-up with the patient every month.
- Monitor the patient's weight loss during each visit.
- Monitor the patient's muscle mass and fat mass using the InBody composition analyzer.
- Monitor the patient's food intake.
- Monitor lab values for albumin, hemoglobin, and hepatitis B virus.
- Monitor the patient's willingness to change his dietary behaviors.
- Monitor the patient's water intake.
- Monitoring the patient's current weight.

CONCLUSION

In this case study, the patient was experiencing a number of conditions, which included NASH, HBV infection, and morbid obesity. The causes of liver cirrhosis and obesity in this case study included poor eating habits and a lack of adequate physical activity. The weight management was achieved through nutritional and medical interventions. For a complete overview of the mind map for this case study, see figure 2. There were significant positive results achieved in this case study in terms of the patient's psychological, physical, and physiological health. Psychologically, he overcame negative feelings he associated with his obesity, enabling him to wear different styles of clothes, overcome his feelings of depression, and feel more satisfied with his body shape. Moreover, through making significant changes to his lifestyle, by consuming healthy foods and becoming more active, the patient was able to become a much healthier person. Although the clinical follow-ups did not occur every month, the patient still managed to adhere to the instructions given to him by the nutritionist. The patient still has liver cirrhosis, but it has been reduced to stage 3, as evidenced by repeating the Fiberoscan at seven months post-treatment, and his BMI has been lowered to 31.62 kg/m^2 (Obesity class I). Additionally, he is living well with his current lifestyle modifications. Notably, as the patient did not bring all of his blood test and Fibroscan results with him every time he visited the nutrition clinic, some information is missing from this case study.

The key message offered by this case study is that with appropriate resources and support, it is possible to make lifestyle changes that may improve one's health status. Additionally, a multidisciplinary clinical team can provide the guidance and monitoring that a patient needs to gradually achieve their goal of losing weight and become healthier. Direct interaction with the patient on a regular basis is a vital component for educating them about how to positively change their lifestyle, which may impact their future health. In closing, educating the patient in an influential manner, motivating them to want to make healthier choices, is the key to achieving a successful outcome.

REFERENCES

Amodio, P., Bemeur, C., Butterworth, R., Cordoba, J., Kato, A., Montagnese, S., Uribe, M., Vilstrup, H., & Morgan, M. Y. (2013). The nutritional management of hepatic encephalopathy in patients with cirrhosis: International society for hepatic encephalopathy and nitrogen metabolism consensus. *Hepatology (Baltimore, Md.)*, *58*(1), 325–336. doi:10.1002/hep.26370 PMID:23471642

Anand, B. S. (1999). Cirrhosis of liver. *The Western Journal of Medicine*, *171*(2), 110–115. PMID:10510657

Bray, G. A., Frühbeck, G., Ryan, D. H., & Wilding, J. P. H. (2016). Management of obesity. *Lancet*, *387*(10031), 1947–1956. doi:10.1016/S0140-6736(16)00271-3 PMID:26868660

Budd, J., & Cusi, K. (2020). Nonalcoholic fatty liver disease: What does the primary care physician need to know? *The American Journal of Medicine*, *133*(5), 536–543. Advance online publication. doi:10.1016/j.amjmed.2020.01.007 PMID:32017891

Kalra, A., & Tuma, F. (2018, December 18). *Physiology, liver.* National Center for Biotechnology Information. https://www.ncbi.nlm.nih.gov/books/NBK535438/

Lab Tests Online. (2019). *Patient education on blood, urine, and other lab tests.* Lab Tests Online. https://labtestsonline.org/

Lee, S. (2014). Non-invasive diagnosis of hepatitis B virus-related cirrhosis. *World Journal of Gastroenterology*, *20*(2), 445. doi:10.3748/wjg.v20.i2.445 PMID:24574713

Mahan, L. K., Escott-Stump, S., & Raymond, J. (2011). *Krause's food & nutrition care process*. Saunders.

Marugán, R. B., & Garzóno, S. G. (2009). DNA-guided hepatitis B treatment, viral load is essential, but not sufficient. *World Journal of Gastroenterology*, *15*(4), 423. doi:10.3748/wjg.15.423 PMID:19152446

Nall, R. (2018, January 11). *Liver fibrosis*. Healthline. https://www.healthline.com/health/liver-fibrosis

Riazi, K., Raman, M., Taylor, L., Swain, M. G., & Shaheen, A. A. (2019). Dietary patterns and components in nonalcoholic fatty liver disease (NAFLD): What key messages can health care providers offer? *Nutrients*, *11*(12), 2878. doi:10.3390/nu11122878 PMID:31779112

Samji, N. S., Heda, R., Kovalic, A. J., & Satapathy, S. K. (2020). Similarities and differences between nonalcoholic steatohepatitis and other causes of cirrhosis. *Gastroenterology Clinics of North America*, *49*(1), 151–164. doi:10.1016/j.gtc.2019.09.004 PMID:32033761

Schiavo, L., Busetto, L., Cesaretti, M., Zelber-Sagi, S., Deutsch, L., & Iannelli, A. (2018). Nutritional issues in patients with obesity and cirrhosis. *World Journal of Gastroenterology*, *24*(30), 3330–3346. doi:10.3748/wjg.v24.i30.3330 PMID:30122874

United States Department of Agriculture. (2019). *What is MyPlate?* Choose My Plate. https://www.choosemyplate.gov/eathealthy/WhatIsMyPlate

U.S. National Library of Medicine. (n.d.). *Entecavir*. MedlinePlus. https://medlineplus.gov/druginfo/meds/a605028.html

Williams, E. J., & Iredale, J. P. (1998). Liver cirrhosis. *Postgraduate Medical Journal, 74*(870), 193–202. doi:10.1136/pgmj.74.870.193 PMID:9683971

Wong, V. W.-S., Chitturi, S., Wong, G. L.-H., Yu, J., Chan, H. L.-Y., & Farrell, G. C. (2016). Pathogenesis and novel treatment options for non-alcoholic steatohepatitis. *The Lancet. Gastroenterology & Hepatology, 1*(1), 56–67. doi:10.1016/S2468-1253(16)30011-5 PMID:28404113

World Health Organization. (2020). *Obesity and overweight*. World Health Organization. https://www.who.int/westernpacific/health-topics/obesity

KEY TERMS AND DEFINITIONS

Bariatric Surgery: A surgical intervention to help patients overcome obesity. There are various types of bariatric surgery, such as a sleeve gastrectomy, gastric bypass, and adjustable gastric band.

Fibroscan: A machine used to determine the stage of liver cirrhosis that a patient is experiencing.

Kabsa Rice: The main dish in Saudi Arabia, usually served at lunch and dinner. It made up of rice, chicken or meat, and mix vegetables.

Morbid Obesity: A type of obesity, characterized by the presence of an excessive amount of fat that negatively affects most of the organs inside the body, such as the heart, brain, kidney, and liver. It may lead to death.

Non-Alcoholic Steatohepatitis: The second stage of fatty liver disease. It involves inflammation of the liver due to untreated fatty liver.

Nutrition Therapy: An essential part of the multidisciplinary team in the hospital to complete the treatment for the patient either by oral or tube feeding.

Nutritional Education: A process of building a trust relationship between the patient and the nutritionist to help them overcome various obstacles related to nutrition and health.

APPENDIX

Table 1. Patient's results pre- and post-treatment for hepatitis B virus DNA real-time by polymerase chain reaction (PCR)

Date	Result
August 15, 2018	22,286,783 IU/ml
June 12, 2019	60.9 IU/ml
September 26, 2019	29 IU/ml

Table 2. Blood test results of a 48-year-old Saudi Arabian male before commencing medical treatment and nutritional intervention

Parameter	Patients Results	Units	Reference Range
Hepatitis B virus	22,286,783 ↑	IU/ml	20 to 170,000,000
Hepatitis C virus	Non-Reactive		Non-reactive
Hemoglobin	14.1	gm/dl	13.3 – 16.5
White blood cell	4.96	10^9/L	3.9 - 11
Red blood cell	4.71	10^{12}/L	4.5 – 5.9
INR	1.19 ↑	ng/ml	0.87- 1.12
Alpha-fetoprotein	14.04 ↑		1 – 10.9
Albumin in serum	3.4 ↓	g/dl	3.5 – 5.2
Aspartate aminotransferase	33.0	U/L	8.0 - 48.0
Alanine aminotransferase	45	U/L	12 - 78
Alkaline phosphatase	80	U/L	45 - 115
Bilirubin (total)	0.54	mg/dl	0.1- 1.2

Table 3. Blood test results of a 48-year-old Saudi Arabian male after one year of medical treatment and nutritional intervention

Parameter	Patients Results	Units	Reference Range
Hepatitis B virus	29	IU/ml	20 to 170,000,000
Hemoglobin	14.4	gm/dl	13.3 - 16.5
White blood cell	5.95	10^9/L	3.9 - 11
Red blood cell	4.86	10^{12}/L	4.5 - 5.9
INR	missing	ng/ml	0.87 - 1.12
Alpha-fetoprotein	missing		1 - 10.9
Albumin in serum	3.8	g/dl	3.5 - 5.2
Aspartate Aminotransferase	38.0	U/L	8.0 - 48.0
Alanine Aminotransferase	66	U/L	12 - 78
Alkaline Phosphatase	84	U/L	45 - 115
Bilirubin (total)	0.3	mg/dl	0.1- 1.2

Table 4. Results of the 24-hour dietary recall for the 47-year-old Saudi Arabian male pre-treatment

Time	Where Consumed?	Meal	Food Items	Quantities
6:00 am	At the restaurant	*Breakfast*	· Two sandwiches with fried eggs · cream cheese · One can of soft drink · One cup of water	Four pieces of toasts Four eggs Three tablespoons 330 ml 250 ml
10:00 am	At work	*Snack*	· One pack of cheddar chips · One cup of tea with white sugar	64 gm Three teaspoons of sugar
3:00 pm	At home	*Lunch*	· White cooked rice · Grilled chicken · Mixed sautéed vegetables · One can of soft drink · One cup of water	Two cups (473 gm) 250 gm One cup (250gm) 330 ml 250 ml
6:00 pm	At home	*Snack*	· One cup of cappuccino (full-fat milk) with white sugar · Cheesecake dessert · One cup of water	Three teaspoons of sugar 125 gm 250 ml
9:30 pm	At home	*Dinner*	· Two sandwiches chicken shawarma · French fries · Mayonnaise · 1 can of soft drink · Fresh fruit · One cup of water	Around 4-6 ounces Around 150 gm Two tablespoons 330 ml One piece 250 ml
11:00 pm	At home	*Snack*	· Three small cups of Arabic coffee · Dried dates	90 ml 7-9 pieces

Figure 1. Weight loss curve over one year of nutritional and medical intervention for a 48-year-old Saudi Arabian male with NAFLD, NASH, and Hepatitis B

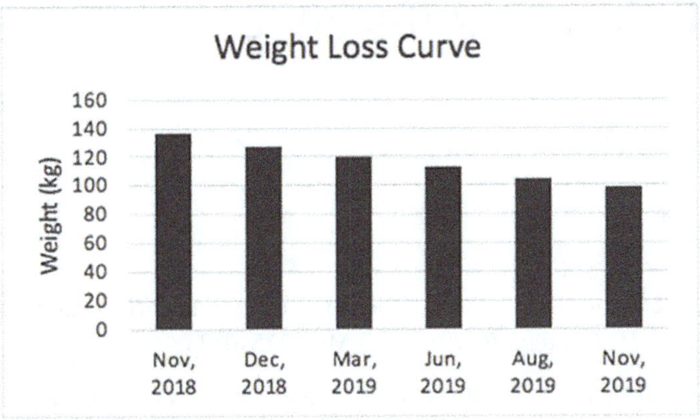

Figure 2. Mind map for the case study.
Source: Khalifah N, (2020)

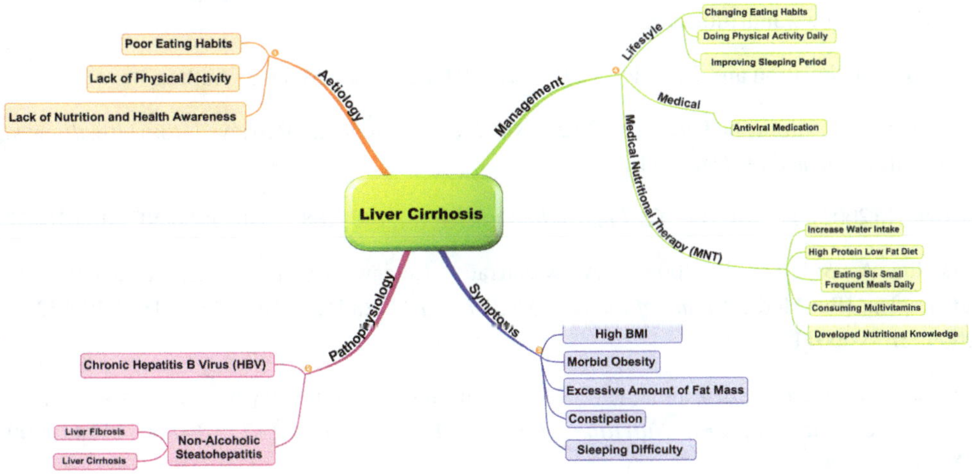

Compilation of References

Abraham, B. P., & Kahn, S. A. (2014). Transition of care in inflammatory bowel disease. *Gastroenterology & Hepatology*, *10*(10), 633. PMID:27540335

Abuzerr, S., Nasseri, S., Yunesian, M., Hadi, M., Mahvi, A. H., Nabizadeh, R., & Abu Mustafa, A. (2019). Prevalence of diarrheal illness and healthcare-seeking behavior by age-group and sex among the population of Gaza strip: A community-based cross-sectional study. *BMC Public Health*, *19*(1), 704. doi:10.118612889-019-7070-0 PMID:31174512

Academy of Nutrition and Dietetics. (2014). Diarrhea. *Nutrition care manual*. Retrieved April 3, 2020 from www.nutritioncaremanual.org

Academy of Nutrition and Dietetics. (2014). eNCPT Reference Manual. Author.

Academy of Nutrition and Dietetics. (2020). *Nutrition care manual*. Retrieved from https://www.nutritioncaremanual.org/?err=NLI

Africa, N. (2002). a 1*501, B 1*02). *English Journal*, *346*(3), 180–188. doi:10.1056/NEJMra010852

Alaedini, A., & Green, P. (2005). Review Narrative Review : Celiac Disease : Understanding a Complex. [PubMed]. *Annals of Internal Medicine*, *142*, 289. doi:10.7326/0003-4819-142-4-200502150-00011

Alastair, F., Emma, G., & Emma, P. (2011). Nutrition in inflammatory bowel disease. *Journal of Parenteral and Enteral Nutrition*, *35*(5), 571–580. doi:10.1177/0148607111413599 PMID:21825089

Alharbi, S. H. (2018). Epidemiology of Irritable Bowel Syndrome in Saudi Arabia. *American Journal of Medicine and Medical Sciences*.

Almadi, M., Almousa, M., Althwainy, A., Altamimi, A., Alamoudi, H., Alshamrani, H., Alharbi, O. R., Azzam, N. A., Sadaf, N., & Aljebreen, A. (2014). Prevalence of symptoms of gastroesopahgeal reflux in a cohort of Saudi Arabians: A study of 1265 subjects. *Saudi Journal of Gastroenterology*, *20*(4), 248–254. doi:10.4103/1319-3767.136982 PMID:25038211

Al-Mofarreh, M. A., & Al-Mofleh, I. A. (2013). Emerging inflammatory bowel disease in Saudi outpatients: a report of 693 cases. *Saudi Journal of Gastroenterology: Official Journal of the Saudi Gastroenterology Association, 19*(1), 16.

Alosaim, M., & Ali, A., & H., R. (2016). Epidemiology of Irritable Bowel Syndrome; A Systematic Review of Literature. *Journal of Health Informatics in Developing Countries, 10*(1).

Alshehri, S. S., Alzahrani, M. A. A., Jan, O. M., Aldughaither, A., Fahad, Alsalem, A. S., ... Alghamdi, A. A. O. (2020). Prevalence, Causes, Risk Factors and Updates of Management of GERD. *EC Microbiology, 16*(2), 1–8.

Alzubaidi, M., & Gabbard, S. (2015). GERD: Diagnosing and treating the burn. *Cleveland Clinic Journal of Medicine, 82*(10), 685–692. doi:10.3949/ccjm.82a.14138 PMID:26469826

Amandeep, K., Robin, S., Ramica, S., & Sunil, K. (2012). Peptic ulcer: A review on etiology and pathogenesis. *IRJP, 3*, 34-38. Retrieved from https://irjponline.com/admin/php/uploads/1161_pdf.pdf

American College of Gastroenterology. (2005). *Updated ACG guidelines for diagnosis and treatment of GERD*. Retrieved April 21, 2020, from https://www.aafp.org/afp/2005/0615/p2376.html

American Dietetic Association. (2011). *International Dietetics and Nutrition Terminology (IDNT) Reference Manual, Standardized Language for the Nutrition Care Process* (3rd ed.). American Dietetic Association.

American Dietetic Association. (2011). *International Dietetics and Nutrition Terminology (IDNT) Reference Manual: Standardized Language for the Nutrition Care Process*. American Dietetic Association.

American Speech-Language Hearing Association (ASHA). (n.d.). *About the CSD Professions*. Retrieved July 15, 2016, from https://www.asha.org/Students/Learn-About-the-CSDProfessions/

Amodio, P., Bemeur, C., Butterworth, R., Cordoba, J., Kato, A., Montagnese, S., Uribe, M., Vilstrup, H., & Morgan, M. Y. (2013). The nutritional management of hepatic encephalopathy in patients with cirrhosis: International society for hepatic encephalopathy and nitrogen metabolism consensus. *Hepatology (Baltimore, Md.), 58*(1), 325–336. doi:10.1002/hep.26370 PMID:23471642

Anand, B. (2020). Peptic Ulcer Disease. *Medscape*. Retrieved from https://emedicine.medscape.com/article/181753-overview

Anand, B. S. (1999). Cirrhosis of liver. *The Western Journal of Medicine, 171*(2), 110–115. PMID:10510657

Ananthakrishnan, A. N. (2015). Epidemiology and risk factors for IBD. *Nature Reviews. Gastroenterology & Hepatology, 12*(4), 205–217. doi:10.1038/nrgastro.2015.34 PMID:25732745

Ananthakrishnan, A. N., Khalili, H., Konijeti, G. G., Higuchi, L. M., de Silva, P., Fuchs, C. S., Willett, W. C., Richter, J. M., & Chan, A. T. (2014). Long-term intake of dietary fat and risk of ulcerative colitis and Crohn's disease. *Gut, 63*(5), 776–784. doi:10.1136/gutjnl-2013-305304 PMID:23828881

Ananthakrishnan, A. N., Khalili, H., Konijeti, G. G., Higuchi, L. M., de Silva, P., Korzenik, J. R., Fuchs, C. S., Willett, W. C., Richter, J. M., & Chan, A. T. (2013). A prospective study of long-term intake of dietary fiber and risk of Crohn's disease and ulcerative colitis. *Gastroenterology*, *145*(5), 970–977. doi:10.1053/j.gastro.2013.07.050 PMID:23912083

Andrews, C. N., & Storr, M. (2011). The pathophysiology of chronic constipation. *Canadian Journal of Gastroenterology*, *25*(suppl b), B16–B21. doi:10.1155/2011/169319 PMID:22114753

Angelis, M. De, Rizzello, C. G., Fasano, A., Clemente, M. G., Simone, C. De, Silano, M., Vincenzi, M. De, Losito, I., & Gobbetti, M. (2006). VSL#3 probiotic preparation has the capacity to hydrolyze gliadin polypeptides responsible for Celiac Sprue. Biochimica et Biophysica Acta - Molecular Basis of Disease, 1762(1), 80–93. https://doi.org/ doi:10.1016/j.bbadis.2005.09.008

Aoki, S., Hosomi, N., Hirayama, J., Nakamori, M., Yoshikawa, M., Nezu, T., Kubo, S., Nagano, Y., Nagao, A., Yamane, N., Nishikawa, Y., Takamoto, M., Ueno, H., Ochi, K., Maruyama, H., Yamamoto, H., & Matsumoto, M. (2016). The multidisciplinary swallowing team approach decreases pneumonia onset in acute stroke patients. *Public Library of Science One*, *11*(5), e0154608. doi:10.1371/journal.pone.0154608 PMID:27138162

Asali, A. M., Alghamdi, M. A., Fallatah, S. A., Alholaily, W. A., Aldandan, R. G., Alnosair, A. H., ... Alharbi, R. A. (2018). Risk factors leading to peptic ulcer disease: Systematic review in literature. *International Journal Of Community Medicine And Public Health*, *5*(10), 4617–4624. doi:10.18203/2394-6040.ijcmph20183869

Ayazi, S., Crookes, P. F., Peyre, C. G., Hagen, J. A., & Leers, J. M. (2007). Objective documentation of the link between GERD and obesity. *The American Journal of Gastroenterology*, *102*, 138–139. doi:10.14309/00000434-200709002-00059

Ayazi, S., Hagen, J. A., Chan, L. S., DeMeester, S. R., Lin, M. W., Ayazi, A., Leers, J. M., Oezcelik, A., Banki, F., Lipham, J. C., DeMeester, T. R., & Crookes, P. F. (2009). Obesity and gastroesophageal reflux: Quantifying the association between body mass index, esophageal acid exposure, and lower esophageal sphincter status in a large series of patients with reflux symptoms. *Journal of Gastrointestinal Surgery*, *13*(8), 1440–1447. doi:10.100711605-009-0930-7 PMID:19475461

Ayers, P., Guenter, P., Holcombe, B., & Plogsted, S. (2014). *ASPEN parenteral nutrition handbook*. American Society for Parenteral and Enteral Nutrition.

Bain, B. J., Lewis, S. M., & Bates, I. (2006). Basic haematological techniques. *Dacie and Lewis Practical Haematology, 4*, 19-46.

Barak, N., Ehrenpreis, E. D., Harrison, J. R., & Sitrin, M. D. (2002). Gastro-oesophageal reflux disease in obesity: Pathophysiological and therapeutic considerations. *Obesity Reviews*, *3*(1), 9–15. doi:10.1046/j.1467-789X.2002.00049.x PMID:12119661

Barkas, F., Liberopoulos, E., Kei, A., & Elisaf, M. (2013). Electrolyte and acid-base disorders in inflammatory bowel disease. *Annals of Gastroenterology*, *26*(1), 23. PMID:24714322

Beaugerie, L., & Itzkowitz, S. H. (2015). Cancers complicating inflammatory bowel disease. *The New England Journal of Medicine*, *372*(15), 1441–1452. doi:10.1056/NEJMra1403718 PMID:25853748

Bernstein, C. N., Blanchard, J. F., Rawsthorne, P., & Yu, N. (2001). The prevalence of extraintestinal diseases in inflammatory bowel disease: A population-based study. *The American Journal of Gastroenterology*, *96*(4), 1116–1122. doi:10.1111/j.1572-0241.2001.03756.x PMID:11316157

Bischoff, S. C., Escher, J., Hébuterne, X., Kłęk, S., Krznaric, Z., Schneider, S., ... Wiskin, A. E. (2020). ESPEN practical guideline: Clinical Nutrition in inflammatory bowel disease. *Clinical Nutrition (Edinburgh, Lothian)*, *39*(3), 632–653. doi:10.1016/j.clnu.2019.11.002 PMID:32029281

Bjarnason, I., Scarpignato, C., Holmgren, E., Olszewski, M., Rainsford, K. D., & Lanas, A. (2018). Mechanisms of Damage to the Gastrointestinal Tract From Nonsteroidal Anti-Inflammatory Drugs. *Gastroenterology*, *154*(3), 500–514. doi:10.1053/j.gastro.2017.10.049 PMID:29221664

Blanař, V., Hödl, M., Lohrmann, C., Amir, Y., & Eglseer, D. (2019). Dysphagia and factors associated with malnutrition risk: A 5-year multicentre study. *Journal of Advanced Nursing*, *75*(12), 3566–3576. doi:10.1111/jan.14188 PMID:31452231

Boullata, J., Brantley, S., Corkins, M., Guenter, P., Krenitsky, J., Lyman, B., . . . Wessel, J. (2009). Enteral Nutrition Practice Recommendations. *Parenteral and Enteral Nutrition, 33*(2).

Bradley, G. M., & Oliva-Hemker, M. (2012). Pediatric ulcerative colitis: Current treatment approaches including role of infliximab Biologics. *Targets and Therapy*, *6*, 125–134. PMID:22740771

Bray, G. A., Frühbeck, G., Ryan, D. H., & Wilding, J. P. H. (2016). Management of obesity. *Lancet*, *387*(10031), 1947–1956. doi:10.1016/S0140-6736(16)00271-3 PMID:26868660

Budd, J., & Cusi, K. (2020). Nonalcoholic fatty liver disease: What does the primary care physician need to know? *The American Journal of Medicine*, *133*(5), 536–543. Advance online publication. doi:10.1016/j.amjmed.2020.01.007 PMID:32017891

Canadian Society of Intestinal Research. (2018). *IBS global impact report 2018*. Retrieved from https://badgut.org/ibs-global-impact-report-2018/

Canavan, C., West, J., & Card, T. (2014). The epidemiology of irritable bowel syndrome. *Clinical Epidemiology*, *6*, 71–80. PMID:24523597

Cardile, S., & Romano, C. (2014, January 7). Current issues in pediatric inflammatory bowel disease-associated arthropathies. *World Journal of Gastroenterology*, *20*(1), 45–52. doi:10.3748/wjg.v20.i1.45 PMID:24415857

Carlsson, A., Axelsson, I., Borulf, S., Bredberg, A., Forslund, M., Lindberg, B., Sjöberg, K., & Ivarsson, S.-A. (1998). Prevalence of IgA-Antigliadin Antibodies and IgA-Antiendomysium Antibodies Related to Celiac Disease in Children With Down Syndrome. *Pediatrics*, *101*(2), 272–275. doi:10.1542/peds.101.2.272

Chang, J., Locke, G. III, McNally, M., Halder, S. L., Schleck, C. D., Zinsmeister, A. R., & Talley, N. J. (2010). Impact of functional gastrointestinal disorders on survival in the community. *The American Journal of Gastroenterology*, *105*(4), 822–832. doi:10.1038/ajg.2010.40 PMID:20160713

Chang, P., & Friedenberg, F. (2014). Obesity and GERD. *Gastroenterology Clinics of North America*, *43*(1), 161–173. doi:10.1016/j.gtc.2013.11.009 PMID:24503366

Chatila, A. T., Nguyen, M. T. T., Krill, T., Roark, R., Bilal, M., & Reep, G. (2020). Natural history, pathophysiology and evaluation of gastroesophageal reflux disease. *Disease-a-Month*, *66*(1), 100848. doi:10.1016/j.disamonth.2019.02.001 PMID:30803725

Chaudhary, A., & Singh, A. (2014). Peptic Ulcer: A Review on Epidemiology, Molecular Mechanism of Pathogenesis and Management. *International Journal of Chemistry and Pharmaceutical Sciences*, *2*, 788–796. http://www.pharmaresearchlibrary.com/wp-content/uploads/2014/04/IJCPS2012.pdf

Chen, N., Li, Y., Fang, J., Lu, Q., & He, L. (2019). Risk factors for malnutrition in stroke patients: A meta-analysis. *Clinical Nutrition (Edinburgh, Lothian)*, *38*(1), 127–135. doi:10.1016/j.clnu.2017.12.014 PMID:29310894

Chey, W. D., Kurlander, J., & Eswaran, S. (2015). Irritable bowel syndrome: A clinical review. *Journal of the American Medical Association*, *313*(9), 949–958. doi:10.1001/jama.2015.0954 PMID:25734736

Chiara, M. M., Franco, S., Marco, P., Antonio, G., & Donato, M. G. A. (2020). Nutrition, IBD and Gut Microbiota: A Review. *Nutrients*, *12*(4), 944. doi:10.3390/nu12040944 PMID:32235316

Cho, S., Lu, Y., & Lee, D.-H. (2013). Dysphagia following anterior cervical spinal surgery: A systematic review. *The Bone & Joint Journal*, *95B*(7), 868–873. doi:10.1302/0301-620X.95B7.31029 PMID:23814234

Choung, R. S., Locke, G. R., Schleck, C. D., Zinsmeister, A. R., & Talley, N. J. (2006). Cumulative incidence of chronic constipation: A population-based study 1988–2003. *Gastroenterology*, *130*, A–508.

Cichero, J. A. Y. (2017). Unlocking opportunities in food design for infants, children, and the elderly: Understanding milestones in chewing and swallowing across the lifespan for new innovations. *Journal of Texture Studies*, *48*(4), 271–279. doi:10.1111/jtxs.12236 PMID:28766752

Cichero, J. A. Y. (2018). Age related changes to eating and swallowing impact frailty: Aspiration, choking risk, modified food texture and autonomy of choice. *Geriatrics*, *3*(4), 69. doi:10.3390/geriatrics3040069 PMID:31011104

Clarke, R. C. (2020). Stress-Induced Gastritis. *Medscape.* Retrieved from https://emedicine.medscape.com/article/176319-overview

Cole, T. J. (1990). The LMS method for constructing normalized growth standards. *European Journal of Clinical Nutrition*, *44*(1), 45–60. PMID:2354692

Conrad, M. A., & Rosh, J. R. (2017). Pediatric inflammatory bowel disease. *Pediatric Clinics, 64*(3), 577–591. PMID:28502439

Continence Foundation of Australia. (2020). *Irritable bowel syndrome (IBS)*. Retrieved from https://www.cedars-sinai.org/health-library/diseases-and-conditions/i/irritable-bowel-syndrome-ibs.html

Cox, S. R., Lindsay, J. O., Fromentin, S., Stagg, A. J., McCarthy, N. E., Galleron, N., . . . Pons, N. (2020). Effects of Low FODMAP Diet on Symptoms, Fecal Microbiome, and Markers of Inflammation in Patients With Quiescent Inflammatory Bowel Disease in a Randomized Trial. *Gastroenterology, 158*(1), 176-188.

Cozma-Petruţ, A., Loghin, F., Miere, D., & Dumitraşcu, D. L. (2017). Diet in irritable bowel syndrome: What to recommend, not what to forbid to patients. *World Journal of Gastroenterology, 23*(21), 3771–3783. doi:10.3748/wjg.v23.i21.3771 PMID:28638217

Crary, M., Humphrey, J. L., Carnaby-Mann, G., Sambandam, R., Miller, L., & Silliman, S. (2013). Dysphagia, nutrition, and hydration in ischemic stroke patients at admission and discharge from acute care. *Dysphagia, 28*(1), 69–76. doi:10.100700455-012-9414-0 PMID:22684924

Cummins, A. G., & Roberts-Thomson, I. C. (2009). Prevalence of celiac disease in the Asia-Pacific region. *Journal of Gastroenterology and Hepatology, 24*(8), 1347–1351. doi:10.1111/j.1440-1746.2009.05932.x

D'Haens, G., Geboes, K., Peeters, M., Baert, F., Ectors, N., & Rutgeerts, P. (1997). Patchy cecal inflammation associated with distal ulcerative colitis: A prospective endoscopic study. *The American Journal of Gastroenterology, 92*, 1275–1279. PMID:9260788

daSilva, J. S. V., Seres, D. S., Sabino, K., Adams, S. C., Berdahl, G. J., Wolfe Citty, S., ... Ayers, P. (2020). ASPEN consensus recommendations for refeeding syndrome. *Nutrition in Clinical Practice, 35*(2), 178–195. doi:10.1002/ncp.10474 PMID:32115791

de Bie, C. I., Buderus, S., Sandhu, B. K., de Ridder, L., Paerregaard, A., & Veres, G. (2005). Inflammatory bowel disease in children and adolescents. Recommendations for diagnosis: the Porto criteria. Medical position paper: IBD working group of the European Society for Paediatric Gastroenterology, Hepatology and Nutrition (ESPGHAN). *Journal of Pediatric Gastroenterology and Nutrition, 41*, 1–7. doi:10.1097/01.MPG.0000163736.30261.82 PMID:15990620

De Giorgi, F., Palmiero, M., Esposito, I., Mosca, F., & Cuomo, R. (2006). Pathophysiology of gastro-oesophageal reflux disease. *Acta Otorhinolaryngologica Italica, 26*(5), 241–246. PMID:17345925

de Onis, M., & .... (2007). Development of a WHO growth reference for school-aged children and adolescents. *Bulletin of the World Health Organization, 85*(09), 660–667. doi:10.2471/BLT.07.043497 PMID:18026621

Delegge, M. H., & Berry, A. (2009). Enteral feeding: Should it be continued in the patient with *Clostridium difficile* enterocolitis? *Practical Gastroenterology, 33*(3), 40–49.

Deng, Y., Misselwitz, B., Dai, N., & Fox, M. (2015). Lactose Intolerance in Adults: Biological Mechanism and Dietary Management. *Nutrients*, *7*(9), 8020–8035. doi:10.3390/nu7095380 PMID:26393648

Dent, J., Becher, A., Sung, J., Zou, D., Agréus, L., & Bazzoli, F. (2012). Systematic Review: Patterns of Reflux-Induced Symptoms and Esophageal Endoscopic Findings in Large-Scale Surveys. *Clinical Gastroenterology and Hepatology*, *10*(8), 863–873.e3. doi:10.1016/j.cgh.2012.02.028 PMID:22401904

Di Cagno, R., De Angelis, M., Auricchio, S., Greco, L., Clarke, C., De Vincenzi, M., Giovannini, C., D'Archivio, M., Landolfo, F., Parrilli, G., Minervini, F., Arendt, E., & Gobbetti, M. (2004). Sourdough Bread Made from Wheat and Nontoxic Flours and Started with Selected Lactobacilli Is Tolerated in Celiac Sprue Patients. [PubMed]. *Applied and Environmental Microbiology*, *70*(2), 1088–1096. doi:10.1128/AEM.70.2.1088-1096.2004

Di Caro, S., Fragkos, K. C., Keetarut, K., Koo, H. F., Sebepos-Rogers, G., Saravanapavan, H., Barragry, Rogers, Mehta, & Rahman, F. (2019). Enteral Nutrition in Adult Crohn's Disease: Toward a Paradigm Shift. *Nutrients*, *11*(9), 2222. doi:10.3390/nu11092222 PMID:31540038

Diaz-Rubio, M., Moreno-Elola-Olaso, C., Rey, E., Locke, G. R., & Rodriguez-Artalejo, F. (2004). Symptoms of gastro-oesophageal reflux: Prevalence, severity, duration and associated factors in a Spanish population. *Alimentary Pharmacology & Therapeutics*, *19*(1), 95–105. doi:10.1046/j.1365-2036.2003.01769.x PMID:14687171

Douglas, L. C., & Sanders, M. E. (2008). Probiotics and prebiotics in dietetics practice. *Journal of the American Dietetic Association*, *108*(3), 510–521. doi:10.1016/j.jada.2007.12.009 PMID:18313433

Drossman, D. A. (2006). The functional gastrointestinal disorders and the Rome III process. *Gastroenterology*, *130*(5), 1377–1390. doi:10.1053/j.gastro.2006.03.008 PMID:16678553

Duffy, J. (2013). *Motor speech disorders: Substrates, differential diagnosis, and management*. Elsevier.

Duro, D., & Duggan, C. (2007). The BRAT diet for acute diarrhea in children: Should it be used? *Practical Gastroenterology*, *31*(6), 60–68.

Eiden, K. A. (2003). Nutritional considerations in inflammatory bowel disease. *Practical Gastroenterology*, *27*(5), 33–54.

El-Serag, H. B., Sweet, S., Winchester, C. C., & Dent, J. (2014). Update on the epidemiology of gastro-oesophageal reflux disease: A systematic review. *Gut*.

El-Serag, H. B., Graham, D. Y., Satia, J. A., & Rabeneck, L. (2005). Obesity is an independent risk factor for GERD symptoms and erosive esophagitis. *The American Journal of Gastroenterology*, *100*(6), 1243–1250. doi:10.1111/j.1572-0241.2005.41703.x PMID:15929752

El-Serag, H. B., Hill, C., & Jones, R. (2009). Systematic review: The epidemiology of gastro-oesophageal reflux disease in primary care, using the UK General Practice Research Database. *Alimentary Pharmacology & Therapeutics*, *29*(5), 470–480. doi:10.1111/j.1365-2036.2008.03901.x PMID:19035977

El-Serag, H. B., Petersen, N. J., Carter, J., Graham, D. Y., Richardson, P., Genta, R. M., & Rabeneck, L. (2004). Gastroesophageal reflux among different racial groups in the United States. *Gastroenterology*, *126*(7), 1692–1699. doi:10.1053/j.gastro.2004.03.077 PMID:15188164

Escott-Stump, S. (2012). Nutrition and Diagnosis-Related Care (7th ed.). Wolters Kluwer: Lippincott Williams & Wilkins.

Escott-Stump, S. (2012). *Nutrition and diagnosis-related care* (7th ed.). Lippinocott Williams & Wilkins, Wolters Kluwer.

Evon, G. P., & Ravikumara, M. (2010, March). Endoscopic and Histologic Findings in Pediatric Inflammatory Bowel Disease. *Gastroenterology & Hepatology*, *6*(3). PMID:20567564

Fashner, J., & Gitu, A. C. (2015). Diagnosis and Treatment of Peptic Ulcer Disease and H. pylori Infection. *American Family Physician*, *91*(4), 236–242. https://www.aafp.org/afp/2015/0215/p236.html PMID:25955624

Fedewa, A., & Rao, S. S. (2014). Dietary fructose intolerance, fructan intolerance and FODMAPs. *Current Gastroenterology Reports*, *16*(1), 370. doi:10.100711894-013-0370-0

Feher, J. (2017). 8.2 - The Stomach. In J. Feher (Ed.), *Quantitative Human Physiology* (2nd ed., pp. 785–795). Academic Press. doi:10.1016/B978-0-12-800883-6.00078-1

Fernández-Bañares, F., Carrasco, A., García-Puig, R., Rosinach, M., González, C., Alsina, M., Loras, C., Salas, A., Viver, J. M., & Esteve, M. (2014). Intestinal intraepithelial lymphocyte cytometric pattern is more accurate than subepithelial deposits of anti-tissue transglutaminase IgA for the diagnosis of celiac disease in lymphocytic enteritis. [PubMed]. *PLoS One*, *9*(7), e101249. Advance online publication. doi:10.1371/journal.pone.0101249

Foley, N. C., Salter, K. L., Robertson, J., Teasell, R. W., & Woodbury, M. G. (2009). Which reported estimate of the prevalence of malnutrition after stroke is valid? *Stroke*, *40*(3), pe66–e74. doi:10.1161/STROKEAHA.108.518910 PMID:19164799

Forbes, A., Escher, J., Hébuterne, X., Kłęk, S., Krznaric, Z., Schneider, S., Shamir, R., Stardelova, K., Wierdsma, N., Wiskin, A. E., & Bischoff, S. C. (2017). ESPEN guideline: Clinical nutrition in inflammatory bowel disease. *Clinical Nutrition (Edinburgh, Lothian)*, *36*(2), 321–347. doi:10.1016/j.clnu.2016.12.027 PMID:28131521

Ford, A. C., Moayyedi, P., Chey, W. D., Harris, L. A., Lacy, B. E., Saito, Y. A., ... Syndrome, A. T. F. M. I. B. (2018). American College of Gastroenterology Monograph on Management of Irritable Bowel Syndrome. *The American Journal of Gastroenterology*, *113*, 1–18. doi:10.103841395-018-0084-x PMID:29950604

Fox, M., Barr, C., Nolan, S., Lomer, M., Anggiansah, A., & Wong, T. (2007). The Effects of Dietary Fat and Calorie Density on Esophageal Acid Exposure and Reflux Symptoms. *Clinical Gastroenterology and Hepatology*, *5*(4), 439–444.e1. doi:10.1016/j.cgh.2006.12.013 PMID:17363334

Freeman, H. J. (2010). Risk factors in familial forms of celiac disease. *World Journal of Gastroenterology*, *16*(15), 1828–1831. doi:10.3748/wjg.v16.i15.1828

Frolkis, A. D., Dykeman, J., Negrón, M. E., deBruyn, J., Jette, N., Fiest, K. M., ... Panaccione, R. (2013). Risk of surgery for inflammatory bowel diseases has decreased over time: A systematic review and meta-analysis of population-based studies. *Gastroenterology*, *145*(5), 996–1006. doi:10.1053/j.gastro.2013.07.041 PMID:23896172

Fujiwara, Y., Machida, A., Watanabe, Y., Shiba, M., Tominaga, K., Watanabe, T., Oshitani, N., Higuchi, K., & Arakawa, T. (2005). Association between dinner-to-bed time and gastroesophageal reflux disease. *The American Journal of Gastroenterology*, *100*(12), 2633–2636. doi:10.1111/j.1572-0241.2005.00354.x PMID:16393212

Geerling, B. J., Badart-Smook, A., Stockbrügger, R. W., & Brummer, R. (1998). Comprehensive nutritional status in patients with long-standing Crohn disease currently in remission. *The American Journal of Clinical Nutrition*, *67*(5), 919–926. doi:10.1093/ajcn/67.5.919 PMID:9583850

Genetics Home Reference. (2020). *Lactose Intolerance*. Retrieved from https://ghr.nlm.nih.gov/condition/lactose-intolerance

Gibson, P. R., & Shepherd, S. J. (2012). Food choice as a key management strategy for functional gastrointestinal symptoms. *The American Journal of Gastroenterology*, *107*(5), 657–666. doi:10.1038/ajg.2012.49 PMID:22488077

Glickman, J. N., Bousvaros, A., Farraye, F. A., Zholudev, A., Friedman, S., Wang, H. H., Leichtner, A. M., & Odze, R. D. (2004). Pediatric patients with untreated ulcerative colitis may present initially with unusual morphologic findings. *The American Journal of Surgical Pathology*, *28*(2), 190–197. doi:10.1097/00000478-200402000-00006 PMID:15043308

Go, A. S., Mozaffarian, D., Roger, V. L., Benjamin, E. J., Berry, J. D., Borden, W. B., ... Turner, M. B. (2012). Heart disease and stroke statistics—2013 update: A report from the American Heart Association. *Circulation*, 2–241. PMID:23239837

Gomes, D. C., & Dantas, R. O. (2014). Acidic and neutral liquid ingestion in patients with gastroesophageal reflux disease. *Arquivos de Gastroenterologia*, *51*(3), 217–220. doi:10.1590/S0004-28032014000300010 PMID:25296082

González-Fernández, M., Humbert, I., Winegrad, H., Cappola, A. R., & Fried, L. P. (2014). Dysphagia in old-old women: Prevalence as determined according to self-report and the 3-ounce Water Swallowing Test. *Journal of the American Geriatrics Society*, *62*(4), 716–720. doi:10.1111/jgs.12745 PMID:24635053

Groher, M. E., & Crary, M. A. (2015). *Dysphagia: Clinical management in adults and children* (2nd ed.). Elsevier.

Growth Charts for Children with Down Syndrome. (n.d.). Retrieved April 21, 2020, from https://www.cdc.gov/ncbddd/birthdefects/downsyndrome/growth-charts.html

Gujral, N., Freeman, H. J., & Thomson, A. B. R. (2012). Celiac disease: Prevalence, diagnosis, pathogenesis and treatment. [PubMed]. *World Journal of Gastroenterology*, *18*(42), 6036–6059. doi:10.3748/wjg.v18.i42.6036

Guo, Q., Goldenberg, J. Z., Humphrey, C., El Dib, R., & Johnston, B. C. (2019). Probiotics for the prevention of pediatric antibiotic-associated diarrhea. *Cochrane Database of Systematic Reviews*, *4*, CD00482.

Gupta, B. (n.d.). Non-steroidal Anti-inflammatory Drugs. *World Federation of Societies of Anaesthesiologists* Retrieved from https://www.wfsahq.org/components/com_virtual_library/media/8ea6b673c075492e525e15016eb2a6b1-Non-steroidal-Anti-inflammatory-Drugs--Update-24-2-2008-.pdf

Hall, J. E. (2011). *Guyton and Hall textbook of medical physiology* (12th ed.). Elsevier.

Halmos, E. P. (2017). When the low FODMAP diet does not work. *Journal of Gastroenterology and Hepatology*, *32*, 69–72. doi:10.1111/jgh.13701 PMID:28244666

Hasler, W. L., & Owyang, C. (2012). Approach to the patient with gastrointestinal disease. In D. L. Longo, A. S. Fauci, D. L. Kasper, S. L. Hauser, J. Jameson, & J. Loscalzo (Eds.), *Harrison's principles of internal medicine* (18th ed.). McGraw-Hill.

Häuser, W., Layer, P., Henningsen, P., & Kruis, W. (2012). Functional bowel disorders in adults. *Deutsches Ärzteblatt International*, *109*(5), 83–94. PMID:22368721

Heidelbaugh, J. J., Nostrant, T. T., Kim, C., & Van Harrison, R. (2003). Management of gastroesophageal reflux disease. *American Family Physician*, *68*(7), 1311–1318. PMID:14567485

Hersberger, L., Bargetzi, L., Bargetzi, A., Tribolet, P., Fehr, R., Baechli, V., . . . Kutz, A. (2019). Nutritional risk screening (NRS 2002) is a strong and modifiable predictor risk score for short-term and long-term clinical outcomes: secondary analysis of a prospective randomized trial. *Clinical Nutrition*.

Hershcovici, T., Mashimo, H., & Fass, R. (2011). The lower esophageal sphincter. *Neurogastroenterology and Motility*, *23*(9), 819–830. doi:10.1111/j.1365-2982.2011.01738.x PMID:21711416

HHS & USDA. (2015). *Dietary guidelines for Americans 2015-2020* (8th ed.). Government Printing Office.

Hodges, J. K., Cao, S., Cladis, D. P., & Weaver, C. M. (2019). Lactose Intolerance and Bone Health: The Challenge of Ensuring Adequate Calcium Intake. *Nutrients*, *11*(4), 718. Advance online publication. doi:10.3390/nu11040718 PMID:30925689

Holick, M. F., & Chen, T. C. (2008). Vitamin D deficiency: A worldwide problem with health consequences. *The American Journal of Clinical Nutrition, 87*(4), 1080s–1086s. doi:10.1093/ajcn/87.4.1080S PMID:18400738

Holloway, R. H., Lyrenas, E., Ireland, A., & Dent, J. (1997). Effect of intraduodenal fat on lower oesophageal sphincter function and gastro-oesophageal reflux. *Gut, 40*(4), 449–453. doi:10.1136/gut.40.4.449 PMID:9176069

Hou, J. K., Abraham, B., & El-Serag, H. (2011). Dietary Intake and Risk of Developing Inflammatory Bowel Disease: A Systematic Review of the Literature. *The American Journal of Gastroenterology, 106*(4), 563–573. doi:10.1038/ajg.2011.44 PMID:21468064

Hyams, J. S. (2005). Inflammatory bowel disease. *Pediatrics in Review, 26*(9), 314–320. doi:10.1542/pir.26-9-314 PMID:16140873

Ibrahim, F., & Stribling, P. (2019). A 5Ad dietary protocol for functional bowel disorders. *Nutrients, 11*(8), E1983.

Itkonen, S. T., Erkkola, M., & Lamberg-Allardt, C. J. E. (2018). Vitamin D Fortification of Fluid Milk Products and Their Contribution to Vitamin D Intake and Vitamin D Status in Observational Studies-A Review. *Nutrients, 10*(8), 1054. Advance online publication. doi:10.3390/nu10081054 PMID:30096919

Jackson, K. A., & Savaiano, D. A. (2001). Lactose maldigestion, calcium intake and osteoporosis in African-, Asian-, and Hispanic-Americans. *Journal of the American College of Nutrition, 20*(2, Suppl), 198s–207s. doi:10.1080/07315724.2001.10719032 PMID:11349943

Jacobson, B. C., Somers, S. C., Fuchs, C. S., Kelly, C. P., & Camargo, C. A. Jr. (2006). Body-Mass Index and Symptoms of Gastroesophageal Reflux in Women. *The New England Journal of Medicine, 354*(22), 2340–2348. doi:10.1056/NEJMoa054391 PMID:16738270

Jameson, J. L., Fauci, A. S., Kasper, D. L., Hauser, S. L., Longo, D. L., & Loscalzo, J. (2018). *Harrison's Principles of Internal Medicine* (20th ed., Vol. 2). McGraw-Hill Education.

Jansen, I., Prager, M., Valentini, L., & Büning, C. (2016). Inflammation-driven malnutrition: A new screening tool predicts outcome in Crohn's disease. *British Journal of Nutrition, 116*(6), 1061–1067. doi:10.1017/S0007114516003044 PMID:27546478

Jarosz, M., & Taraszewska, A. (2014). Risk factors for gastroesophageal reflux disease: The role of diet. *Przegląd Gastroenterologiczny, 9*(5), 297–301. doi:10.5114/pg.2014.46166 PMID:25396005

John Hopkins Medicine. (2020). *Irritable bowel syndrome (IBS).* Retrieved from https://www.hopkinsmedicine.org/health/conditions-and-diseases/irritable-bowel-syndrome-ibs

Johnson-Wimbley, T. D., & Graham, D. Y. (2011). Diagnosis and management of iron deficiency anemia in the 21st century. *Therapeutic Advances in Gastroenterology, 4*(3), 177–184. doi:10.1177/1756283X11398736 PMID:21694802

Jung, H., Choung, R. S., & Talley, N. J. (2010). Gastroesophageal Reflux Disease and Sleep Disorders: Evidence for a Causal Link and Therapeutic Implications. *Journal of Neurogastroenterology and Motility, 16*(1), 22–29. doi:10.5056/jnm.2010.16.1.22 PMID:20535322

Kahrilas, P. J. (2003). GERD pathogenesis, pathophysiology, and clinical manifestations. *Cleveland Clinic Journal of Medicine, 70*(SUPPL. 5), S4–S19. doi:10.3949/ccjm.70.Suppl_5.S4 PMID:14705378

Kahrilas, P. J., & Gupta, R. R. (1990). Mechanisms of acid reflux associated with cigarette smoking. *Gut, 31*(1), 4–10. doi:10.1136/gut.31.1.4 PMID:2318431

Kahrilas, P. J., Lin, S., Chen, J., & Manka, M. (1999). The effect of hiatus hernia on gastro-oesophageal junction pressure. *Gut, 44*(4), 476–482. doi:10.1136/gut.44.4.476 PMID:10075953

Kalra, A., & Tuma, F. (2018, December 18). *Physiology, liver.* National Center for Biotechnology Information. https://www.ncbi.nlm.nih.gov/books/NBK535438/

Kaltenbach, T., Crockett, S., & Gerson, L. B. (2006). Are lifestyle measures effective in patients with gastroesophageal reflux disease? An evidence-based approach. *Archives of Internal Medicine, 166*(9), 965–971. doi:10.1001/archinte.166.9.965 PMID:16682569

Katz, P. O., Gerson, L. B., & Vela, M. F. (2013). Guidelines for the Diagnosis and Management of Gastroesophageal Reflux Disease. *The American Journal of Gastroenterology, 108*(3), 308–328. doi:10.1038/ajg.2012.444 PMID:23419381

Kelly, D. G., & Nadeau, J. (2004). Oral rehydration solution: A "low-tech" oft neglected therapy. *Practical Gastroenterology, 28*(10), 51–62.

Khan, A. M., Sarker, S. A., Alam, N. H., Hossain, M. S., Fuchs, G. J., & Salam, M. A. (2005). Low osmolar oral rehydration salts solution in the treatment of acute watery diarrhea in neonates and young infants: A randomized, controlled clinical trial. *Journal of Health, Population and Nutrition, 23*(1), 52. PMID:15884752

Kondrup, J., Rasmussen, H. H., & Hamberg, O. (2003). Nutritional risk screening (NRS 2002): A new method based on an analysis of controlled clinical trials. *Clinical Nutrition (Edinburgh, Lothian), 22*(3), 321–336. doi:10.1016/S0261-5614(02)00214-5 PMID:12765673

Kowalska, J., Bojko, E., Szczepańska-Gieracha, J., Rymaszewska, J., & Rożek-Piechura, K. (2015). Occurrence of depressive symptoms among older adults after a stroke in the nursing home facility. *Rehabilitation Nursing, 41*(2), 112–119. doi:10.1002/rnj.203 PMID:25772117

Kugathasan, S., Judd, R. H., Hoffmann, R. G., Heikenen, J., Telega, G., Khan, F., ... Yaffe, M. (2003). Epidemiologic and clinical characteristics of children with newly diagnosed inflammatory bowel disease in Wisconsin: A statewide population-based study. *The Journal of Pediatrics, 143*(4), 525–531. doi:10.1067/S0022-3476(03)00444-X PMID:14571234

Kulshreshtha, M., Srivastava, G., & Singh, M. (2017). Pathophysiological status and nutritional therapy of peptic ulcer: An update. *Environmental Disease, 2*(3), 76–86. doi:10.4103/ed.ed_11_17

Lab Tests Online. (2019). *Patient education on blood, urine, and other lab tests*. Lab Tests Online. https://labtestsonline.org/

Lacy, B. E., Mearin, F., Chang, L., Chey, W. D., Lembo, A. J., Simren, M., & Spiller, R. (2016). Bowel Disorders. *Gastroenterology*, *150*(6), 1393–1407.e1395. doi:10.1053/j.gastro.2016.02.031 PMID:27144627

Lacy, B. E., & Patel, N. K. (2017). Rome criteria and a diagnostic approach to irritable bowel syndrome. *Journal of Clinical Medicine*, *6*(11), E99. doi:10.3390/jcm6110099 PMID:29072609

Laffolie, J. D., Laass, M. W., Scholz, D., Zimmer, K. P., & Buderus, S.CEDATA-GPGE Study Group. (2017). Prevalence of anemia in pediatric IBD patients and impact on disease severity: Results of the pediatric IBD-registry CEDATA-GPGE®. *Gastroenterology Research and Practice*, 2017. PMID:29358946

Laharie, D. (2017). Towards therapeutic choices in ulcerative colitis. *Lancet*, *390*(10090), 98–99. doi:10.1016/S0140-6736(17)31263-1 PMID:28527707

Lee, J. J., Escher, J. C., Shuman, M. J., Forbes, P. W., Delemarre, L. C., Harr, B. W., Kruijer, M., Moret, M., Allende-Richter, S., & Grand, R. J. (2010). Final adult height of children with inflammatory bowel disease is predicted by parental height and patient minimum height Z-score. *Inflammatory Bowel Diseases*, *16*(10), 1669–1677. doi:10.1002/ibd.21214 PMID:20127995

Lee, S. (2014). Non-invasive diagnosis of hepatitis B virus-related cirrhosis. *World Journal of Gastroenterology*, *20*(2), 445. doi:10.3748/wjg.v20.i2.445 PMID:24574713

Lee, T. H., Choi, S. C., Park, M. I., Park, K. S., Shin, J. E., Kim, S. E., Jung, K. W., Koo, H. S., Kim, W. J., Cho, Y. K., Kim, Y. S., Lee, J. S., & and. (2014). Constipation misperception is associated with gender, marital status, treatment utilization and constipation symptoms experienced. *Journal of Neurogastroenterology and Motility*, *20*(3), 379–387. doi:10.5056/jnm14011 PMID:24935009

Leffler, D. A., Dennis, M., Hyett, B., Kelly, E., Schuppan, D., & Kelly, C. P. (2007). {A figure is presented}Etiologies and Predictors of Diagnosis in Nonresponsive Celiac Disease. [PubMed]. *Clinical Gastroenterology and Hepatology*, *5*(4), 445–450. doi:10.1016/j.cgh.2006.12.006

Lehrer, J. K. (2019). *Irritable bowel syndrome (IBS): practice essentials, background, pathophysiology*. Retrieved from https://emedicine.medscape.com/article/180389-overview

Leung, F. W. (2007). Etiologic factors of chronic constipation: Review of the scientific evidence. *Digestive Diseases and Sciences*, *52*(2), 313–316. doi:10.100710620-006-9298-7 PMID:17219073

Levesque, B. G., & Sandborn, W. J. (2012). Infliximab versus ciclosporin in severe ulcerative colitis. *Lancet*, *380*(9857), 1887–1888. doi:10.1016/S0140-6736(12)61259-8 PMID:23063315

Levine, J.S., & Burakoff, R. (2011). Extraintestinal Manifestations of Inflammatory Bowel Disease. *Gastroenterology & Hepatology*, *7*(4).

Li, L. F., Chan, R. L., Lu, L., Shen, J., Zhang, L., Wu, W. K., Wang, L., Hu, T., Li, M. X., & Cho, C. H. (2014). Cigarette smoking and gastrointestinal diseases: The causal relationship and underlying molecular mechanisms. *International Journal of Molecular Medicine*, *34*(2), 372–380. doi:10.3892/ijmm.2014.1786 PMID:24859303

Lo, B., Holm, J. P., Vester-Andersen, M. K., Bendtsen, F., Vind, I., & Burisch, J. (2020). Incidence, Risk Factors and Evaluation of Osteoporosis in Patients With Inflammatory Bowel Disease: A Danish Population-Based Inception Cohort With 10 Years of Follow-Up. *Journal of Crohn's and Colitis*.

Lohsiriwat, S., Puengna, N., & Leelakusolvong, S. (2006). Effect of caffeine on lower esophageal sphincter pressure in Thai healthy volunteers. *Diseases of the Esophagus*, *19*(3), 183–188. doi:10.1111/j.1442-2050.2006.00562.x PMID:16722996

Lomer, M. C. (2011). Dietary and nutritional considerations for inflammatory bowel disease. *The Proceedings of the Nutrition Society*, *70*(3), 329–335. doi:10.1017/S0029665111000097 PMID:21450124

Longstreth, G. F., Thompson, W. G., Chey, W. D., Houghton, L. A., Mearin, F., & Spiller, R. C. (2006). Functional bowel disorders. *Gastroenterology*, *130*(5), 1480–1491. doi:10.1053/j.gastro.2005.11.061 PMID:16678561

Ludvigsson, J. F., & Fasano, A. (2012). Timing of introduction of gluten and celiac disease risk. [PubMed]. *Annals of Nutrition & Metabolism*, *60*(s2), 22–29. doi:10.1159/000335335

Macdonald, S. (2007). Sarah Macdonald. 90–124.

Madoff, R. D. (2012). Chronic constipation: From evaluation to treatment. *International Foundation for Functional Gastrointestinal Disorders*, *02*, G1075–G1084.

Mahan, L. K., Escott-Stump, S., & Raymond, J. (2011). *Krause's food & nutrition care process*. Saunders.

Mahan, L. K., & Raymond, J. L. (2016). *Krause's food & the nutrition care process-e-book*. Elsevier Health Sciences.

Mahan, L. K., & Raymond, J. L. (2017). *Krause's Food & the Nutrition Care Process* (14th ed.). Elsevier.

Mahan, L. K., & Raymond, J. L. (2017). *Krause's food & the nutrition care process*. Elsevier.

Mahan, L. K., & Raymond, J. L. (2017). *Krause's Food and the Nutrition Care Process* (14th ed.). Elsevier.

Mamula, P., Markowitz, J. E., & Baldassano, R. N. (2013). *Pediatric inflammatory bowel disease* (2nd ed.). Springer Science of Business Media. doi:10.1007/978-1-4614-5061-0

Manhan, K., & Janice, R. (2017). *Krause's Food & Nutrition Care Process* (14th ed.). ELSEVIER.

Mann, G., Hankey, G., & Cameron, D. (2000). Swallowing disorders following acute stroke: Prevalence and diagnostic accuracy. *Cerebrovascular Diseases (Basel, Switzerland)*, *10*(5), 380–386. doi:10.1159/000016094 PMID:10971024

Martino, R., Foley, N., Bhogal, S., Diamant, N., Speechley, M., & Teasell, R. (2005). Dysphagia after stroke: Incidence, diagnosis, and pulmonary complications. *Stroke*, *36*(12), 2756–2763. doi:10.1161/01.STR.0000190056.76543.eb PMID:16269630

Marugán, R. B., & Garzóno, S. G. (2009). DNA-guided hepatitis B treatment, viral load is essential, but not sufficient. *World Journal of Gastroenterology*, *15*(4), 423. doi:10.3748/wjg.15.423 PMID:19152446

Matlik, L., Savaiano, D., McCabe, G., VanLoan, M., Blue, C. L., & Boushey, C. J. (2007). Perceived milk intolerance is related to bone mineral content in 10- to 13-year-old female adolescents. *Pediatrics*, *120*(3), e669–e677. doi:10.1542/peds.2006-1240 PMID:17766507

Mattar, R., de Campos Mazo, D. F., & Carrilho, F. J. (2012). Lactose intolerance: Diagnosis, genetic, and clinical factors. *Clinical and Experimental Gastroenterology*, *5*, 113–121. doi:10.2147/CEG.S32368 PMID:22826639

Matysiak-Budnik, T., Candalh, C., Cellier, C., Dugave, C., Namane, A., Vidal-Martinez, T., Cerf-Bensussan, N., & Heyman, M. (2005). Limited efficiency of prolyl-endopeptidase in the detoxification of gliadin peptides in celiac disease. [PubMed]. *Gastroenterology*, *129*(3), 786–796. doi:10.1053/j.gastro.2005.06.016

Mayo Clinic Organization. (2020). *Lactose Intolerance*. Retrieved May 26, 2020, from https://www.mayoclinic.org/diseases-conditions/lactose-intolerance/symptoms-causes/syc-20374232

Mayo Clinic. (2018). *Irritable bowel syndrome - symptoms and causes*. Retrieved from https://www.mayoclinic.org/diseases-conditions/irritable-bowel-syndrome/symptoms-causes/syc-20360016

McCullough, G. H., Rosenbeck, J. C., Wertz, R. T., McCoy, S., Mann, G., & McCullough, K. (2005). Utility of clinical swallowing examination measures for detecting aspiration post-stroke. *Journal of Speech, Language, and Hearing Research*, *48*, 1280-1293. doi: 1092-4388/05/4806-1280

McDonald, L. C., Gerding, D. N., Johnson, S., Bakken, J. S., Carroll, K. C., Coffin, S. E., Dubberke, E. R., Garey, K. W., Gould, C. V., Kelly, C., Loo, V., Shaklee Sammons, J., Sandora, T. J., & Wilcox, M. H. (2018). Clinical Practice Guidelines for Clostridium difficile Infection in Adults and Children: 2017 Update by the Infectious Diseases Society of America (IDSA) and Society for Healthcare Epidemiology of America (SHEA). *Clinical Infectious Diseases*, *66*(7), e1–e48. doi:10.1093/cid/cix1085 PMID:29462280

Meining, A., & Classen, M. (2000). The role of diet and lifestyle measures in the pathogenesis and treatment of gastroesophageal reflux disease. *The American Journal of Gastroenterology*, *95*(10), 2692–2697. doi:10.1111/j.1572-0241.2000.03175.x PMID:11051337

Miele, E., Shamir, R., Aloi, M., Assa, A., Braegger, C., Bronsky, J., ... Koletzko, S. (2018). Nutrition in pediatric inflammatory bowel disease: A position paper on behalf of the Porto Inflammatory Bowel Disease Group of the European Society of Pediatric Gastroenterology, Hepatology and Nutrition. *Journal of Pediatric Gastroenterology and Nutrition*, *66*(4), 687–708. doi:10.1097/MPG.0000000000001896 PMID:29570147

Mifflin, M. D., St Jeor, S. T., Hill, L. A., Scott, B. J., Daugherty, S. A., & Koh, Y. O. (1990). new predictive equation for resting energy expenditure in healthy individuals. *The American Journal of Clinical Nutrition*, *51*(2), 241–247. doi:10.1093/ajcn/51.2.241 PMID:2305711

Mishori, R., Otubu, A., & Jones, A. A. (2011). The dangers of colon cleansing. *The Journal of Family Practice*, *60*(8), 454–457. PMID:21814639

Mittal, R. K., Lange, R. C., & McCallum, R. W. (1987). Identification and mechanism of delayed esophageal acid clearance in subjects with hiatus hernia. *Gastroenterology*, *92*(1), 130–135. doi:10.1016/0016-5085(87)90849-3 PMID:3781181

Miwa, H., Igarashi, A., Teng, L., Uda, A., Deguchi, H., & Tango, T. (2019). Systematic review with network meta-analysis: Indirect comparison of the efficacy of vonoprazan and proton-pump inhibitors for maintenance treatment of gastroesophageal reflux disease. *Journal of Gastroenterology*, *54*(8), 718–729. doi:10.100700535-019-01572-y PMID:30919071

Moayyedi, P., Mearin, F., Azpiroz, F., Andresen, V., Barbara, G., Corsetti, M., Emmanuel, A., Hungin, A. P. S., Layer, P., Stanghellini, V., Whorwell, P., Zerbib, F., & Tack, J. (2017). Irritable bowel syndrome diagnosis and management: A simplified algorithm for clinical practice. *United European Gastroenterology Journal*, *5*(6), 773–788. doi:10.1177/2050640617731968 PMID:29026591

Montalto, M., Nucera, G., Santoro, L., Curigliano, V., Vastola, M., Covino, M., Cuoco, L., Manna, R., Gasbarrini, A., & Gasbarrini, G. (2005). Effect of exogenous β-galactosidase in patients with lactose malabsorption and intolerance: A crossover double-blind placebo-controlled study. *European Journal of Clinical Nutrition*, *59*(4), 489–493. doi:10.1038j.ejcn.1602098 PMID:15674309

Morelli, L., Amrani, N., Goulet, O., & Lukito, W. (2019). Lactose Intolerance: Clinical Symptoms, Diagnosis and Treatment. *Global Dabetes Open Access Journal*, *1*(1), 1–10.

Morely, J. E. (1997). Anorexia of aging: Physiologic and pathologic. *The American Journal of Clinical Nutrition*, *66*(4), 760–773. doi:10.1093/ajcn/66.4.760 PMID:9322549

Morozov, S., Isakov, V., & Konovalova, M. (2018). Fiber-enriched diet helps to control symptoms and improves esophageal motility in patients with non-erosive gastroesophageal reflux disease. *World Journal of Gastroenterology*, *24*(21), 2291–2299. doi:10.3748/wjg.v24.i21.2291 PMID:29881238

Mueller, C. M. (2017). *The ASPEN Adult Nutrition Support Core Curriculum* (3rd ed.). American Society for Parenteral and Enteral Nutrition.

Nahikian-Nelms, M., Sucher, K., & Lacey, K. (2016). *Nutrition therapy and pathophysiology* (3rd ed.). Cengage Learning.

Nall, R. (2018, January 11). *Liver fibrosis*. Healthline. https://www.healthline.com/health/liver-fibrosis

Namasivayam-Macdonald, A. M., Barbon, C. E., & Steele, C. M. (2018). A review of swallow timing in the elderly. *Physiology & Behavior, 184*, 12–26. doi:10.1016/j.physbeh.2017.10.023 PMID:29101012

Narula, N., Dhillon, A., Zhang, D., Sherlock, M. E., Tondeur, M., & Zachos, M. (2018). Enteral nutritional therapy for induction of remission in Crohn's disease. *Cochrane Database of Systematic Reviews*, 4. doi:10.1002/14651858.CD000542.pub3 PMID:29607496

National Institute of Diabetes and Digestive and Kidney Diseaes. (2014). *Eating, Diet, & Nutrition for GER & GERD*. Retrieved April 17, 2020, from https://www.niddk.nih.gov/health-information/digestive-diseases/acid-reflux-ger-gerd-adults/eating-diet-nutrition

National Institute of Health. (2020). *Irritable bowel syndrome (IBS)*. Retrieved from https://www.niddk.nih.gov/health-information/digestive-diseases/irritable-bowel-syndrome

Neri, L., & Iovino, P. (2016). Bloating is associated with worse quality of life, treatment satisfaction, and treatment responsiveness among patients with constipation-predominant irritable bowel syndrome and functional constipation. *Neurogastroenterology and Motility, 28*(4), 581–591. doi:10.1111/nmo.12758 PMID:26867677

Newberry, C., & Lynch, K. (2019). The role of diet in the development and management of gastroesophageal reflux disease: Why we feel the burn. *Journal of Thoracic Disease, 11*(S12), S1594–S1601. doi:10.21037/jtd.2019.06.42 PMID:31489226

Nilsson, M., Johnsen, R., Ye, W., Hveem, K., & Lagergren, J. (2004). Lifestyle related risk factors in the aetiology of gastrooesophageal reflux. *Gut, 53*(12), 1730–1735. doi:10.1136/gut.2004.043265 PMID:15542505

Norman, K., Pichard, C., Lochs, H., & Pirlich, M. (2008). Prognostic impact of disease-related malnutrition. *Clinical Nutrition (Edinburgh, Lothian), 27*(1), 5–15. doi:10.1016/j.clnu.2007.10.007 PMID:18061312

O'Keefe, S. J. (2008). Nutrition and colonic health: The critical role of the microbiota. *Current Opinion in Gastroenterology, 24*(1), 51–58. doi:10.1097/MOG.0b013e3282f323f3 PMID:18043233

O'Sullivan, M., & O'Morain, C. (2006). Nutrition in inflammatory bowel disease. *Best Practice & Research. Clinical Gastroenterology, 20*(3), 561–573. doi:10.1016/j.bpg.2006.03.001 PMID:16782529

Oak, S. J., & Jha, R. (2019). The effects of probiotics in lactose intolerance: A systematic review. *Critical Reviews in Food Science and Nutrition, 59*(11), 1675–1683. doi:10.1080/10408398.2018.1425977 PMID:29425071

Okuyama, M., Takaishi, O., Nakahara, K., Iwakura, N., Hasegawa, T., Oyama, M., Inoue, A., Ishizu, H., Satoh, H., & Fujiwara, Y. (2017). Associations among gastroesophageal reflux disease, psychological stress, and sleep disturbances in Japanese adults. *Scandinavian Journal of Gastroenterology*, *52*(1), 44–49. doi:10.1080/00365521.2016.1224383 PMID:27571846

Papas, A., Palmer, C., Rounds, M. C., & Russell, R. M. (1998). The effect of denture status on nutrition. *Special Care in Dentistry*, *18*(1), 17–25. doi:10.1111/j.1754-4505.1998.tb01354.x PMID:9791303

Papathanasiou, I., & Coppens, P. (2017). *Aphasia and related neurogenic communication disorders*. Jones & Bartlett Learning.

Pappa, H. M., Gordon, C. M., Saslowsky, T. M., Zholudev, A., Horr, B., Shih, M. C., & Grand, R. J. (2006). Vitamin D status in children and young adults with inflammatory bowel disease. *Pediatrics*, *118*(5), 1950–1961. doi:10.1542/peds.2006-0841 PMID:17079566

Peery, A. F., Crockett, S. D., Barritt, A. S., Dellon, E.S., Eluri, S., Gangarosa, L.M., Jensen, E.T., Lund, J.L., Pasricha, S,, Runge, T., Schmidt, M., Shaheen N.J., Sandler, R.S. (2015). Burden of gastrointestinal, liver, and pancreatic diseases in the United States. *Gastroenterology, 149*(7), 1731–1741.

Perry, S. E., Huckabee, M. L., Tomkins, G., & Milne, T. (2020). The association between oral bacteria, the cough reflex and pneumonia in patients with acute stroke and suspected dysphagia. *Journal of Oral Rehabilitation*, *47*(3), 386–394. doi:10.1111/joor.12903 PMID:31698513

Peyrin-Biroulet, L., Panés, J., Sandborn, W. J., Vermeire, S., Danese, S., Feagan, B. G., . . . Rycroft, B. (2016). Defining disease severity in inflammatory bowel diseases: current and future directions. *Clinical Gastroenterology and Hepatology, 14*(3), 348-354.

Peyton, L., & Greene, J. (2014). Irritable bowel syndrome: current and emerging treatment options. *P & T: A Peer-Reviewed Journal for Formulary Management, 39*(8), 567-578.

Piesman, M., Hwang, I., Maydonovitch, C., & Wong, R. K. H. (2007). Nocturnal Reflux Episodes Following the Administration of a a standardized meal. Does timing matter? *The American Journal of Gastroenterology*, *102*(10), 2128–2134. doi:10.1111/j.1572-0241.2007.01348.x PMID:17573791

Plummer, M. P., Blaser, A. R., & Deane, A. M. (2014). Stress ulceration: Prevalence, pathology and association with adverse outcomes. *Critical Care (London, England)*, *18*(2), 213–213. doi:10.1186/cc13780 PMID:25029573

Pointer, S. D., Rickstrew, J., Slaughter, J. C., Vaezi, M. F., & Silver, H. J. (2016). Dietary carbohydrate intake, insulin resistance and gastro-oesophageal reflux disease: A pilot study in European- and African-American obese women. *Alimentary Pharmacology & Therapeutics*, *44*(9), 976–988. doi:10.1111/apt.13784 PMID:27582035

Pray, W. (2000). Lactose Intolerance: The Norm Among the World's Peoples. *American Journal of Pharmaceutical Education*, *64*, 205–207.

Pronsky, Z. M., Elbe, D., & Ayoob, K. (2015). *Food-Medication Interactions* (18th ed.). Food-Medication Interactions.

Quigley, E. M. M. (2012). Prebiotics and probiotics: Their role in the management of gastrointestinal disorders in adults. *Nutrition in Clinical Practice*, *27*(2), 195–200. doi:10.1177/0884533611423926 PMID:22127952

Ramakrishnan, K., & Salinas, R. C. (2007). Peptic Ulcer Disease. *American Family Physician*, *76*(7), 1005–1012. https://www.aafp.org/afp/2007/1001/p1005.html PMID:17956071

Rassow, J. (2011). Helicobacter pylori vacuolating toxin A and apoptosis. *Cell Communication and Signaling*, *9*(1), 26. doi:10.1186/1478-811X-9-26 PMID:22044628

Riazi, K., Raman, M., Taylor, L., Swain, M. G., & Shaheen, A. A. (2019). Dietary patterns and components in nonalcoholic fatty liver disease (NAFLD): What key messages can health care providers offer? *Nutrients*, *11*(12), 2878. doi:10.3390/nu11122878 PMID:31779112

Robayo-Torres, C. C., & Nichols, B. L. (2007). Molecular Differentiation of Congenital Lactase Deficiency from Adult-Type Hypolactasia. *Nutrition Reviews*, *65*(2), 95–98. doi:10.1111/j.1753-4887.2007.tb00286.x PMID:17345962

Rosenbek, J. C., Robbins, J. A., Roecker, E. B., Coyle, J. L., & Wood, J. L. (1996). A penetration-aspiration scale. *Dysphagia*, *11*(2), 93–98. doi:10.1007/BF00417897 PMID:8721066

Rostami, K., Malekzadeh, R., Shahbazkhani, B., Akbari, M. R., & Catassi, C. (2004). Coeliac disease in Middle Eastern countries: A challenge for the evolutionary history of this complex disorder? [PubMed]. *Digestive and Liver Disease*, *36*(10), 694–697. doi:10.1016/j.dld.2004.05.010

Sabater-Molina, M., Larqué, E., Torrella, F., & Zamora, S. (2009). Dietary fructooligosaccharides and potential benefits on health. *Journal of Physiology and Biochemistry*, *65*(3), 315–328. doi:10.1007/BF03180584 PMID:20119826

Saeed, A., Assiri, A., Assiri, H., Ullah, A., & Rashid, M. (2017). Celiac disease in Saudi children: Evaluation of clinical features and diagnosis. [PubMed]. *Saudi Medical Journal*, *38*(9), 895–899. doi:10.15537mj.2017.9.20808

Said, H. (2009). Cell and molecular aspects of human intestinal biotin absorption. *The Journal of Nutrition*, *139*(1), 158–162. doi:10.3945/jn.108.092023 PMID:19056639

Samji, N. S., Heda, R., Kovalic, A. J., & Satapathy, S. K. (2020). Similarities and differences between nonalcoholic steatohepatitis and other causes of cirrhosis. *Gastroenterology Clinics of North America*, *49*(1), 151–164. doi:10.1016/j.gtc.2019.09.004 PMID:32033761

Sams, A., & Hawks, J. (2014). Celiac disease as a model for the evolution of multifactorial disease in humans. [PubMed]. *Human Biology*, *86*(1), 19–36. doi:10.3378/027.086.0102

Sawczenko, A., & Sandhu, B. K. (2003). Presenting features of inflammatory bowel disease in Great Britain and Ireland. *Archives of Disease in Childhood*, *88*(11), 995–1000. doi:10.1136/adc.88.11.995 PMID:14612366

Schiavo, L., Busetto, L., Cesaretti, M., Zelber-Sagi, S., Deutsch, L., & Iannelli, A. (2018). Nutritional issues in patients with obesity and cirrhosis. *World Journal of Gastroenterology*, *24*(30), 3330–3346. doi:10.3748/wjg.v24.i30.3330 PMID:30122874

Schiffman, S. S., & Graham, B. G. (2000). Taste and smell perception affect appetite and immunity in the elderly. *European Journal of Clinical Nutrition*, *54*(3), S54–S63. doi:10.1038j.ejcn.1601026 PMID:11041076

Schiller, L. R., Pardi, D. S., & Sellin, J. H. (2017). Chronic diarrhea: Diagnosis and management. *Clinical Gastroenterology and Hepatology*, *15*(2), 182–193.e3. doi:10.1016/j.cgh.2016.07.028 PMID:27496381

Schlottmann, F., Andolfi, C., Herbella, F. A., Rebecchi, F., Allaix, M. E., & Patti, M. G. (2018). GERD: Presence and Size of Hiatal Hernia Influence Clinical Presentation, Esophageal Function, Reflux Profile, and Degree of Mucosal Injury. *The American Surgeon*, *84*(6), 978–982. doi:10.1177/000313481808400651 PMID:29981634

Schmid, A., & Walther, B. (2013). Natural Vitamin D Content in Animal Products. *Advances in Nutrition*, *4*(4), 453–462. doi:10.3945/an.113.003780 PMID:23858093

Schorr-Lesnick, B., & Brandt, L. J. (1988). Selected rheumatologic and dermatologic manifestations of inflammatory bowel disease. *The American Journal of Gastroenterology*, *83*, 216–223. PMID:3278591

Shaukat, A., Levitt, M., Taylor, B., MacDonald, R., Shamliyan, T., Kane, R., & Wilt, T. (2010). Systematic Review: Effective Management Strategies for Lactose Intolerance. *Annals of Internal Medicine*, *152*(12), 797–803. doi:10.7326/0003-4819-152-12-201006150-00241 PMID:20404262

Shaw, V. (2014). *Clinical Paediatric Dietetics* (4th ed.)., doi:10.1002/9781118915349

Shi, Y., Xiang, Y., Yang, Y., Zhang, N., Wang, S., Ungvari, G., ... Zhao, X. (2015). Depression after minor stroke: Prevalence and predictors. *Journal of Psychosomatic Research*, *79*(2), 143–147. doi:10.1016/j.jpsychores.2015.03.012 PMID:25868687

Singh, P., Arora, A., Strand, T. A., Leffler, D. A., Catassi, C., Green, P. H., Kelly, C. P., Ahuja, V., & Makharia, G. K. (2018). Global Prevalence of Celiac Disease: Systematic Review and Meta-analysis. [PubMed]. *Clinical Gastroenterology and Hepatology*, *16*(6), 823–836.e2. doi:10.1016/j.cgh.2017.06.037

Slavin, J. L. (2008). Position of the American Dietetic Association: Health implications of dietary fiber. *Journal of the American Dietetic Association*, *108*(10), 1716–1731. doi:10.1016/j.jada.2008.08.007 PMID:18953766

Sleisenger, M. H., Feldman, M., Friedman, L. S., & Brandt, L. J. (2006). *Sleisenger & Fordtran's gastrointestinal and liver disease: Pathophysiology, diagnosis, management* (8th ed.). Saunders.

Soda, A., Midha, V., Sood, N., & Bhatia, A. S. (2003). Incidence and prevalence of ulcerative colitis in Punjab, North India. *Gut*, *52*(11), 1587–1590. doi:10.1136/gut.52.11.1587 PMID:14570727

Song, J. H., Chung, S. J., Lee, J. H., Kim, Y. H., Chang, D. K., Son, H. J., Kim, J. J., Rhee, J. C., & Rhee, P. L. (2011). Relationship between gastroesophageal reflux symptoms and dietary factors in Korea. *Journal of Neurogastroenterology and Motility*, *17*(1), 54–60. doi:10.5056/jnm.2011.17.1.54 PMID:21369492

Stanford Health Care. (2020) *Low FODMAP diet*. Retrieved from https://stanfordhealthcare.org/medical-treatments/l/low-fodmap-diet.html

Stefanidis, D., Hope, W. W., Kohn, G. P., Reardon, P. R., Richardson, W. S., & Fanelli, R. D.SAGES Guidelines Committee. (2010). Guidelines for surgical treatment of gastroesophageal reflux disease. *Surgical Endoscopy*, *24*(11), 2647–2669. doi:10.100700464-010-1267-8 PMID:20725747

Stringer, D. A. (1987). Imaging inflammatory bowel disease in the pediatric patient. *Radiologic Clinics of North America*, *25*, 93–113. PMID:3823396

Surawicz, C. M. (2010). Mechanisms of diarrhea. *Current Gastroenterology Reports*, *12*(4), 236–241. doi:10.100711894-010-0113-4 PMID:20532705

Surdea-Blaga, T., Negrutiu, D. E., Palage, M., & Dumitrascu, D. L. (2017). Food and Gastroesophageal Reflux Disease. *Current Medicinal Chemistry*, *26*(19), 3497–3511. doi:10.2174/0929867324666170515123807 PMID:28521699

Su, Y., Yuki, M., Hirayama, K., Sato, M., & Han, T. (2020). Denture wearing and malnutrition risk among community-dwelling older adults. *Nutrients*, *12*(1), 151. doi:10.3390/nu12010151 PMID:31948104

Sverdén, E., Agréus, L., Dunn, J. M., & Lagergren, J. (2019). Peptic ulcer disease. *BMJ (Clinical Research Ed.)*, *367*, l5495. doi:10.1136/bmj.l5495 PMID:31578179

Swagerty, D., Walling, A., & Klein, R. (2002). Lactose Intolerance. *American Family Physician*, *65*(9), 1845–1851. PMID:12018807

Sylvester, J. (2019). Nonsteroidal Anti-inflammatory Drugs. *World Federation of Societies of Anaesthesiologists* Retrieved from https://www.wfsahq.org/components/com_virtual_library/media/a1363aaa0a41f691d0c5335673055a10-atow-405-00.pdf

Tanaka, N., Nohara, K., Kotani, Y., Matsumura, M., & Sakai, T. (2013). Swallowing frequency in elderly people during daily life. *Journal of Oral Rehabilitation*, *40*(10), n/a. Advance online publication. doi:10.1111/joor.12085 PMID:23855718

Tarasconi, A., Coccolini, F., Biffl, W. L., Tomasoni, M., Ansaloni, L., Picetti, E., Molfino, S., Shelat, V., Cimbanassi, S., Weber, D. G., Abu-Zidan, F. M., Campanile, F. C., Di Saverio, S., Baiocchi, G. L., Casella, C., Kelly, M. D., Kirkpatrick, A. W., Leppaniemi, A., Moore, E. E., ... Catena, F. (2020). Perforated and bleeding peptic ulcer: WSES guidelines. *World Journal of Emergency Surgery; WJES*, *15*(1), 3–3. doi:10.118613017-019-0283-9 PMID:31921329

Ternent, C. A., Bastawrous, A. L., Morin, N. A., Ellis, C. N., Hyman, N. H., & Buie, W. D. (2007). Standards practice task force of the American Society of Colon and Rectal Surgeons. Practice parameters for the evaluation and management of constipation. *Diseases of the Colon and Rectum, 50*(12), 2013–2022. doi:10.100710350-007-9000-y PMID:17665250

The International Dysphagia Diet Standardisation Initiative. (2016). *Complete IDDSI framework detailed definitions.* The International Dysphagia Diet Standardisation Initiative 2016. https://iddsi.org/framework/

Thierfelder, W., Dortschy, R., Hintzpeter, B., Kahl, H., & Scheidt-Nave, C. (2008). Biochemical measures in the German Health Interview and Examination Survey for Children and Adolescents (KiGGS) 1. *Laboratoriumsmedizin (Berlin), 32*(2), -. doi:10.1515/JLM.2008.010et

Trost, L. B., Bergfeld, W. F., & Calogeras, E. (2006). The diagnosis and treatment of iron deficiency and its potential relationship to hair loss. *Journal of the American Academy of Dermatology, 54*(5), 824–844. doi:10.1016/j.jaad.2005.11.1104 PMID:16635664

Tuck, C. J., & Vanner, S. J. (2018). Dietary therapies for functional bowel symptoms: Recent advances, challenges, and future directions. *Neurogastroenterology and Motility, 30*(1), e13238. doi:10.1111/nmo.13238 PMID:29094792

U.S. Department of Health and Human Services. (2013, September 10). *Digestive diseases statistics for the United States.* National Digestive Diseases Information Clearinghouse. Retrieved May 1, 2020 from http://digestive.niddk.nih.gov/statistics/statistics.aspx#specific

U.S. National Library of Medicine. (n.d.). *Entecavir.* MedlinePlus. https://medlineplus.gov/druginfo/meds/a605028.html

UCSF. (2008). Food Exchange Lists. Choose Your Foods: Exchange Lists for Diabetes, 1–17. https://dtc.ucsf.edu/pdfs/FoodLists.pdf

United States Department of Agriculture. (2019). *What is MyPlate?* Choose My Plate. https://www.choosemyplate.gov/eathealthy/WhatIsMyPlate

United States Department of Agriculture. (n.d.). Retrieved April 24, 2020, from https://fdc.nal.usda.gov/

Vakil, N., Van Zanten, S. V., Kahrilas, P., Dent, J., Jones, R., Bianchi, L. K., & Cesario, K. B. (2006). The Montreal definition and classification of gastroesophageal reflux disease: A global evidence-based consensus. *American Journal of Gastroenterology, 101*(8), 1900–20.

Van Gossum, A., Cabre, E., Hebuterne, X., Jeppesen, P., Krznaric, Z., Messing, B., Powell-Tuck, J., Staun, M., & Nightingale, J. (2009). ESPEN guidelines on parenteral nutrition: Gastroenterology. *Clinical Nutrition (Edinburgh, Lothian), 28*(4), 415–427. doi:10.1016/j.clnu.2009.04.022 PMID:19515465

Van Limbergen, J., Russell, R. K., Drummond, H. E., Aldhous, M. C., Round, N. K., Nimmo, E. R., Smith, L., Gillett, P. M., McGrogan, P., Weaver, L. T., Bisset, W. M., Mahdi, G., Arnott, I. D., Satsangi, J., & Wilson, D. C. (2008). Definition of phenotypic characteristics of childhood-onset inflammatory bowel disease. *Gastroenterology, 135*(4), 1114–1122. doi:10.1053/j.gastro.2008.06.081 PMID:18725221

Veauthier, B., & Hornecker, J. R. (2018). Crohn's Disease: Diagnosis and Management. *American Family Physician, 98*(11), 661–669. PMID:30485038

Vege, S. S., Ziring, B., Jain, R., Moayyedi, P., Adams, M. A., Dorn, S. D., Dudley-Brown, S. L., Flamm, S. L., Gellad, Z. F., Gruss, C. B., Kosinski, L. R., Lim, J. K., Romero, Y., Rubenstein, J. H., Smalley, W. E., Sultan, S., Weinberg, D. S., & Yang, Y.-X. (2015). American gastroenterological association institute guideline on the diagnosis and management of asymptomatic neoplastic pancreatic cysts. [PubMed]. *Gastroenterology, 148*(4), 819–822. doi:10.1053/j.gastro.2015.01.015

Vesa, T. H., Marteau, P., & Korpela, R. (2000). Lactose Intolerance. *Journal of the American College of Nutrition, 19*(sup2), 165S-175S. doi:10.1080/07315724.2000.10718086

Visser, M., Heijenbrok-Kal, M., van't Spijker, A., Oostra, K., Busschbach, J., & Ribbers, G. (2015). Coping, problem solving, depression, and health-related quality of life in patients receiving outpatient stroke rehabilitation. *Archives of Physical Medicine and Rehabilitation, 96*(8), 1492–1498. doi:10.1016/j.apmr.2015.04.007 PMID:25921980

Volta, U., & Villanacci, V. (2011). Celiac disease: Diagnostic criteria in progress. [PubMed]. *Cellular & Molecular Immunology, 8*(2), 96–102. doi:10.1038/cmi.2010.64

Vomero, N. D., & Colpo, E. (2014). Nutritional care in peptic ulcer. *Arquivos brasileiros de cirurgia digestiva: ABCD =. Arquivos Brasileiros de Cirurgia Digestiva, 27*(4), 298–302. doi:10.1590/S0102-67202014000400017 PMID:25626944

Wajed, S. A., Streets, C. G., Bremner, C. G., & DeMeester, T. R. (2001). Elevated body mass disrupts the barrier to gastroesophageal reflux. *Archives of Surgery, 136*(9), 1014–1019. doi:10.1001/archsurg.136.9.1014 PMID:11529823

Walsh, A. J., Bryant, R. V., & Travis, S. P. (2016). Current best practice for disease activity assessment in IBD. *Nature Reviews. Gastroenterology & Hepatology, 13*(10), 567–579. doi:10.1038/nrgastro.2016.128 PMID:27580684

Walsh, J., Meyer, R., Shah, N., Quekett, J., & Fox, A. T. (2016). Differentiating Milk Allergy (IgE and Non-IgE Mediated) from Lactose Intolerance: Understanding the Underlying Mechanisms and Presentations. *The British Journal of General Practice, 66*(649), e609–e611. doi:10.3399/bjgp16X686521 PMID:27481986

Web, M. D. (2020). *Irritable bowel syndrome.* Retrieved from https://www.webmd.com/ibs/guide/digestive-diseases-irritable-bowel-syndrome#3

Whitney, E. N., & Rolfes, S. R. (2016). *Understanding nutrition.* Cengage Learning.

Whyte, L. A., & Jenkins, H. R. (2012). Pathophysiology of diarrhea. *Paediatrics & Child Health*, *22*(10), 443–447. doi:10.1016/j.paed.2012.05.006

Width, M., & Reinhard, T. (2018). *The Essential Pocket Guid for Clinical Nutrition*. Second.

Width, M., & Reinhard, T. (2018). *The Essential Pocket Guide for Clinical Nutrition* (2nd ed.). Wolters Kluwer Health.

Wienbeck, M., & Babnert, J. (1989). Epidemiology of reflux disease and reflux esophagitis. *Scandinavian Journal of Gastroenterology*, *24*(sup156, S156), 7–13. doi:10.3109/00365528909091032 PMID:2662390

Williams, C. B., & Nicholls, S. (1994). Endoscopic features of chronic inflammatory bowel disease in childhood. *Bailliere's Clinical Gastroenterology*, *8*(1), 121–131. doi:10.1016/S0950-3528(06)80022-9 PMID:8003739

Williams, E. J., & Iredale, J. P. (1998). Liver cirrhosis. *Postgraduate Medical Journal*, *74*(870), 193–202. doi:10.1136/pgmj.74.870.193 PMID:9683971

Wong, V. W.-S., Chitturi, S., Wong, G. L.-H., Yu, J., Chan, H. L.-Y., & Farrell, G. C. (2016). Pathogenesis and novel treatment options for non-alcoholic steatohepatitis. *The Lancet. Gastroenterology & Hepatology*, *1*(1), 56–67. doi:10.1016/S2468-1253(16)30011-5 PMID:28404113

World Health Organization. (2017). *Diarrhoeal disease. Fact Sheet No. 330.* World Health Organization Website. Retrieved May 1, 2020 from http://www.who.int/mediacentre/factsheets/fs330/en/

World Health Organization. (2020). *Obesity and overweight*. World Health Organization. https://www.who.int/westernpacific/health-topics/obesity

Yeoh, K. G., Ho, K. Y., Guan, R., & Kang, J. Y. (1995). How Does Chili Cause Upper Gastrointestinal Symptoms? *Journal of Clinical Gastroenterology*, *21*(2), 87–90. doi:10.1097/00004836-199509000-00004 PMID:8583092

Zaninotto, G., DeMeester, T. R., Schwizer, W., Johansson, K. E., & Cheng, S. C. (1988). The lower esophageal sphincter in health and disease. *American Journal of Surgery*, *155*(1), 104–111. doi:10.1016/S0002-9610(88)80266-6 PMID:3341525

Zheng, Z., Nordenstedt, H., Pedersen, N. L., Lagergren, J., & Ye, W. (2007). Lifestyle Factors and Risk for Symptomatic Gastroesophageal Reflux in Monozygotic Twins. *Gastroenterology*, *132*(1), 87–95. doi:10.1053/j.gastro.2006.11.019 PMID:17241862

About the Contributors

Elham Aljaaly is an Associate Professor at the Clinical Nutrition Department of King Abdulaziz University, Saudi Arabia and a Consultant in Clinical Nutrition (SCFHS). A member in different organizations e.g. "American Society for Nutrition and "The Canadian Obesity Network". An editorial member in the Arab Journal of Nutrition and Exercise (AJNE) and the Journalism of mass communication. A regular reviewer for many institutions/organizations & Journals including e.g. the Bulletin of the World Health Organization; King Abdulaziz City for Science and Technology (KACST). Dr. Aljaaly is the first graduate Saudi Dietitian from the King Saud Clinical Nutrition Programme in Riyadh, SA who practiced the profession. Holding a M.Sc. in Human Nutrition from University of Sheffield, UK and PhD in Community Nutrition, Media Nutrition and International Health & Development from University College London (UCL), UK. Elham also done Post-Doctoral Fellowships Programs: In Clinical Nutrition at GOSH and in Nutrition & Public Health (University of Westminster). Has a house of Experience: "The Professionalism for Clinical Nutrition".

Rouba Khalil Naaman, MSc, PhD, is an assistant professor at the Clinical Nutrition Department at King Abdulaziz University. Her research interests involve assessing the effect of dietary interventions on health related problems and investigating nutritional and lifestyle factors influencing healthy aging. She is interested in identifying action steps that individuals can take to maintain their health and function as they get older. Dr. Naaman earned her Masters and PhD degrees in clinical nutrition from the University of Glasgow, United Kingdom. She has worked in coordinating and delivering lectures on Medical Nutrition Therapy for clinical nutrition students since 2018. Dr. Naaman has several publications in peer-reviewed journals in the field of nutrition and dietetics.

Manar Abduljalil Bakhsh is a lecturer in the Clinical Nutrition Department at King Abdulaziz University, Saudi Arabia. She has been involved in teaching many courses including Nutrition During Life Cycle and Medical Nutrition Therapy.

Mrs. Bakhsh holds a MSc degree from the University of Toronto, Canada and a diploma in holistic nutrition from the Canadian School of Natural Nutrition, Canada. She spent her training years in the Division of Gastroenterology, Hepatology, and Nutrition, and the Neonatal Intensive Care Unit at the Hospital for Sick Children, Canada. Her research interests include pediatric, neonatal, and maternal nutrition.

* * *

Albatool Abumunaser is a registered dietitian in Saudi Arabia. Received her bachelor degree in Clinical Nutrition from King Abdulaziz University with first honors.

Sarah M. Ajabnoor, MSc, Ph.D., RD, is an assistant professor in Clinical Nutrition Departement at King Abdulaziz University. Her clinical specialty and research interests include the nutritional management of gastrointestinal diseases. Her Ph.D. was focused on investigating the role of nutrition in the aetiopathogenesis and treatment of inflammatory bowel diseases. She earned her master and Ph.D. degrees from University College London and University of East Anglia, UK. Dr. Sarah has many peer-reviewed publications in the field of clinical nutrition.

Shoug Alashmali is an assistant professor in the Department of Clinical Nutrition at King Abdul Aziz University in Jeddah, Saudi Arabia. She earned her MSc and PhD degrees in Nutrition from the University of Manitoba and University of Toronto, respectively. Dr. Alashmali has been recognized internationally for her excellence in the graduate research conducted in the field of nutrition. Her area of interests and research focuses on understanding the effect of diet on the underlying neuroinflammatory processes which is a risk factor for many neurological and psychological disorders. She is a member of the Dietitians of Canada and Saudi Society for Clinical Nutrition. In 2020, she became a Certified Bariatric Educator from Obesity Canada. Dr. Alashmali has contributed to many publications in high quality journals in the field of nutrition.

Eram A. Albajri, MSc, PhD, RDN, IBCLC, is an Assistant Professor at the Clinical Nutrition Department of King Abdulaziz University in Jeddah, Saudi Arabia. Dr. Albajri is a Senior Specialist in Clinical Nutrition (SCFHS) in Saudi Arabia and a Registered Dietitian Nutritionists in the United States. She earned her MSc in Human Nutrition and PhD in Nutrition Sciences from Drexel University, USA. In 2019, she became an International Board-Certified Lactation Consultant. During her PhD, she was involved in many research projects and publications. Dr. Albajri has been recognized for her excellence in graduate research and her PhD dissertation was nominated for the Outstanding Dissertation Award. Her area of interest and research focuses on food intake regulation, brain and food intake, neuroimaging technique and food intake, weight management, and prevention and treatment of obesity.

Jomanah A. Bakhsh is an instructor in the Clinical Nutrition Department at King Abdulaziz University in Saudi Arabia. She earned her bachelor's degree in Clinical Nutrition in 2018 from King Abdulaziz University. She was awarded The University President's Award for Scientific Excellence for attaining the highest grade among all medical graduates. Afterwards, she completed a one-year dietetic internship in three public hospitals in Saudi Arabia. As of 2020, she is a master's student in the Leonard Davis School of Gerontology at the University of Southern California in the United States.

Naglaa Elsayed is a diagnostic radiologist and academic professor with over 25 years experience at Cairo and King Abdulaziz universities & hospitals. Having excellent experience in reporting and interpreting medical imaging in different modalities including X Ray, CT, MRI and Ultrasonography. Having excellent experience in teaching, accreditation and research with about 30 researches concerning Radiology published in prestigious international journals. Able to use and apply new technologies in teaching and have excellent experience in teaching under and postgraduate subjects. Energetic, talented and highly committed to work independently and within teams. Having excellent organization and communication skills. Research interests include diagnostic radiology and related subjects.

Almoutaz Hashim obtained his bachelor degree in medicine and surgery in the Faculty of Medicine at King Abdulaziz University, Jeddah, Saudi Arabia, 2003. He successfully complete his fellowship at the Royal College of Physicians of Canada, Ottawa, Canada, 2008. Subsequently, Dr. Hashim attended the University of British Columbia in Vancouver, Canada, to receive his certification by the American Board of Internal Medicine in 2008. He completed the fellowship at the Royal College of Physicians of Canada in 2010, where he later completed another fellowship program in Liver Transplant in 2012. In addition, Dr. Hashim acquired his gastroenterology certification by the American Board of Internal Medicine in 2012. Dr. Hashim worked as a Consultant in Liver Transplant at King Faisal Specialist Hospital & Research Centre in Riyadh, Saudi Arabia, between 2012 and 2014. At the present time, he is a Consultant Gastroenterology and Hepatology in Doctor Soliman Fakeeh Hospital (DSFH, Jeddah, Saudi Arabia). Dr. Hashim is a Vice dean of quality and improvement at the University of Jeddah. He is also working as an assistant professor of Gastroenterology and Hepatology at the Faculty of Medicine at the University of

Jeddah, Saudi Arabia. In addition, he is a board member of the Saudi association of the study of liver disease and liver transplant (SASLT).

Hebah M. Najeeb Khayat, MS, RD, is a registered dietitian with a Masters Degree in Dietetics and Nutrition from Florida International University. She has been working at King Abdulaziz University Hospital since 2014 dealing with patients suffering from different diseases such as diabetes, obesity and gastrointestinal diseases. Hebah has also been counseling people with inflammatory bowel diseases for 5 years. She is a member of the Nutrition Support Multidisciplinary Team and the Inflammatory Bowel Disease Multidisciplinary Team.

Manal A. Naseeb, MSc, PhD, RDN, IBCLC, is an Assistant Professor at the Clinical Nutrition Department of King Abdulaziz University in Jeddah, Saudi Arabia, and Specialist in Clinical Nutrition (SCFHS). She is a Registered Dietitian Nutritionists in the United States. Dr. Naseeb earned her MSc in Human Nutrition and PhD in Nutrition Sciences from Drexel University, USA. In 2018, she became an International Board-Certified Lactation Consultant. She is a member of the Academy of Nutrition and Dietetics in the United States. Her areas of interest and research include micronutrient intake, various type of diabetes especially type 2 diabetes in children and adolescents, and lactation. Dr. Naseeb has contributed to many publications in the field of nutrition. She has published articles on sarcopenia, type 2 diabetes in children, and Master athletes.

Heba Sanousi is a Registered Dietitian obtained the Bachelor degree in Nutrition and Food Science from King Abdulaziz University, Jeddah, Saudi Arabia, 2006. In addition, she completed the Master degree in Applied Human Nutrition from Mount Saint Vincent University, Halifax, Canada, 2015. In addition, Heba is a Certified Specialist-Nutrition from Saudi Commission for Health Specialities. Heba has been a clinical dietitian with experience for almost 10 years, working in Doctor Soliman Fakeeh Hospital (DSFH, Jeddah), and King Abdullah University Of Science And Technology (KAUST Health, Thuwal). She has been providing nutritional counseling to all patients with different conditions in inpatient care and outpatient care as well. For instance; she is covering the burn, renal dialysis, ICU, pediatric, oncology and cardiology units. She works with a team of Bariatric Surgeons in DSFH. An expert and interested in bariatric surgeries, using the International proved guidelines such as ASPEN and ESPEN. Heba is providing a full training program for students who wants to complete the internship in DSFH. She is a speaker in nutrition and dietetics in Almutaweroon Health Training Center which is a citified education center, providing an educational lectures about the updated studies and guideline in medical nutrition therapy for students, dietitians, and all medical staff.

Haalah Shaaker believes that a good teacher must be able to put herself in the place of those who find learning hard. This is her third year at King Abdulaziz University (KSA) teaching clinical nutrition students as a teaching assistant. So far, Clinical rotation in medical nutrition therapy is her favorite subject to teach. She had spent one year working as a registered clinical dietitian at the National guard health affairs (KSA). Haalah is passionate about researching and working in the scope of renal nutrition, she overcame many challenges in conducting her bachelor's project in 14 private and governmental hospitals to assess the dietetic practice, nutritional services, and patient satisfaction within the scope of Chronic Kidney Diseases.

Maryanne Weatherill holds the Certificate of Clinical Competence in Speech-Language Pathology (CCC-SLP) from the American Speech-Language-Hearing Association. She received her M.S. degree from Auburn University, and her Ph.D. from the University of Georgia, in the United States. Dr. Weatherill has been evaluating and treating adults with dysphagia as part of an interdisciplinary team in hospital settings since 1992.

Index

E

F

G

H

I

K

L

T

U

V

W

www.ingramcontent.com/pod-product-compliance
Lightning Source LLC
LaVergne TN
LVHW081520300926
849161LV00006B/1242
* 9 7 8 1 7 9 9 8 3 8 0 2 9 *